The Lymphoproliferative Disorders

Seasons Greetings

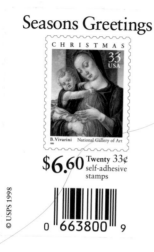

CHRISTMAS
33
USA

B. Vivarini   National Gallery of Art

$6.60 Twenty 33¢
self-adhesive
stamps

© USPS 1998

0 663800 9

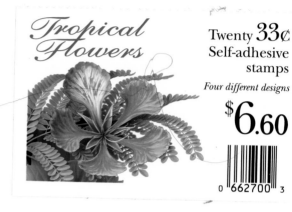

Tropical
Flowers

Twenty 33¢
Self-adhesive
stamps

Four different designs

$6.60

0 662700 3

The Lymphoproliferative Disorders

Handbook of Diagnosis, Investigation & Management

J A Child
Consultant Haematologist

A S Jack
Consultant Haematopathologist

G J Morgan
Leukaemia Research Fund Senior Lecturer

The General Infirmary
Great George Street
Leeds
United Kingdom

CHAPMAN & HALL MEDICAL
London · Weinheim · New York · Tokyo · Melbourne · Madras

Published by Chapman & Hall, 2–6 Boundary Row, London SE1 8HN, UK

Thomson Science, 2–6 Boundary Row, London SE1 8HN, UK

Thomson Science, 115 Fifth Avenue, New York, NY 10003, USA

Thomson Science, Suite 750, 400 Market Street, Philadelphia, PA 19106, USA

Thomson Science, Pappelallee 3, 69469 Weinheim, Germany

First edition 1998

© 1998 Chapman & Hall

Thomson Science is an imprint of International Thomson Publisishing I(T)P'

Typeset in 11½/14 Adobe Garamond by Genesis Typesetting, Rochester, Kent

Printed in the United Kingdom at the University Press, Cambridge

ISBN 0 412 58030 6

A catalogue record for this book is available from the British Library

Library of Congress Catalog Card Number: 97-77658

⊗ Printed on acid free text paper,manufactured in accordance with ANSI/NISO Z39.48–1992 (Permanence of Paper)

Contents

Contributors

Additional contributions from:

The General Infirmary at Leeds:
Ms S. Barrans (Chapter 2)
   Senior Medical Laboratory Scientific Officer
Mr D. Blythe (Chapter 2)
   Chief Medical Laboratory Scientific Officer
Dr A. G. Chalmers (Chapter 3)
   Consultant Radiologist
Dr K. Kerr (Chapter 4)
   Consultant Microbiologist
Dr S. Misbah (Chapter 11)
   Consultant Immunologist
Dr D. R. Norfolk
   Consultant Haematologist
Ms S. J. O'Connor (Chapter 2)
   Clinical Scientist
Dr S. Richards (Chapters 2 and 9)
   Clinical Scientist
Dr B. E. Roberts (Chapter 8)
   Consultant Haematologist
Dr C. Shiach (Chapter 4)
   Consultant Paediatric Haematologist
Dr G. M. Smith (Chapter 4)
   Consultant Haematologist

Yorkshire Radiotherapy Centre, Cookridge Hospital, Leeds:
Dr D. Gilson (Chapter 4)
   Consultant Clinical Oncologist

St James's University Hospital, Leeds:
Dr S. Kinsey (Chapter 4)
   Consultant Paediatric Haematologist

Preface

The past few years have been a time of great progress in haematological oncology. The growing understanding of the cellular and molecular pathology of lymphoproliferative disorders is causing a re-evaluation of many of the basic concepts of diagnosis and treatment. The use of antibody-based cell markers and molecular biological techniques are now essential for the accurate diagnosis of lymphoproliferative disorders and have an increasing role in detecting very low levels of residual disease following therapy. The delivery of high-dose chemotherapy has been transformed by the ability to collect and manipulate peripheral blood stem cells. The range of therapeutic options is also increasing with the introduction of new drugs, cytokines and therapeutic monoclonal antibodies. In the near future methods of manipulating the immune response and gene transfer techniques are likely to find a clinical role. Developments in imaging technology have greatly improved the ability to accurately stage and monitor patients without recourse to invasive techniques. These changes mean that it is no longer possible to consider diagnosis in isolation from treatment or to separate basic science from clinical practice.

The many technical and conceptual changes that have occurred has made the study of lymphoproliferative disorders appear at times rather daunting to those new to haematological oncology. We have written this book as a guide to current practice and new developments, which we hope will allow the reader to place the ever-increasing primary literature of the subject in its proper context. The first section begins with a short overview of the normal lymphoid system and is followed by chapters on the principles and basic techniques of laboratory diagnosis, imaging and therapy. The second section is a systematic account of the lymphoproliferative disorders. The terminology used is based on the Revised European–American Lymphoma (REAL) classification. One of the most useful features of this classification is the emphasis on disease entities, which are defined in terms of both their cellular and clinical features. However, for reasons of clarity and continuity of the text we have not closely followed the order in which the entities are listed in the published version of the REAL classification. Each chapter has a list of suggested further reading. This is not intended to be comprehensive but instead contains a range of recent review articles and papers covering areas of current interest.

We hope that this book will be of value to those undertaking higher specialist training in haematology, pathology or oncology or to those in established posts who require a concise review of the subject. Research workers, specialist nurses and laboratory staff may also find the book useful in providing a broader perspective for their professional work.

The contributions which a number of colleagues made to specific chapters are listed above. We are also very grateful to Professor W. Cunliffe, Dr M. Wilkinson, Dr G. Stables, Mr M. Menage, Mr H. Sue-Ling and Dr B. Carey, who provided a number of the clinical photographs and radiographs. Dr F. Davies, Dr A. Haynes and Dr P. Da Costa kindly read the manuscript and made helpful comments. We would also like to thank Ms J. Hamblin for secretarial support, Mr S. Toms for expert assistance in photography and Ms J. Koster of Chapman & Hall for her encouragement. Finally we wish to acknowledge the support of our clinical colleagues and collaborators throughout Yorkshire and beyond.

J. A. Child
A. S. Jack
G. J. Morgan
Leeds, September 1997

Part One

Principles of Diagnosis and Treatment

The structure of the lymphoid system

1

The growth in knowledge of the lymphoproliferative disorders can be attributed at least in part to the rapid expansion of understanding of the normal immune system. The classification of lymphoid tumours is increasingly based on the lineage and pathways of differentiation of normal lymphoid cells and the diagnosis of many types of tumour depends heavily on recognizing abnormalities of the microarchitecture of lymphoid organs. In the near future it is expected that novel therapies will be based on modification of the intercellular interactions between neoplastic and normal lymphoid cells using cytokines, monoclonal antibodies and gene transfer techniques. This chapter is a brief outline of the structure of the normal lymphoid system which will serve a basis for the discussion of diagnosis and management of individual lymphoproliferative disorders.

1.1 Classification of lymphoid organs

Lymphoid organs are classified as primary and secondary

The primary lymphoid organs are the sites of production of lymphocytes and in mammals this includes the bone marrow and the thymus. Secondary (or peripheral) lymphoid organs are where lymphocytes encounter antigens and undergo antigen-driven proliferation and differentiation. Secondary lymphoid organs include lymph nodes, spleen, bone marrow, Peyer's patches, Waldeyer's ring and acquired lymphoid tissue, which develops in the stomach, skin or respiratory tract in response to local antigenic stimuli. The organs of the lymphoid system are integrated by the various pathways of lymphocyte circulation.

1.2 Primary lymphoid organs

1.2.1 The bone marrow

The pathways of cellular differentiation of the normal bone marrow have been extensively studied *in vitro*. The organization of the marrow is based on a small number of pluripotent stem cells which, when they divide, give rise to a cell that becomes committed to a specific lineage of differentiation – erythroid, myeloid, lymphoid, monocyte or mega-karyocyte. The pluripotent stem cells and their immediate lineage-committed progeny are contained within the CD34$^+$ mononuclear cell fraction. It is not yet possible to accurately count true pluripotent stem cells in clinical samples using cell surface markers, and the closest approximation for application clinically is counting CD34$^+$ cells using a flow cytometer. These cells can be further subdivided using a range of cell surface markers and the immunophenotype that most closely defines a pluripotent stem cell appears to be CD34$^+$, Thy-1$^+$, CD38$^-$ without specific lineage markers.

A considerable effort is being made to develop techniques to expand pluripotent haemopoietic stem cells *in vitro* but to date these have not been successful. A population of cells can be identified in normal marrow by their ability to initiate long-term haemopoiesis on bone marrow stroma (long-term culture initiating cells); however these cells are not able to sustain self-renewal, which is the key property of true pluripotent stem cells. Committed progenitor cells derived from long-term culture or fresh marrow can be identified by their ability to form differentiated colonies in semi-solid agar. These colonies are classified according to the lineages present and the results from this assay have formed the basis of current model of bone marrow function.

In vivo the bone marrow consists of a specialized stroma, which can support the proliferation and differentiation of committed progenitor cells produced by stem cell division in response to demand for peripheral blood cells. The stroma consists of adipocytes, myofibroblasts, endothe-lium, pericytes and bone-forming cells. These may be derived from a common stromal CD34$^+$ stem cell although this has not been fully characterized. There is growing evidence that the progeny of this stem cell may migrate and repopulate connective cells in other organs. The cells of each haemopoietic lineage tend to localize within specific areas of stroma. Myeloid progenitors are found adjacent to the surface of bone trabeculae with more differentiated granulocytes within the central area of the marrow close to blood vessels. Erythroid progenitors form colonies in association with iron-containing macrophages in the central area of the marrow. These colonies produce a group of red blood cells which are then discharged into the blood stream. Evidence from culture studies indicate that erythroid colonies and seams of myeloid differentiation are transient structures, which expand to produce a defined number of red cell or granulocytes before being dissipated by the terminal maturation of all the cells (Figure 1.1).

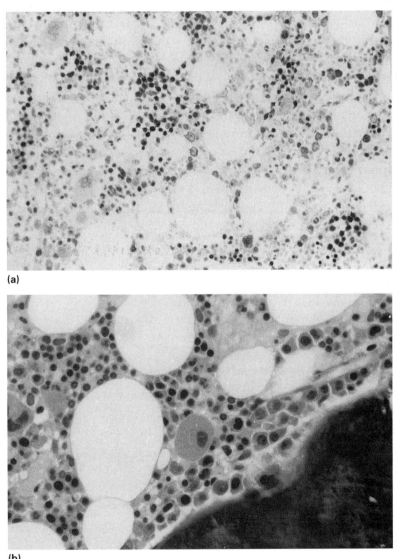

(a)

(b)

Figure 1.1 Normal bone marrow. In the normal bone marrow committed erythroid progenitors form colonies in association with iron-containing macrophages. The more immature erythroid cells are found at the centre of the colony with more mature cells showing smaller more densely staining nuclei at the periphery (a). Early myeloid precursors are found adjacent to bone (b).

Committed lymphoid progenitors that give rise to B-cells, NK cells, T-cells and possibly some antigen-presenting cells are usually present in very small numbers in comparison to the other cell lines. B-cell progenitors, which complete their development in the marrow, appear to be associated with stroma close to the endosteal surface of bone. They can be identified by the expression of CD19, CD38, the surface endopeptidase CD10 and nuclear Tdt and lack of surface immunoglobulin. As with myeloid and erythroid progenitors each cell is able to give rise to a limited number of mature progeny; in the case of B-cells this is probably about 64 cells. The central event in B-cell maturation is rearrangement of the immunoglobulin genes to produce a functioning antigen receptor. This is a very inefficient process with many cells failing to carry out a productive Ig gene rearrangement. These cells undergo apoptosis in the bone marrow. Following chemotherapy, increased numbers of B-cell progenitors may be found in the marrow and may sometimes be confused with residual B-lineage acute lymphoblastic leukaemia (Figure 1.2).

Figure 1.2 The organization and recombination of the immunoglobulin heavy chain locus.

The bone marrow is also the site of production of lymphoid accessory cells such as the antigen-presenting interdigitating reticulin cells of the lymph node paracortex. It is likely that these cells share a common progenitor with peripheral monocytes and other mononuclear

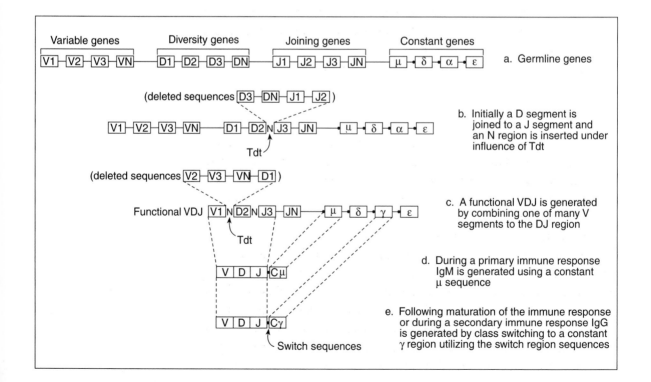

phagocytes. The exception may be follicular dendritic cells of the germinal centre. These cells may differentiate from local connective cell precursors in lymph nodes and other organs.

As well as being the site of production of precursor lymphocytes the bone marrow also acts as a secondary lymphoid organ. T-lymphocytes have an interstitial distribution between adipocytes. In addition to their immune functions, T-cells may have an important role in supporting normal haemopoiesis through the production of IL-3 and probably other cytokines. The bone marrow is a major site of long-term immunoglobulin production, with preplasma cells migrating to the marrow from lymph nodes. Bone marrow plasma cells are usually closely related to blood vessels. Aggregates of B-cells are not uncommonly seen in the marrow the incidence increasing with age, but their significance is uncertain and in some cases may represent occult lymphoma. Lymphoid follicles with germinal centres can be found in the marrow, usually in association with immune-mediated systemic disorders such as rheumatoid disease, but are very rare.

A feature of many neoplastic disorders of the marrow is the loss of organized microarchitecture. In myelodysplastic syndrome the structure of the erythroid colonies may be lost and early myeloid progenitors are seen at abnormal sites within the marrow. In myeloma, the neoplastic plasma cells are not localized around blood vessels but are distributed in small groups between fat cells which later coalesce to form more diffuse areas of infiltration. Most other lymphoproliferative disorders that involve the marrow have a characteristic pattern of infiltration.

1.2.2 The thymus

The thymus is a combined epithelial and lymphoid organ. The epithelial elements are derived from the third and fourth pharyngeal pouches in the early embryo and these are then colonized by marrow-derived stem cells destined to become committed to T-cell development. Histological examination of an H&E-stained section of thymus shows a darkly staining cortex and a less densely cellular medullary region within each of the thymic lobules (Figure 1.3).

External to the cortex is the subcapsular region, which is the point of arrival of stem cells from the marrow. Only after entering the thymus do these cells become committed T-cell progenitors; the earliest evidence that these cells show of commitment to T-cell differentiation is the expression of CD7 and Tdt. These lymphoblasts are highly proliferative and give rise to cells that enter the thymic cortex and begin the complex process of T-cell maturation. A distinctive form of epithelial nurse cell

Figure 1.3 Normal thymus. The thymus consists of two main functional zones – the cortex and medulla. The cortex contains densely staining lymphoblasts which migrate into the medulla as immunocompetent T-lymphocytes prior to entering the peripheral circulation (a). Within the medulla clusters of epithelial cells form Hassall's corpuscles; these are probably degenerate structures. Lymphoblasts express Tdt (b), which is a key enzyme involved in T-cell receptor gene rearrangement and the generation of diversity.

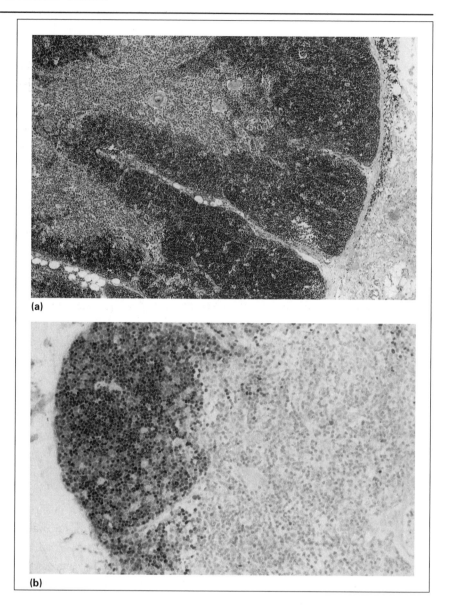

(a)

(b)

present within the subcapsular zone is responsible for regulating this process.

Cells entering the thymic cortex undergo rearrangement of the T-cell gamma and delta gene but almost all cells subsequently rearrange the alpha and beta genes (TCR2) leaving only a few gamma/delta (TCR1)-expressing cells (Figure 1.4). It is likely that a considerable proportion of cells die at this stage by apoptosis, having failed to produce a functioning receptor. Cells that survive this process differentiate into

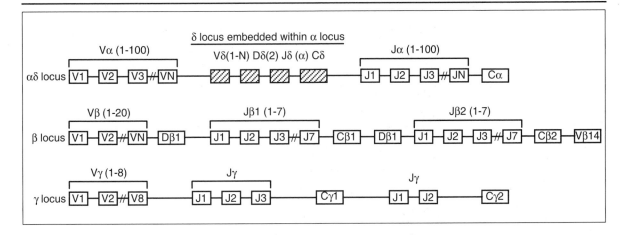

common thymocytes. These cells express TCR2 in conjunction with CD3 and coexpress CD4 and CD8. They are also distinguished by the expression of CD1 and continue to have nuclear Tdt. The TCR2 is essentially a receptor that recognizes MHC molecules in association with antigens, and during random rearrangements of the TCR genes cells are produced that can strongly bind to self MHC molecules without antigens present. These are potentially self-reactive T-cells. Alternatively, cells are produced that have a minimal capacity to associate with MHC molecules with or without antigens. These would be non-functional. Both these groups of cells are eliminated in the thymic cortex by direct cell to cell contact with the dense network of interdigitating reticulum cells and thymic cortical epithelial cells. The remaining cells leave the thymic cortex and enter the medulla, where they lose expression of CD1a, Tdt and either CD4 or CD8. The final stage in the process is the expression of adhesion molecules such as L-selectin and CD44, which allow the cell to pass through the specialized endothelium lining medullary blood vessels and enter the circulation (Figure 1.5).

A distinctive feature of the thymic medulla is the presence of Hassall's corpuscles, which are large aggregates of epithelial cells. These cells are thought to be degenerate and non-functioning. The thymic medulla also has a specialized population of B-cells, which may undergo expansion, with the formation of B-cell follicles with germinal centres. These may be prominent in some autoimmune conditions, such as myasthenia gravis, although the normal function of this population is not known. It is possible that these cells may be the cells of origin of mediastinal B-cell lymphoma.

Figure 1.4 The organization of the T-cell receptor locus.

Figure 1.5 T-cell development in the thymus. Circulating stem cells enter the thymus from the peripheral blood and become committed to the T-cell lineage. The earliest evidence of lineage commitment is expression of CD7. The main events in the thymus are rearrangement of the *TCR1* (gamma/delta) genes and subsequently the *TCR2* (alpha/beta) gene. In each case diversity is increased by the action of Tdt in adding and deleting bases. Cells expressing either *TCR1* or *TCR2* undergo positive selection and clonal expansion by interaction with thymic epithelium. Cells with receptors that do not have a moderate affinity for MHC molecules are deleted. Negative selection for strong self-reactivity is mediated by macrophages. Surviving cells pass into the thymic medulla and then into the peripheral blood as immunocompetent T-cells.

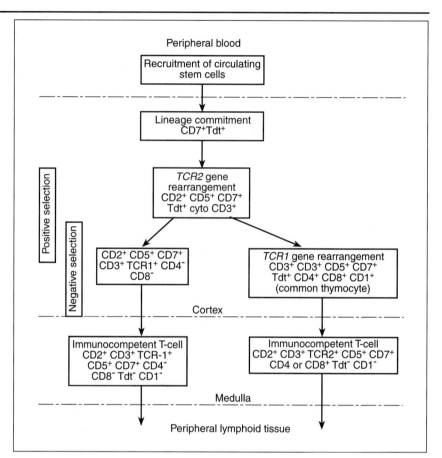

1.3 Secondary lymphoid organs

1.3.1 The lymph nodes

The framework of a lymph node consists of a fibrous capsule which is attached to fine connective tissue septa radiating towards the hilum of the node. The capsule is penetrated by a number of afferent lymphatic vessels, which discharge in the subcapsular sinus. The subcapsular sinus is in continuity with the nodal sinuses, which are partly lined by histiocytes and converge on the efferent lymphatic vessel in the hilum of the node. This structure acts as a filter removing particulate material from the lymph. Lymph nodes also have a microvascular circulation with specialized venular endothelium providing the point of entry of lymphoid cells into the node (Figure 1.6).

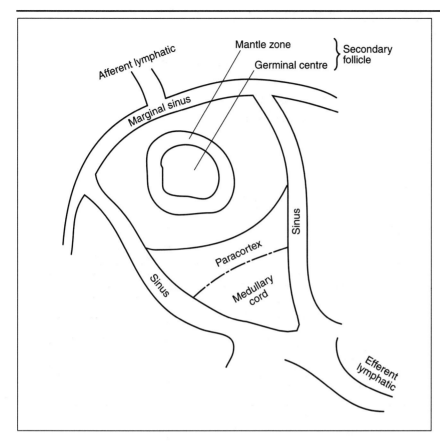

Figure 1.6 Lymph node microarchitecture. The basic structure of a lymph node consists of a marginal sinus which collects lymph from the afferent lymphatic and discharges into the centrally radiating sinuses which collect together to form the efferent lymphatic. The lymphoid tissue lying between the sinuses is divided into three main functional zones. The cortex which contains the B-cell follicles, the paracortex which is the main T-cell area and the medullary cords which contains transformed lymphoid cells and developing plasma cells.

The lymphoid tissue is associated with specialized connective tissue lying between the sinuses and is organized into three functional zones. The cortex of the node is the B-cell area, the paracortex is the T-cell area and the cords of tissue that lie between the medullary sinuses are rich in plasma cells. In its unstimulated state the cortex consists of primary follicles of sIgM/IgD$^+$ virgin B-cells. In the adult this will include a small proportion of CD5$^+$ B-cells (B$_1$-cells), which appear to be a separate B-cell lineage. These cells, which are more numerous in young animals, appear to respond to non-T-cell-dependent antigens by producing low-affinity IgM antibodies. There has been much speculation on the role of these cells in early defence against common bacterial infection and stimulation of anti-idiotype network. B$_1$-cells also seem to be the source of many IgM autoantibodies.

The paracortex contains a complex mixture of cells. The T-cell population may include normal peripheral lymphocytes, activated cells with larger more irregular nuclei and usually relatively small numbers of proliferating large blast cells. The ratio of CD4:CD8 shows a wider range than in the peripheral blood. Antigen-presenting interdigitating dendritic cells are present and can be identified by S100 and CD1a expression and by their highly characteristic cleft along the long axis of the nucleus. Phagocytic macrophages and small numbers of B-cells and plasma cells may also be found within the paracortex (Figure 1.7).

A wide spectrum of structural change occurs in the node during the normal immune response. The initiation of a T-cell-dependent B-cell

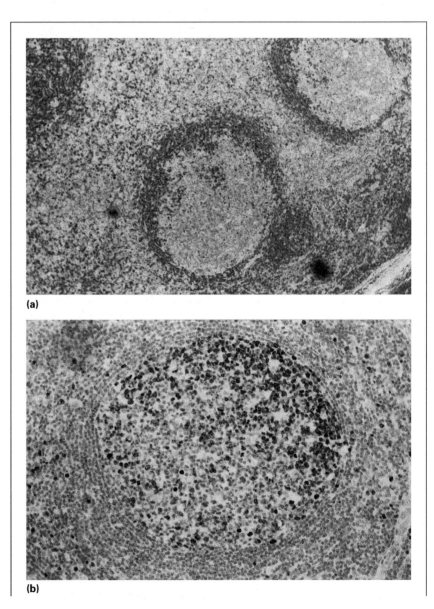

Figure 1.7 Reactive lymph node. **(a)** In this reactive node the follicular mantle zones surrounding the reactive germinal centres are identified using the antibody MT2 (CD45RA). **(b)** A reactive germinal centre with the cells in cycle identified by the marker Ki67. The germinal centre is polarized, with the majority of the cycling cells being contained within the centroblast rich zone.

(a)

(b)

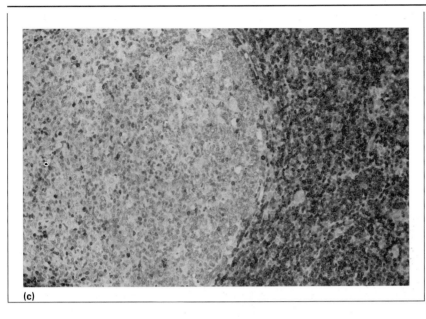

(c)

Figure 1.7 (c) The distribution of Bcl-2 expression in a reactive B-cell follicle. There is strong expression by most of the mantle zone cells but almost all of the germinal centre cells are negative. The induction of Bcl-2 expression is a key event in preventing the apoptosis of centrocytes which have been selected by the affinity for antigen of their surface immunoglobulin.

response leads to the formation of germinal centres within the follicle with the remaining cells forming the follicular mantle zone. Germinal centres are seeded by a small number of activated B-cells, which differentiate into centroblasts and undergo a rapid phase of oligoclonal expansion. These cells exit from the cell cycle to become centrocytes. During this process, the immunoglobulin genes undergo somatic hypermutation. The immunoglobulin molecule produced by the mutated genes is expressed on the cell surface and tested for reactivity against antigen bound to the network of follicular dendritic cells present with the centrocyte-rich zone of the germinal centre. Class switching from IgM to IgG or IgA production may also occur. A high proportion of B-cells no longer react with antigen and undergo apoptosis and are phagocytosed by macrophages. Cells with high affinity for antigen are rescued by receiving survival signals from T-cells that inhibit apoptosis by induction of Bcl-2 expression. The most powerful of these signals is the binding of CD40 on the B-cell surface to its ligand expressed on T-cells. The rescued cell is then diverted to becoming either a memory B-cell or a plasma cell precursor which migrates to the bone marrow. The structure of the germinal centre is of great importance in understanding the morphological changes of follicle centre lymphoma. The marginal zone, which is a common feature of splenic or gut-associated lymphoid tissue, is usually poorly developed in lymph node. When present it consists of a population of slightly larger cells with increased amounts of cytoplasm;

these cells express IgM without IgD and often have 'late' B-cell markers such as CD25 and CD11c. Variable number of macrophages are also present. Recent data suggest that the marginal zone may represent a pool of post-germinal-centre non-recirculating memory B-cells. These cells show evidence of somatic hypermutation of immunoglobulin genes but have not undergone class switching. On re-exposure to antigen these cells can switch to IgG or IgA production and differentiate to plasma cells (Figure 1.8).

T-cell stimulation causes paracortical expansion with proliferation of T-cells and antigen presenting cells. Activated T-cells show increased morphological heterogeneity and the expression of markers of activation

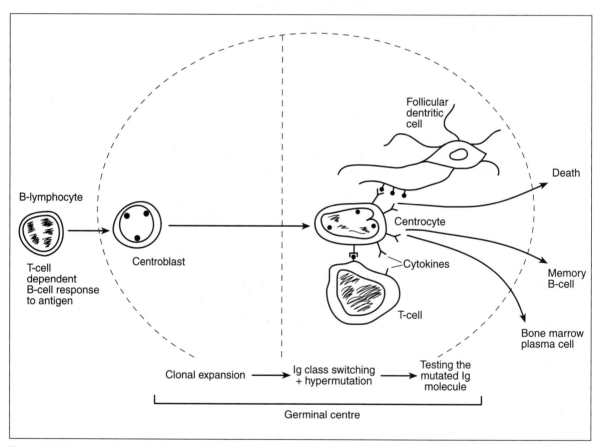

Figure 1.8 The normal germinal centre. The formation of a germinal centre is initiated by several B-cells responding to antigen. Within the germinal centres there is a proliferating compartment consisting of centroblasts in which clonal expansion occurs. Cells exit from the cell cycle and become centrocytes. During this process the immunoglobulin genes undergo mutation. The functional activity of the mutated immunoglobulin molecule is tested against antigen presented by follicular dendritic cells. The binding affinity of sIg, together with T-cell signals and cytokines, determines whether the cell survives to become a memory cell or a plasma cell. Cells destined to become plasma cells switch from IgM to IgG or IgA production by transferring the VDJ region to an α or γ constant region gene.

such as HLA-DR and CD25 (IL-2R). Depending on the nature of the stimulus, CD4$^+$ T-cells may differentiate to T$_H$1- or T$_H$2-cells, which are distinguished by their profile of cytokine secretion. T$_H$1-cells promote the development of cytotoxic T-cell responses and T$_H$2-cells are involved in the stimulation of antibody production. CD8$^+$ cells may become activated cytotoxic cells which have large granular lymphocyte morphology. Following contact with antigen T-cells switch CD45 isoform from CD45RA to CD45RO.

Many agents may induce reactive hyperplasia of lymph nodes producing clinically apparent lymphadenopathy

The patterns of cellular reactivity produced within the lymph node are relatively few and in most cases there are no specific morphological features that allow the cause to be identified. In the majority of cases the lymph node will show expansion of the B-cell population with germinal centre formation, paracortical hyperplasia and increased numbers of sinus-lining phagocytic histiocytes in varying proportions. There are a number of variations on this basic pattern, which may give rise to diagnostic difficulties. In young adults massive follicular hyperplasia may occur with large irregular germinal centres affecting only part of the node with the remaining normal tissue being compressed at one pole of the node. In infectious mononucleosis the reactive paracortex may be so large as to displace the follicles and sinuses, giving an appearance suggestive of destruction of normal nodal architecture. Knowledge of the clinical features, the highly polymorphic cellular content of the paracortex and the demonstration, by marker studies if necessary, of the compressed follicles and sinuses will prevent the erroneous diagnosis of lymphoma in these circumstances. Lymphadenopathy may occur in association with almost any type of skin disorder. This dermatopathic reaction involves paracortical hyperplasia, which includes macrophages containing melanin pigment and large numbers of interdigitating cells. In a few cases areas of paracortex become T-cell-depleted and consist mainly of cohesive sheets of interdigitating cells which should not be confused with Langerhans cell histiocytosis (Figure 1.9).

In addition to expansion of normal nodal elements the presence of granulomas is a relatively common feature of non-neoplastic lymphadenopathy. Although the differential diagnosis is wide, the morphology and distribution of the granuloma may give useful information as to the probable cause. In tuberculosis and other types of mycobacterial infection the node is usually replaced by large granulomas with prominent giant

Figure 1.9 Dermatopathic reaction. **(a)** In dermatopathic lymphadenopathy there is massive expansion of the T-cell zone (paracortex). In this section the paracortex is delineated by identifying the hyperplastic interdigitating reticulin cells using anti-S100. The elliptical regions without S100-positive cells are areas of B-cell cortex. **(b)** In this case of dermatopathic lymphadenopathy the paracortex is almost completely replaced by pale staining interdigitating cells with relative T-cell depletion.

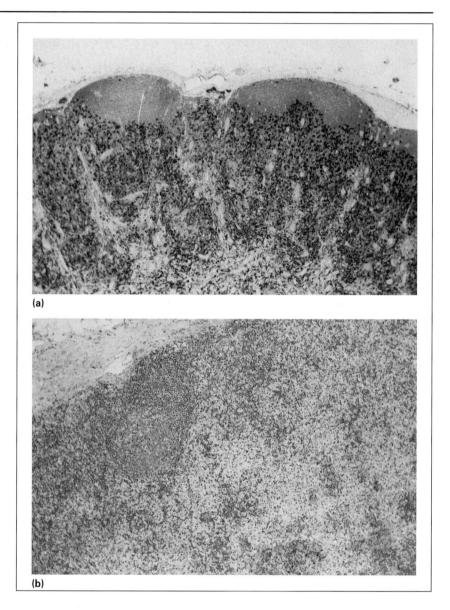

(a)

(b)

cells and necrosis with caseation. Conventional direct ZN stains are very insensitive and where this diagnosis is suspected it is essential that fresh tissue is cultured. Where this is not possible, PCR techniques may be used to identify the organism although this does not provide information on drug sensitivity. In sarcoidosis the node is also usually completely replaced but, in contrast to tuberculosis, the granulomas are smaller and more regular in shape, show only minimal necrosis and have a relatively small reactive T-cell component. The presence of non-necrotizing

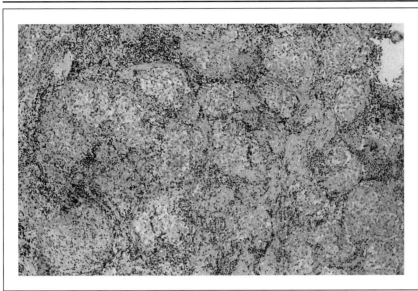

Figure 1.10 Nodal sarcoidosis. This node is almost completely replaced by granulomas, which consist of epithelioid macrophages and do not show necrosis. Sarcoidosis is one of the commonest of many granulomatous disorders that affect lymph nodes.

microgranulomas closely related to reactive germinal centres should suggest the possibility of toxoplasmosis. When large necrotizing granulomas heavily infiltrated by granulocytes are present within a reactive node this should suggest the possibility of Chlamydia or Yersinia infection or cat scratch disease, depending on the site of the node and clinical history. In cases where there is extensive paracortical or more generalized nodal necrosis with large amounts of nuclear debris but few granulocytes the possibility of Kikuchi's lymphadenitis should be considered. This condition has a very high female predominance, mainly causes self-limiting cervical lymphadenopathy and is possibly caused by a bacterial infection. It is difficult to distinguish this from the pattern seen in nodal disease due to SLE; in all cases serological studies should be performed (Figure 1.10).

1.3.2 The spleen

The detailed microanatomy of the spleen has long been a subject of debate. Basically the spleen consists of arterioles, which discharge into splenic sinuses, which in turn join to form venules. The sinuses are lined mainly by endothelium and are separated by cords of connective tissue which may contain a variety of cell types including phagocytes, activated T-cells and plasma cells. A reticulin stain shows that the sinuses are encircled by collagen fibres. It is believed that the splenic sinuses have a major role in trapping damaged red blood cells from the circulation,

Figure 1.11 Periarteriolar splenic lymphoid tissue. Lymphoid tissue in the spleen is organized around arterioles. The main arteriole is surrounded by the T-zone and separate branches enter the B-cell area. In splenic lymphoid tissue the marginal zone of the B-cell area is usually more prominent than in lymph nodes. After passing through the lymphoid tissue the arterioles discharge into the splenic sinuses, which collect to form the splenic vein.

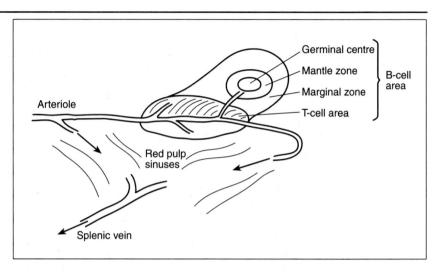

although there is uncertainty as to the precise mechanisms which discriminate between normal and abnormal red cells (Figure 1.11).

The splenic lymphoid tissue is organized around arterioles. The T-cell area of the spleen surrounds the main arteriole, which may then branch further to supply the B-cell areas. The B-cell areas consist of primary and secondary follicles with germinal centres but, unlike lymph nodes, a wide marginal zone is often a prominent feature of reactive lymphoid tissue in the spleen. The reason why the marginal zone is much more commonly expanded in the spleen compared to lymph nodes is not understood. Vascular loops associated with lymphoid tissue also discharge into the red pulp sinuses. In the spleen lymphocytes enter the periarteriolar lymphoid tissue through the arteriole walls and most cells probably leave by passing through the sinuses into the venous system (Figure 1.12).

1.3.3 Lymphoid tissue associated with mucosal surfaces

The main sites of organized mucosal-associated lymphoid tissue in the aerodigestive tract are the nasopharynx and Peyer's patches

The palatine tonsils are covered by squamous epithelium, which is folded into deep crypts. At the base of these crypts the epithelial lining becomes attenuated and closely associated with lymphoid cells. The lymphoid tissue in the tonsil is organized in a similar way to the other secondary lymphoid organs with defined B- and T-cell zones. A large plasma cell population is often present, underlying the epithelial surface, which is involved in secretion of immunoglobulin into the lumen. In other parts of the pharynx

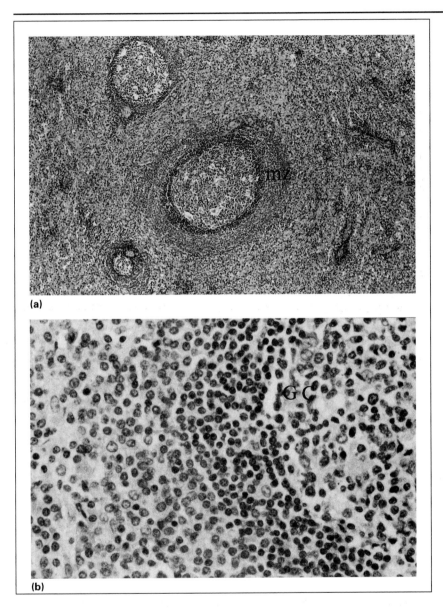

(a)

(b)

Figure 1.12 Normal spleen. (a) A section of spleen removed at the time of gastric surgery. In the centre of the photograph there is a large reactive germinal centre surrounded by a darkly stained mantle zone and expanded outer marginal zone (mz). (b) This high-power view of para-arteriolar lymphoid tissue shows the edge of the germinal centre separated from the marginal zone by the mantle zone, which consists mainly of small darkly staining lymphocytes. The germinal centre (GC) consists of a mixture of centrocytes and centroblasts. The marginal zone is more polymorphic with so-called monocytoid B-cells, plasmacytoid cells and moderate numbers of macrophages.

less clearly defined nodules of organized lymphoid tissue may be present in association with either respiratory-type or squamous epithelium.

The Peyer's patches of the small intestine consist of nodules of organized lymphoid tissue associated with specialized surface epithelium. The epithelium lacks mucin-secreting goblet cells and consists mainly of specialized absorptive M-cells thought to be involved in antigen transport from the lumen of the intestine. The B-cell area consists of a series of follicles with their base around the level of the muscularis mucosae.

Between the follicle and specialized epithelium there is a 'dome' which consists of IgM$^+$ IgD$^-$ B-cells, plasma cells and macrophages analogous to the marginal zone of spleen and lymph nodes. Cells in the marginal zone may infiltrate the adjacent epithelium and this should not be confused with the destructive lymphoepithelial lesions of marginal zone lymphoma. The T-cells lie in the interfollicular area and are similar in composition to the paracortex of lymph nodes.

Activated Peyer's patch B-cells, which are committed to plasma cell differentiation, enter the circulation *via* the lymphatics and colonize the lamina propria of the intestine and possibly other mucosal sites, such as the respiratory and genitourinary tract. IgA produced by these cells is transported across the epithelium into the lumen of the bowel. In addition to the Peyer's patches, the small intestine has a large T-cell population, which includes intraepithelial lymphocytes and lamina propria T-cells. There is evidence that lymphoid progenitors from the bone marrow may enter the small intestine and develop into T-cells, with the intestinal epithelium assuming the same function as the thymic epithelial cells. T-cells that develop in the small intestine can be distinguished from their thymic counterparts by the subtype of CD8 expressed.

The stomach normally contains very few lymphoid cells but, in the presence of chronic *Helicobacter* infection, organized lymphoid tissue may develop in the gastric antrum. This is important in the pathogenesis of gastric lymphoma and is discussed in Chapter 10.

The secondary lymphoid organs are linked by migrating lymphocytes

The efficiency of the immune system depends on the continual circulation of lymphocytes between secondary lymphoid organs. This allows the maximum concentration of reactive cells at the site of antigenic stimulation. The circulation of lymphocytes is dependent on the adhesive interaction between lymphocytes and endothelial cells. At least four lymphocyte cell-surface molecules participate in this interaction. These include L-selectin, which binds to mannose 6-phosphate containing polysaccharides, CD44, which mediates adhesion to hyaluronic acid, and the integrins LFA-1 and VLA-4. Specialized endothelial cells in lymph nodes and mucosal surface express unique addresin molecules, which results in partial separation of the lymphocyte populations circulating between lymph nodes and those that localize primarily to mucosal lymphoid tissue. The induction of expression of VCAM1 and ICAM1 and 2 on endothelial cells serves to recruit activated lymphocytes into sites of inflammation. The retention of lymphocytes within the stroma depends on subsequent adhesive interactions with the extracellular matrix and other cell types present.

1.4 Key references

Dunn-Walters, D. K., Isaacson, P. G. and Spencer, J. (1995) Analysis of mutations in immunoglobulin heavy chain variable genes in microdissected marginal zone (MGZ) B-cells suggests that the MGZ of the human spleen is a reservoir of memory B-cell. *Journal of Experimental Medicine*, **182**, 559–566.

Krause, D. S., Fackler, M. J., Civin, C. I. and May, W. S. (1996) CD34: structure, biology and clinical utility. *Blood*, **87**, 1–13.

Maclennan, I. C. M. (1994) Germinal centers. *Annual Revue of Immunology*, **12**, 117–139.

Shivdasani, R. A. and Orkin, S. H. (1996) The transcriptional control of hematopoiesis. *Blood*, **87**, 4025–4039.

Spits, H., Lanier, L. L. and Phillips, J. H. (1995) Development of human T and natural killer cells. *Blood*, **85**, 2654–2670.

Stewart, K. A. and Schwartz, R. S. (1994) Immunoglobulin V regions and the B-cell. *Blood*, **83**, 1717–1730.

Thorbecke, G. J., Amin, A. R. and Tsiabge, V. K. (1994) Biology of germinal centers in lymphoid tissue. *FASEB Journal*, **8**, 832–840.

2 Laboratory methods for the diagnosis and classification of lymphoproliferative disorders

Although the morphological examination of conventional H&E- or Giemsa-stained cytological preparations or histological sections remains important, the use of antibody-based methods and molecular biology techniques are now essential to the provision of a high standard of diagnosis of lymphoproliferative disorders.

2.1 Morphology, cytochemistry and immunohistology

The initial handling of specimens is critical to accurate diagnosis

Many diagnostic problems in lymphoid pathology are attributable to failures in the way specimens are taken and their initial handling in the laboratory. The removal of a normal or reactive node is a simple procedure but removal of a node involved by lymphoma that is infiltrating the surrounding tissues and is associated with fibrosis requires a higher level of surgical skill. Once removed, lymph node specimens should always be sent unfixed to the laboratory by the fastest possible route. If any delay is likely a suitable transport medium should be used and the specimen should be kept at 4°C. Such unfixed tissue offers the greatest flexibility in investigation with the possibility of disaggregation of the tissue for flow cytometric immunophenotypical studies, marker studies on cryostat sections and the extraction of both good-quality RNA and DNA. The rapid receipt of fresh tissues is also of great value in ensuring the correct fixation and processing of tissue for routine paraffin histology. Placing a large node, especially when there is fibrosis, in a small volume of fixative for an indeterminate period will inevitably result in poor-quality tissue preservation. In some cases only a thin rim of properly fixed tissue will be obtained because of poor penetration of the fixative. In order to obtain optimal fixation an unfixed node should be sliced along its long axis in 3 mm slices using a very sharp blade before immersion in the fixative (Figure 2.1).

Numerous fixatives have been advocated as being of special value in processing lymphoid tissue but 10% formaldehyde in tap water gives satisfactory results without the need for more complicated preparations. It is simple to prepare, stable and gives a good balance between morphological and antigenic preservation. Formaldehyde, like all aldehyde fixatives, acts by the formation of methylene cross-links between basic amino acids such as lysine. Lymphoid tissue should be fixed for 24–48 h (except for endoscopic or very small biopsies). A particular fixation problem is splenic tissue, which allows very slow penetration of fixative.

Once fixed, tissues are processed by stepwise replacement of the water with graded alcohols, which are then replaced by chloroform or xylene.

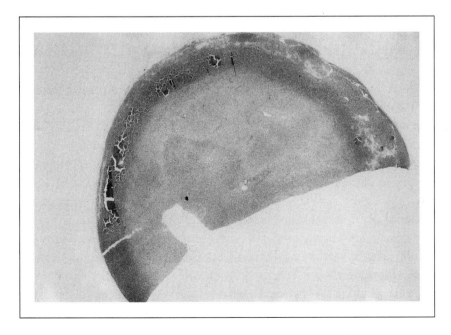

Figure 2.1 The effects of inadequate fixation on nodal tissue. This is a greatly enlarged node that was placed intact in a small volume of fixative. Most of the centre of the node is autolytic, with only a thin rim of fixed tissue at the edge.

This allows permeation by paraffin wax which is formed into a block surrounding the tissue. The process takes about 16 h, although very small fragments of tissue can be processed in 3–4 h.

Bone marrow biopsies require special processing

Bone is much harder than paraffin wax, so specimens of bone processed as described above would be impossible to cut and would cause damage to conventional microtomes. This can be overcome by removing the calcium from the bone using EDTA or formic acid or by using a much harder embedding medium. In each the final tissue block has a uniform degree of hardness. For either method the specimen should be fixed in 10% formalin for 24 h.

Resin sections provide a higher level of morphological detail than is achievable with decalcified specimens and allow detailed assessment of marrow architecture. Minor degrees of nuclear atypia, such as those that occur in red cell precursors in myelodysplasia, and minimal lymphoid infiltrates are more readily identified. Specimens can be processed in 48 h with an additional day for marker studies. The use of a modified methyl methacrylate resin has the major advantage of being soluble in xylene, which allows all the resin to be removed before conventional or immunohistological staining. Resin embedding is now the technique of choice.

A wide range of cell markers can be demonstrated on fixed tissues embedded in paraffin wax or resin

The past few years have seen a considerable increase in the range of markers that can be demonstrated in fixed tissues, together with a major improvement in the consistency and reliability of the results. The technique of choice at the present time is the streptavidin–biotin complex method (StrABC). In this method the tissue section is incubated with an unlabelled specific antibody and then with a biotinylated anti-immunoglobulin. The high sensitivity of the StrABC method is based on the use of a streptavidin–enzyme complex to demonstrate binding of the primary antibody to the cells. This complex consists of an optimum ratio of biotinylated enzyme with the high-affinity biotin binding protein streptavidin, which is formulated to maximize the number of enzyme molecules and hence the final signal at the site of antibody binding (Figure 2.2).

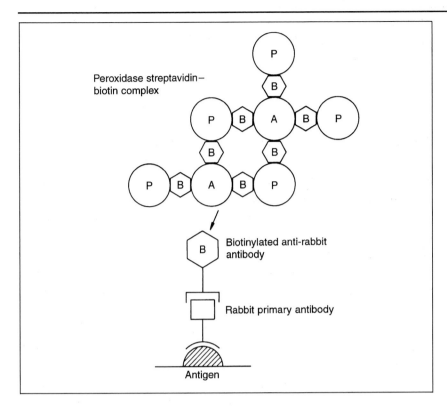

Peroxidase streptavidin–
biotin complex

Biotinylated anti-rabbit
antibody

Rabbit primary antibody

Antigen

Figure 2.2 The avidin–biotin complex method. In this method specific antibody–antigen binding is detected using an biotinylated anti-immunoglobulin antibody, which is then visualized by the addition of a complex of streptavidin linked to biotinylated horseradish peroxidase. The complex is formulated to maximize the ratio of enzyme molecules to molecules of bound primary antibody.

In some tissues, such as kidney, it may necessary to block endogenous biotin with free avidin. Horseradish peroxidase is the most commonly used enzyme with diaminobenzidine (DAB) as the chromogen. This gives a brown colour following development. In fixed tissues endogenous peroxidase can be readily blocked by hydrogen peroxide in methanol.

Alkaline phosphatase is a commonly used alternative, which can be used on fresh cells and tissues where endogenous peroxidase levels are high (Figure 2.3).

Further amplification may be obtained using biotinylated tyramide. On activation by hydrogen peroxide this agent reacts with the bound complex of antibodies, increasing the number of sites to which streptavidin peroxidase can be attached. This procedure allows the more economical use of a number of antibodies and the demonstration of weak antigens in paraffin sections.

The range of antigens that can be demonstrated in fixed tissues is considerably less than in fresh tissues. Some of these antigens are lost during processing but many are concealed by formalin-induced cross-linking. A number of techniques are now available to remove cross-links and expose the concealed antigens. These use enzyme digestion, heat

Figure 2.3 Alkaline phosphatase – antialkaline phosphatase method. This technique is most commonly used on cytological preparations. In this method the primary specific antibody is linked to a complex of the enzyme alkaline phosphatase and anti-alkaline phosphatase using a bridging antibody.

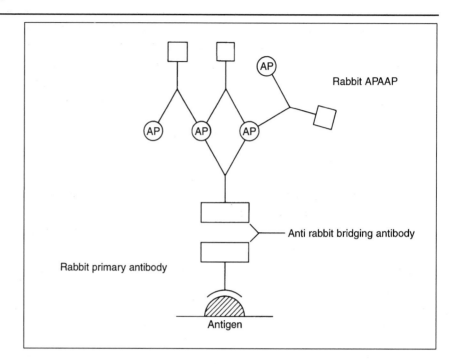

Rabbit APAAP

Anti rabbit bridging antibody

Rabbit primary antibody

Antigen

treatment or a combination of both. The most commonly used enzyme method is incubation of tissue sections with trypsin but it is important to prevent over- or underdigestion, which can abolish reactivity, cause non-specific binding and destroy morphological detail. Heat-mediated antigen retrieval using a domestic microwave oven has improved the consistency and range of antigens demonstrable by immunocytochemistry. It is not as difficult to control as enzyme digestion and is less dependent on the fixation time and processing method. However it is essential to use slides coated with an adhesive agent to prevent loss of the section during processing.

2.2 Flow cytometry

Specimens for flow cytometry are relatively robust

Specimens of blood or bone marrow intended for flow cytometric analysis should be collected into containers with EDTA anticoagulant. In this form the cells are relatively stable and good-quality results can be obtained up to 24 h after the specimen was taken, allowing specimens to be sent by mail or routine specimen delivery services. However, there are two qualifications to this statement. Firstly, if any delay is anticipated, fresh smears made at the time of specimen collection should be sent with the EDTA samples. Cells kept in EDTA are unsuitable for morphological analysis and the fresh smears are also preferred for routine cytochemical investigations. Secondly, if the specimen is going to be used for RNA extraction it is essential that it be sent by the fastest possible route to limit RNA degradation.

Specimens of cerebrospinal fluid (CSF) or serous effusions usually do not require anticoagulation but, when the sample is very cellular, a small amount of preservative-free heparin may be helpful. Solid tissue specimens should remain unfixed and be sent to the laboratory as quickly as possible. In some cases simply shaking small fragments of tumour vigorously in a few millilitres of isotonic medium will liberate enough cells for analysis. In others a piece of tissue can be gently injected with small volumes of cell culture medium through a fine bore needle and then chopped into small pieces with a scalpel blade.

Before analysis the white blood cell fraction needs to be separated from the red cells. This can be carried out in one of two ways. If the objective is the immunophenotypical characterization of a neoplastic population it is usual to separate the cells by density gradient centrifugation. However, this method leads to unpredictable loss of white cell fractions and if quantitation of lymphocyte subsets is required a whole blood lysis method should be used.

Flow cytometers analyse cells according to their light scattering and fluorescence properties

All flow cytometers have five essential components – the fluid system, light sources, optical system, detectors and software (Figure 2.4).

The power of flow cytometric systems depends on their ability to make multiple measurements on large numbers of single cells. To do this it is essential that a single cell stream passes through the light source and detection system. Most flow cytometers operate on the principle of hydrodynamic focusing. The aspirated cell suspension is injected into the centre of a channel through which sheath fluid is flowing. The sheath fluid flow is retarded by viscous drag where it is in contact with the channel walls. This has the effect of creating a gradient of flow rate, which increases towards the centre of the channel. Cells are drawn towards the centre of the stream, ultimately producing a single cell stream for analysis.

Figure 2.4 Schematic representation of a flow cytometer. The main components of a flow cytometer form a hydrodynamic focussing system, which produces a single file of cells passing through the flow cell. The cells pass through a laser, which excites fluorescent dyes attached to the cell. The fluorescent emissions are collected by detectors for analysis. The pattern of scattering of the laser light also gives information about the size and granularity of the cell. Filters are used to measure the intensity of emission from a particular fluorochrome.

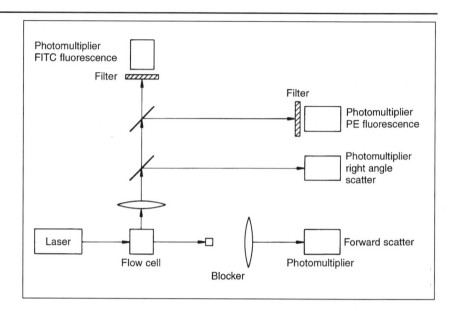

Almost all flow cytometers use one or more lasers as their light source. Laser light is produced by using a high current to excite electrons in an ionized gas. The output of the laser is coherent light at a number of wavelengths characteristic of the element used. In a flow cytometer a prism is used to separate the components of the laser light to produce a beam of a single wavelength. In most flow cytometers in routine use the primary light source is the 488 nm emission of an argon laser. A number of fluorochromes will absorb light at this wavelength. By choosing dyes that differ in their emission spectrum it is possible for a single laser instrument to analyse cells labelled with two or three different monoclonal antibodies. The fluorochromes most commonly used are fluorescein isothiocyanate (FITC), phycoerythrin (PE) and its derivative Cy5.

The detection system of a flow cytometer is a combination of lenses, filter and photomultiplier tubes. In most instruments forward scattered light is collected between 1 and 20° off the beam. To be effective in measuring cell size this system must be designed to exclude stray light from the primary source. A more complex detection system is orientated at 90° to the stream. This collects both the side-scattered laser light and the fluorescent emissions, which are then separated into their component parts by a series of coloured filters. The intensity of each component is measured by a photomultiplier tube. The output of the flow cytometer is a record of each cell passing through the detection system and consists of a sequence of numbers corresponding to the intensity of light detected by the various photomultipliers. For example, if a population of cells has been stained with an FITC- and a PE-labelled antibody, each cell will be specified by four numbers corresponding to the FSC, SSC and fluorescent emissions of the FITC and PE antibodies.

The forward and side scatter pattern of light diffraction is used to define specific cell populations

The starting point for an immunophenotypical analysis is to collect data from several thousand cells and plot a scattergram in which each cell is represented by its forward scatter (size) and side scatter (granularity). In normal peripheral blood or marrow samples the scattergram has a predictable pattern, with areas corresponding to the main normal cell types – granulocytes, lymphocytes, etc. (Figure 2.5).

The presence of abnormal populations such as leukaemic blast cells may be apparent on the forward/side scatter plot. The cell population of interest is defined by drawing around an area on the scattergram using a screen cursor. The fluorescent data, usually representing the binding of labelled antibodies, can then be displayed for the cells that fall within this gate. For a single antibody this data is displayed as a frequency distribution histogram of fluorescent intensity. In most cases this histogram has two distinct and separate peaks corresponding to non-specific binding and positive staining of cells. Examination of this

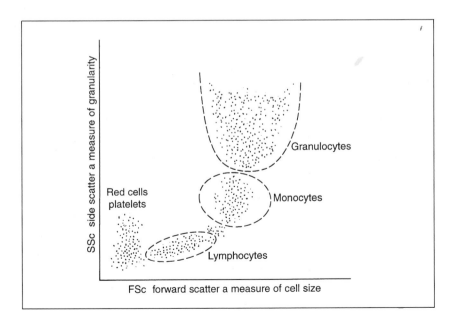

Figure 2.5 The use of light scatter characteristics. This scatter plot shows the distribution of forward and side scatter in a normal peripheral blood sample. On the basis of size and granularity it is possible to make a preliminary distinction between lymphocytes, monocytes and granulocytes. Electronic gates can then be set to specifically analyse immunophenotypical features of these individual populations.

histogram allows a fluorescent intensity to be selected for each antibody that will separate positive and negative cells.

There are several problems that may be encountered at this stage of the analysis. A large amount of cell debris may make it difficult to separate live from dead cells. The presence of dead cells leads to a high level of non-specific binding of antibody and erroneous results. This can be corrected by analysing an aliquot of the sample stained with the dye propidium iodide which is only taken up by dead cells. This allows a gate to be defined in which only data from live cells is collected. A similar problem is found in older samples, where swelling of red blood cells leads to their inclusion in the lymphocyte and other populations as defined by forward and side scatter. Again, this can at least in part be compensated for by staining an aliquot of the sample with an antibody to a red cell antigen such as glycophorin A. A further difficult problem may arise with antibodies with relatively low binding affinity in which there is lack of clear separation between positive and negative populations – the distinction may be subjective and rather arbitrary.

In the investigation of neoplastic cells it is not sufficient to rely only on physical characteristics to define the cell population of interest. The lymphocyte gate defined in this way will contain variable numbers of T- and B-cells and probably some macrophages. For this reason analyses are always carried out by double or sometimes triple labelling. For example, in the investigation of a suspected B-cell malignancy all the relevant antibodies such as Ig light chain, CD5, CD23, CD20, etc. would be analysed in conjunction with a pan-B-cell marker such as CD19. This is essential to eliminate effects caused by non-specific binding and because few antibodies are truly lineage specific – for example CD5 and CD38 may be found on both B- and T-cells. These results can be expressed as a scattergram in which the position of each cell is defined by the fluorescent intensity of staining with each antibody. The intensity value for each antibody distinguishing positive and negative cells is then used to divide the plot into four quadrants containing cells positive with both antibodies, cells positive with one or other of the antibodies or negative for both (Figure 2.6).

The final results are usually expressed as the proportion of the cells reacting positively with the reference antibody which express the test marker, e.g. in B-cell CLL the proportion of the lymphocytes positive with CD19 (pan-B-cell) that also express CD5. The mean fluorescence intensity of the test antibody should also be reported. Some applications may require the use of three antibodies, each labelled with different fluorochromes.

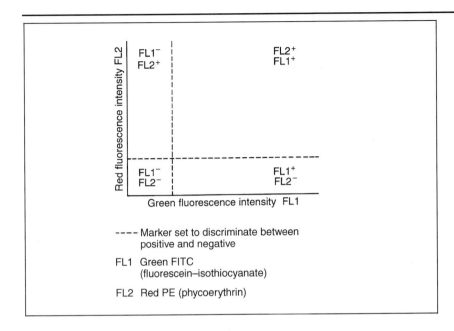

Figure 2.6 Flow cytometry quadrant analysis. In almost all diagnostic applications in haematological oncology it is essential to use at least double labelling. For each antibody a marker is set using cells stained with a isotype-matched control antibody to discriminate positive from negative cells. The scattergram is then analysed in quadrants to determine the numbers of dual- and single-labelled cells and negative cells.

The major application of flow cytometry is in the demonstration of cell surface antigens. Antibodies that recognize cell surface determinants are sufficient for a detailed phenotypical characterization of most haematological malignancies but there are circumstances where the demonstration of cytoplasmic or nuclear markers is important, the main examples being cytoplasmic immunoglobulin in plasma cells or cytoplasmic IgM or CD3 in leukaemias of precursor B- or T-lymphocytes. It is possible to demonstrate cytoplasmic markers by flow cytometry but the staining technique is more difficult and non-specific binding is a greater problem. In general these techniques are not yet sufficiently robust for routine use and cytoplasmic antigens are usually demonstrated by slide-based methods either on a smear or an accompanying biopsy.

Panels of antibodies should be selected for routine use in both flow cytometry and immunocytochemistry

There are a number of general principles that should be used in selecting panels of antibodies for routine flow cytometric immunophenotyping. The aim is to select antibodies which, either alone or in combination, define major subsets of leukaemia or lymphoma. The immunophenotypical investigations should complement the morphological examination of the specimen. The concordance of morphological, cytochemical and immunophenotypical investigations is a major element in achieving a high level of diagnostic accuracy and discordance of any of these elements should be an indication for further investigation. It is usual to devise a screening panel which consists of a small number of antibodies and a series of panels designed for specialist tasks such as the investigation of acute leukaemias, B-cell malignancy, T-cell malignancy and immuno-logical disorders (Figure 2.7).

Figure 2.7 Antibody panel for the investigation of B-cell lymphoproliferative disorders. This flow cytometry worksheet illustrates an approach to investigating B-cell lymphoproliferative disorders. The expression of all cell surface markers is determined in relation to the pan-B cell marker CD19 by two colour flow cytometry. The results are expressed as the percentage of positive cells and the mean fluorescent intensity. In this protocol the expression of cytoplasmic immunoglobulins, Tdt and Ki67 are demonstrated by direct immunofluorescence.

Name   Specimen   HMDS No

B Lymphoproliferative Disorders Worksheet

Tag	11	12	13	14	15	16	17	18	19	20	21	22
Fitc	CD3	Kappa	Lambda	CD11a	CD20	FMC7	CD10	CD19	CD19	CD19	CD19	CD19
PE	CD19	CD19	CD19	CD19	CD19	CD19	CD19	CD3	CD5	CD22	CD23	CD38
% pos												
mean Fl int												
mean Fl of whole peak	control							control				

Fitc +/- marker set at
PE +/- marker set at   <20%, - : 21- 49% +/-: >50% +   Carried out by: _____.

Hairy Cell/SLVL Panel Tag 023-025

Tube	23	24	25
Fitc	CD103	CD11c	CD19
PE	CD19	CD19	CD25
% pos			
mean Fl int			

Carried out by: _____.

Cytoplasmic Immunoglobulins

κ	λ	G	A	M	D

Carried out by: _____.

Ki67	Tdt		

Carried out by: _____.

Results	CD19	SIgκ	SIgλ	CD5	CD11a	CD20	FMC7	CD10	CD22	CD23	CD38
composite phenotype											
strength											

	CD103	CD25	CD11c						%CD3	%CD19
strength									% of total lymphocyte gate/BM or PBMC	

Phenotypic Diagnosis _____

Lab Comments _____

Flow cytometry can also be used to assess cell proliferation and cell death

There are a variety of methods available for measuring cell proliferation by flow cytometry. The simplest methods use estimation of cellular DNA content in whole cells or isolated nuclei liberated from tissues by pepsin digestion and centrifugation. A dye such as propidium iodide is used which has stoichometric binding to DNA. The fluorescent signal is in direct proportion to the DNA content of the cell. Cells in G_0/G_1 phases of the cell cycle have a normal diploid content of DNA, cells in G_2 have double the amount of DNA and cells in S phase have quantities intermediate between G_1 and G_2. A DNA histogram is produced and standard curve fitting and integration methods can be used to calculate the proportion of cells in each of these categories (Figure 2.8).

This is a simple and effective technique which has two main limitations. As in other malignancies, a proportion of leukaemias and lymphomas are aneuploid and contain a mixture of clones with varying DNA content. In these cases complex histograms are produced

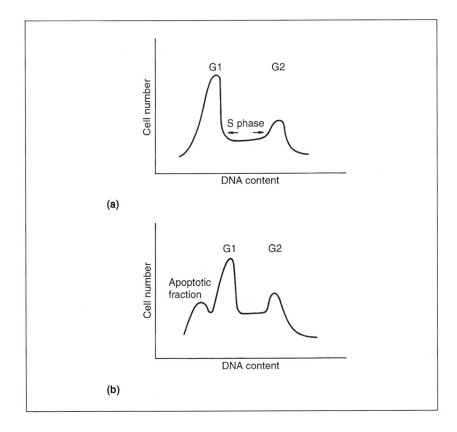

(a)

(b)

Figure 2.8 Determination of DNA content by flow cytometry. **(a)** The fluorescent dye propidium iodide binds to DNA and, when excited by a laser, the intensity of the emitted light is proportional to the DNA content of the nucleus. Cells in G_2 phase of the cell cycle that have replicated their DNA will have twice the concentration of DNA of those in G_1/G_0 phase. Cells in S-phase will have a concentration that varies between these two values. By integration of curves values can be obtained for the proportion of cells in each phase of the cycle. **(b)** If a significant number of the cells in the sample are apoptotic, a further peak will be seen to the left of the G_1 peak. This represents cells in the early stage of cell death, which have lost a proportion of their fragmenting DNA.

from which it is difficult to calculate the proportion in each phase of the cell cycle. A related problem applies mainly to nuclei extracted from fixed tissue. Degradation of DNA often results in wide peaks in which it may be impossible to distinguish the effects of poor sample quality from the presence of a mixed diploid and aneuploid population. Consequently, the reliability of cell cycle calculations may be poor.

Cell cycle markers such as Ki67, which identifies the proportion of cells actively cycling, can be used in flow cytometric systems. The most specific, but most difficult, method is to prelabel the cell with bromodeoxyuridine and then demonstrate labelled DNA using an antibody conjugate. This provides the most direct measurement of S-phase fraction but requires the use of fresh samples and carefully defined labelling protocols.

There is increasing interest in the mechanisms of cell death and how these relate to response to cytotoxic chemotherapy. Several flow cytometric methods are available for the determination of the proportion of cells in a sample undergoing programmed cell death (apoptosis). The simplest of these use a DNA stain as described above. A key feature of programmed cell death is fragmentation of DNA, some of which may be lost from the cell following permeabilization of the membrane. The cell DNA content will then be less than the normal diploid amount and this will be apparent on a DNA histogram. In practice this is a difficult technique to standardize. An alternative method uses the enzyme Tdt to add biotin-labelled nucleotide bases to any free ends of DNA fragments. The enzyme and the labelled nucleotides are introduced into the cell by permeabilizing the membrane. Newly synthesized labelled DNA is then demonstrated using FITC-conjugated streptavidin. The method can be combined with surface membrane markers to define the lineage of the apoptotic cell (Figure 2.9).

Cell sorting allows flow cytometry to be combined with cell collection

In standard flow cytometry the cells are discarded after analysis. However, a number of instruments are available that allow collection of viable cells, which are defined by their flow cytometric features. In simple instruments this is an electromechanical device which removes the defined cells from the single cell stream after passing through the detector. This is a relatively slow process, with collection of only several hundred cells per minute. In more complex and expensive instruments

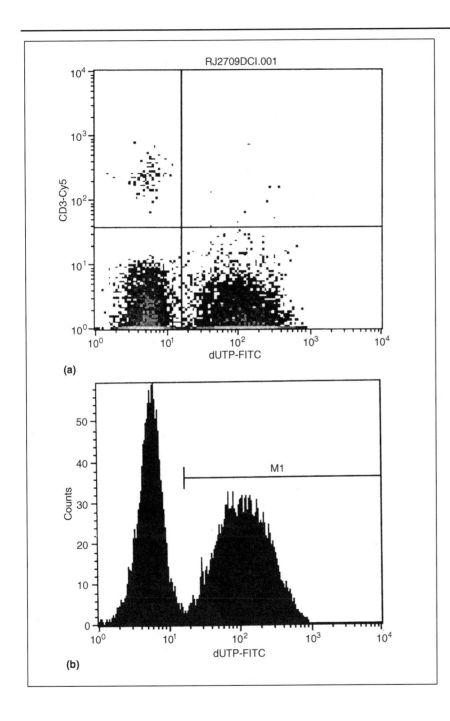

RJ2709DCI.001

(a)

(b)

Figure 2.9 Flow cytometric detection of apoptosis by DNA end-labelling. A key step in apoptosis is the fragmentation of DNA. The enzyme Tdt can be added to permeabilized cells and will add fluorescently labelled bases to broken DNA strands. This technique can be carried out in cells which are labelled with antibodies to allow the apoptotic fraction in a specific cell population to be identified. In plot A the CD3- cells show dUTP end labelling. In histogram B the M1 region represents B-CLL cells in culture in which Tdt-mediated end labelling has occurred.

cells are carried within an electrically charged droplet, which can be diverted into a collection chamber by altering the charge on a system of electrodes. These systems are much faster and can sort many thousands of cells per minute.

2.3 Molecular biological methods

There have been great advances in molecular biology techniques in recent years and techniques have now become a routine and indispensable part of the investigation of haematological malignancy. It is anticipated that, as they become more fully applied, classifications will rely heavily on the combination of morphological, immunophenotypical and molecular biological features.

The development of Southern blotting was a major landmark in molecular biology

To perform Southern blotting DNA is extracted and digested with a restriction endonuclease, which cuts DNA molecules at specific points and results in a range of fragments of different size. The digested DNA is then separated by fragment size using electrophoresis and the fragments are subsequently transferred to a nylon or nitrocellulose membrane. The fragment on which specific sequences are located can then be determined by hybridizing the membrane with a labelled DNA probe. After washing in salt solutions to remove non-specifically-bound probe the fragments of interest are visualized by autoradiography (Figure 2.10). For many applications Southern blotting remains the definitive technique but in the investigation of diagnostic samples it is often limited by the need for large amounts of high-quality DNA and it is also a relatively labour-intensive and slow method.

The polymerase chain reaction can provide an easy, rapid diagnostic test

The polymerase chain reaction (PCR) is a technique for the amplification of specific DNA sequences and for many applications is replacing Southern blotting. Short DNA primer sequences are synthesized which are complementary to the ends of the sequence of interest. The test DNA is mixed with these primer sequences, nucleotides and a thermostable DNA polymerase in a thermal cycler instrument. This is programmed to heat and cool the mixture through a preset number of cycles. In each cycle the primers initiate the synthesis of new DNA strands, which are then separated by heating. The repeated process results in a chain reaction that exponentially synthesizes large numbers of copies of the sequence of interest. These

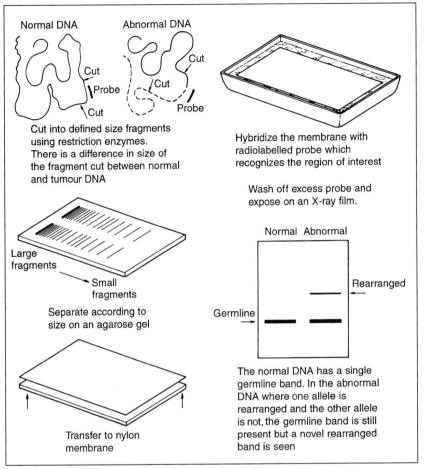

Figure 2.10 Southern blotting. To perform a Southern blot DNA is digested using one or more restriction enzymes and the resulting fragments are separated on the basis of size using gel electrophoresis. The separated fragments are then blotted from the gel on to a membrane. Specific fragments can then be identified by hybridizing the membrane with labelled DNA probes, which bind to the sequences of interest and which are then visualized by autoradiography.

fragments are so abundant that their size can be determined following electrophoresis merely by staining with ethidium bromide and using UV illumination (Figure 2.11). The sensitivity of detection can be improved by labelling the PCR product with either radioisotopes or fluorescent dyes.

RNA can also be analysed by the PCR but in this case it is essential to use reverse transcriptase to synthesize DNA copies of the RNA. Any RNA based technique is limited by the sensitivity of the expressed sequences to degradation by ribonucleases in isolated cells or tissues.

In some cases it may be necessary to determine the sequence of a PCR product

Figure 2.11 The polymerase chain reaction. This is a method of making large numbers of copies of short DNA sequences defined by pairs of primers that hybridize to opposite DNA strands at either end of the target sequence. Copying is achieved by cycles of denaturation, primer binding and strand extension in the presence of a thermostable DNA polymerase.

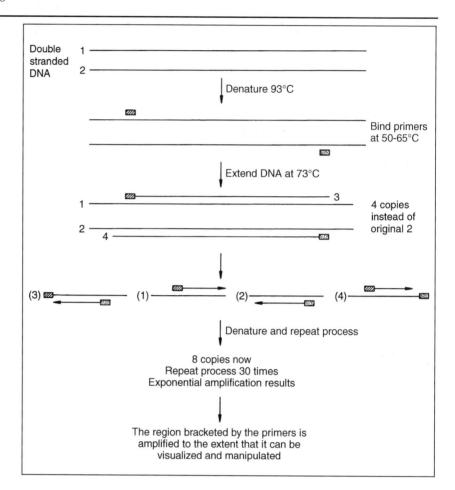

Sequencing can be done by synthesizing further DNA strands in the presence of small amounts of a modified nucleotide which, when incorporated, will block further extension. Electrophoresis of the products of this reaction on a high resolution gel will demonstrate fragments of varying length corresponding to the point at which the blocking nucleotide was incorporated. In order to perform a sequencing reaction this procedure is carried out with terminating nucleotides corresponding to each of the four DNA bases. If a radiolabel is used, four individual reactions have to be carried out with either an A, G, C or T terminator. The sequence is obtained by running the four reactions side by side. Fluorescent sequencing uses a different colour label for each of the bases and so the sequence can be read from a single lane according to the sequence of coloured peaks (Figure 2.12).

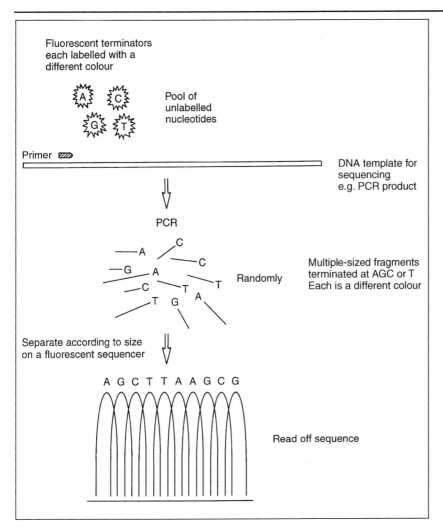

Fluorescent terminators each labelled with a different colour

Pool of unlabelled nucleotides

Primer

DNA template for sequencing e.g. PCR product

PCR

Multiple-sized fragments terminated at AGC or T
Each is a different colour

Randomly

Separate according to size on a fluorescent sequencer

A G C T T A A G C G

Read off sequence

Figure 2.12 Fluorescent cycle sequencing. To determine a DNA sequence by this method single-stranded DNA is copied in the presence of modified A, C, T, G nucleotides which when incorporated into the growing strand will terminate further synthesis. Each type of modified nucleotide is labelled with a different fluorescent dye. This produces a set of DNA molecules which differ in length by one base and end in a fluorescently labelled base. After electrophoresis, which separates the fragments by size, the sequence can be read in a fluorescent sequencer.

Detection of lymphocyte monoclonality

Analysis of the immunoglobulin or T-cell receptor genes is the major method of detecting lymphocyte monoclonality

During normal lymphocyte development, diversity of antigen specificity is generated by genetic recombination. Recombination occurs between more or less randomly selected V, D and J region genes, which combine with the constant region gene to form a functioning immunoglobulin or T-cell receptor gene. During this process the enzyme Tdt both adds and deletes variable numbers of bases between the recombining segments and so produces further diversity. The enormous range of possible combinations makes the antigen receptor genes powerful clonal markers, which can be detected by Southern blotting or PCR (Figures 2.13, 2.14).

In a normal polyclonal population of lymphocytes the recombined Ig or TCR genes will vary considerably in size. Restriction enzyme digestion and hybridization with probes to the constant region of TCR or Ig genes will produce a banding pattern corresponding to the genes in germline configuration, as would be found in non-lymphoid cells. The rearranged sequences present in a polyclonal B-cell population are below the level of sensitivity of the test and are therefore not seen. If a clone is present that is greater than about 5–10% of the total cells in the sample, a further band or bands will be seen corresponding to the size of the rearranged fragment carried by the clone. In general, results should be confirmed using a second enzyme digest to exclude normal polymorphisms and false-positive results.

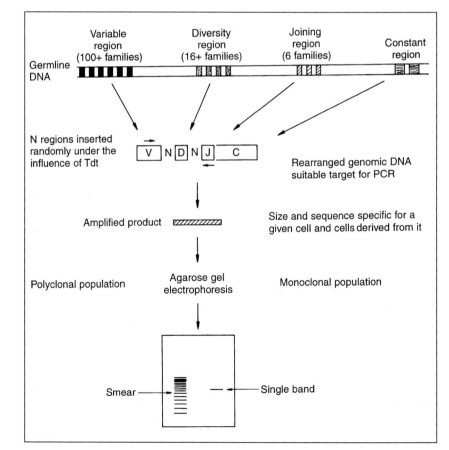

Figure 2.13 Detection of B-cell monoclonality by PCR of IgH gene rearrangements. As immunoglobulin V, D and J regions are rearranged to form a functioning immunoglobulin molecule the enzyme Tdt adds a variable number of bases to the joining regions. Amplification of this region by PCR shows a normal distribution of size of the region containing the added bases (N region). In a clonal B-cell population all the cells will have N regions of the same size. In interpreting the results it is important to remember that cells belonging to different clones with different IgH genes may generate PCR products of the same size. The specificity and sensitivity can be improved by sequencing the amplified fragment and repeating the PCR with specific primers (allele-specific oligonucleotides).

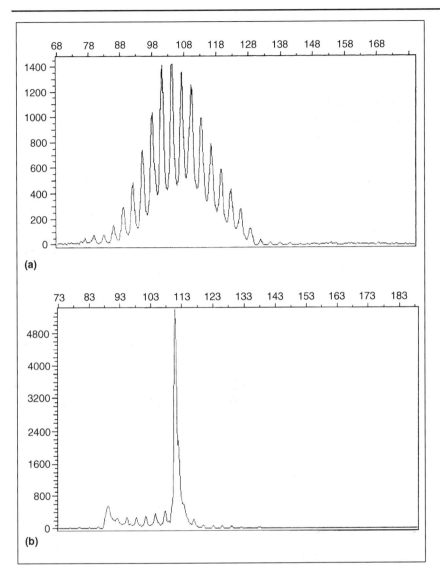

Figure 2.14 Detection of clonal IgH rearrangements by fluorescent PCR. The detection of IgH gene rearrangements by PCR can be improved using fluorescent primer and laser scanning gene sequencer. A polyclonal population gives a typical 'hedgehog' pattern **(a)**. The presence of a monoclonal population is shown by a single large peak **(b)**. Although the areas under the peak can be readily determined they cannot be used to quantify individual clones.

PCR-based techniques amplify the region spanning the join between the V and J genes of the TCR or IgH. The size of this region will vary according to the number of bases added or deleted by Tdt during development. A polyclonal lymphoid population will give either a smear or ladder pattern depending on the electrophoresis conditions and detection system used. Again clonal populations appear as a dense single or double band, though it is also possible to see a clonal band within a polyclonal background. In these cases it is more difficult to assign clonality definitively.

Most methods for the detection of B-cell monoclonality use a combination of a primer that recognizes a consensus sequence in the IgH J gene and a consensus sequence common to all V genes in the framework 3 region. This technique will demonstrate clonality in approximately 60–70% of B-cell tumours; a further 10% will be shown to be monoclonal if a further PCR is carried out using framework 1 regions that cover all of the IgH V region families.

The detection of T-cell clones uses the same principle but is based on primers that recognize consensus sequences in the T-cell receptor genes. The most common technique uses sequences in the TCR-Vgamma together with TCR-Jgamma. The TCR-gamma genes rearrange before the most commonly expressed TCR-alpha and beta genes and because of this the test is more generally applicable and will detect clonal populations of precursor T-cells in which rearrangement TCR-beta or alpha has not occurred.

Fluorescent PCR, when used in combination with a laser scanning system, is able to detect smaller clones than with Southern blotting. However, all PCR methods have a significant false negative rate which is higher than that seen with Southern blotting. PCR reactions are more likely to be disrupted by the presence of chromosomal abnormalities or simply by failure of the DNA to amplify.

Lymphocyte monoclonality is not a specific marker of malignancy

Monoclonality and neoplasia are closely associated. Almost all malignant lymphoproliferations are monoclonal and demonstration of mono-clonality is an integral part of diagnosis. However, it must be stressed that, although most lymphomas are monoclonal, not all monoclonal populations are neoplastic. When sensitive methods are used, mono-clonal T-cell or B-cell populations may be seen in infective and inflammatory disorders such as infective mononucleosis or *Helicobacter*-associated gastritis. The detection of monoclonality alone should never be used to make a diagnosis of malignancy.

The detection of mutations and chromosomal abnormalities

There are a number of tests that can be used as screening tests for mutations

Sequencing is a slow process and in order to detect mutations in tumour tissue a screening test is useful to reduce the amount of DNA sequencing required. One example is the detection of single-stranded conformational polymorphisms. When DNA is denatured the single strands fold into a secondary structure, which is determined by the sequence of bases and which has a predictable electrophoretic mobility in a non-denaturing gel.

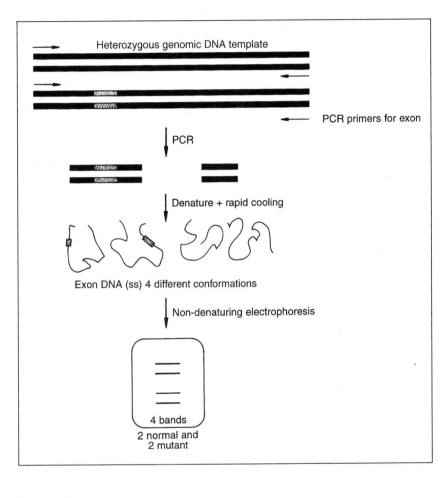

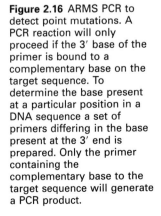

Figure 2.15 PCR single-stranded conformational polymorphism analysis. When denatured DNA is allowed to cool rapidly base pairing within single strands leads to the formation of a secondary conformation. The conformation will be affected by the presence of mutations and deletion and the different conformations are detectable by electrophoresis. PCR amplification allows this property to be exploited to screen small segments of target DNA for mutations.

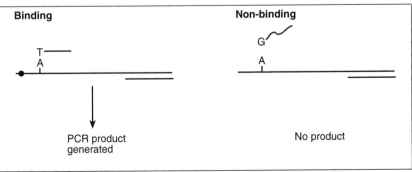

Figure 2.16 ARMS PCR to detect point mutations. A PCR reaction will only proceed if the 3′ base of the primer is bound to a complementary base on the target sequence. To determine the base present at a particular position in a DNA sequence a set of primers differing in the base present at the 3′ end is prepared. Only the primer containing the complementary base to the target sequence will generate a PCR product.

Figure 2.17 The detection of allele imbalance. Very large numbers of microsatellites consisting of repetitive DNA sequences are scattered throughout the genome. The size of these microsatellites is highly polymorphic in the human population. DNA primers that bind at each end of the microsatellite can be used to amplify the sequence by PCR and measure its length. A panel of primer sets can be used to amplify a range of microsatellites, e.g. those adjacent to tumour suppresser genes in both tumour and normal DNA from the same patient. At loci where the patient is heterozygous for microsatellite size the ratio of the alleles can be compared between the tumour and normal tissue. Imbalance in the ratio, as in this case, suggests that a deletion or amplification has occurred at this locus in the tumour. This can be used to screen for deletions at particular loci or as a general index of genetic abnormality. In this case the ratio in the normal tissue N1/N2 is 1.3 whereas in the tumour tissue (T1/T2) it is 0.53, showing the presence of allele imbalance.

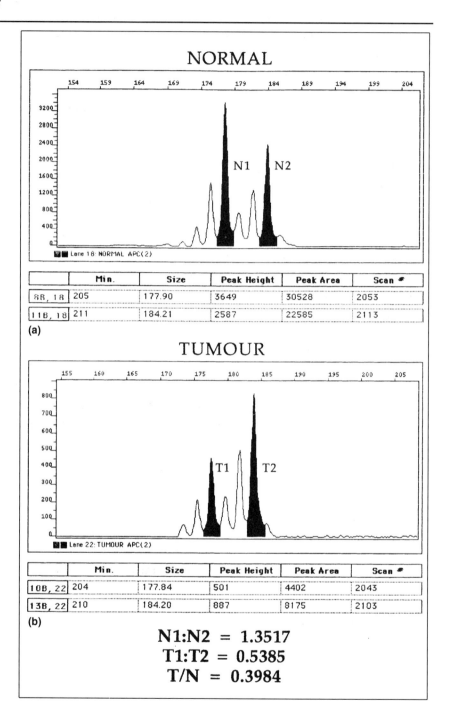

NORMAL

	Min.	Size	Peak Height	Peak Area	Scan #
8B, 18	205	177.90	3649	30528	2053
11B, 18	211	184.21	2587	22585	2113

(a)

TUMOUR

	Min.	Size	Peak Height	Peak Area	Scan #
10B, 22	204	177.84	501	4402	2043
13B, 22	210	184.20	887	8175	2103

(b)

$$N1:N2 = 1.3517$$
$$T1:T2 = 0.5385$$
$$T/N = 0.3984$$

Changes in the base sequence by mutation may alter the secondary structure and can be detected by a change in mobility of the fragment after electrophoresis. An alternative is to carry out a PCR reaction in which one of the primers has a 3′ nucleotide that will only hybridize to a mutated gene and only result in an amplified product when this mutation is present (Figures 2.15–2.16).

Many chromosomal abnormalities can be detected by a combination of PCR and *in situ* hybridization techniques

Non-random chromosomal abnormalities are a central feature of the pathogenesis of many types of leukaemia and lymphoma. Translocations may result in the deregulation of gene expression when the gene is brought under the influence of a new promoter that is constitutively activated in a particular cell. The major examples are when c-*myc* or *bcl-2* become associated with the immunoglobulin heavy-chain promoter on chromosome 14. Other translocations result in the synthesis of a new fusion protein, which may disrupt normal cell growth, the best known example being the Bcr–Abl protein produced as a result of the t(9;22). This is known as the Philadelphia translocation and is characteristic of both chronic myeloid leukaemia and ALL (Tables 2.1–2.3).

The detection of chromosomal abnormalities is already a standard feature of the diagnosis and classification of acute leukaemia and it is likely that this will soon be extended to the full range of lymphoproliferative disorders. The standard technique for the detection of chromosomal

Table 2.1 Examples of genetic abnormalities in lymphoproliferative disorders

Chromosomal translocations		
Fusion genes	t(9;22)	*abl*
	t(4;11)	*HRX*
Deregulation	t(14;18)	*bcl-2*
	t(8;14)	*myc*
Mutations		
Activating	*ras*	
Inactivating	*rb1*	
Increase rate of mutation	*p53*	
Deletions		
Loss of tumour suppressor genes	13q–	
Amplification		
Oncogene overexpression	trisomy 12	

Table 2.2 Examples of genes deregulated by translocation into the immunoglobulin loci

Immunoglobulin genes	Locus	Deregulated gene	Locus	Function
IgH	14q32	*bcl-1*	11q13	Cyclin D1 cell-cycle regulator
IgLλ	22q11	*bcl-2*	18q21	Antiapoptotic
IgLκ	2p12	*bcl-6*	3q27	Transcription factor
		myc	8q24	Transcription factor

Table 2.3 Examples of genes deregulated by translocation to the T-cell receptor loci

T cell receptor genes	Locus	Deregulated gene	Locus
TCR αδ	(14q11)	TCL 1	10q24
TCR γ	(7p15)	TCL 2	11p13
TCR β	(7q35)	TCL3	14q32
		LIM1	11p15
		Lyl 1	19p13

abnormalities has been cytogenetic analysis. This requires the examination of metaphase spreads using high-resolution banding of chromosomes either by conventional techniques or by DNA *in situ* hybridization. Metaphase preparations may by obtained from direct smears of highly proliferative cells or by culture and mitogen stimulation of more slowly growing cells. Unfortunately, it is often not possible to obtain sufficient numbers of metaphase cells in many cases of lymphomas, which can lead to high rates of false-negative examinations.

It is now becoming clear that a relatively small number of specific non-random abnormalities are important in the classification of lymphoproliferative disease. This more limited range of abnormalities can be readily detected by either PCR or *in situ* hybridization techniques. This approach is more rapid, often more sensitive and obviates the need for metaphase preparations. When a translocation has relatively constant breakpoints it may be detected by conventional DNA PCR using primers that bind to sites on each side of the breakpoint. The t(14;18) is a frequent lymphoid translocation that can be detected in this way. The majority of breakpoints occur in the major breakpoint region MBR but a minority cluster in a second region, the minor cluster region MCR, and if rearrangements in both of the regions are to be detected, two separate reactions are required. When a fusion protein is produced the problem of variable breakpoints at the DNA level can be overcome by the use of an RT (reverse transcriptase) PCR technique. Translocations detectable by this technique include t(9;22), t(2;5) and t(1;19) (Figure 2.18).

A number of important translocations and numerical chromosomal abnormalities are not readily detectable by PCR techniques

Fluorescent *in situ* hybridization on isolated metaphases prepared from whole cells or nuclei is readily applicable to cases where PCR or Southern blotting is not possible. Using probes to the centromeric repetitive DNA,

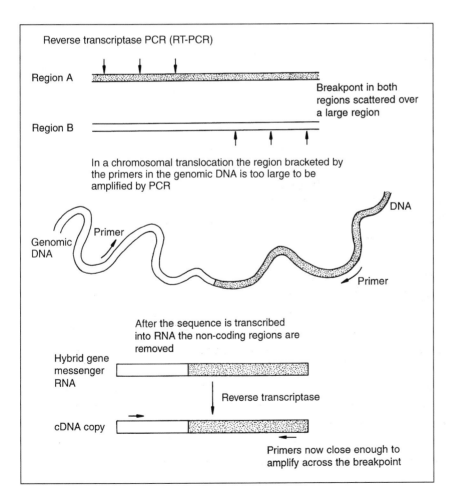

Figure 2.18 Reverse transcriptase PCR. This technique is used where a translocation results in the transcription of a hybrid gene. It is of most value where the translocation breakpoints are variable and the region may in many cases be too large for DNA PCR amplification. The transcribed RNA will be shorter because of removal of introns. The RNA is transcribed to DNA and PCR is performed by the standard method. RT–PCR is also used to detect the presence of specific mRNA molecules especially where the transcribed protein is difficult to localize with antibodies.

it is readily possible to detect important numerical abnormalities such as monosomy 7 or trisomy 12. Translocations can also be detected by *in situ* hybridization and there are at least three basic approaches to its use. The first uses a combination of two probes that recognize sequences close to the chromosomal breakpoints. These probes are labelled with different-coloured fluorescent dyes and in a normal cell four independent signals will be detectable. A translocation is detected by the opposition of the two different-coloured signals. One problem with this technique is that dots can be opposed either by chance or by the orientation of the cell, giving a false-positive result. Such events limit the sensitivity of the test for detecting residual disease (Table 2.4).

An alternative technique is to use a long sequence of DNA from the translocated region which includes all the possible breakpoints. These probes can either be yeast artificial chromosomes (YACs) or contiguous cosmid sequences. Using this technique two signals will be seen in a normal cell but, where a translocation is present and a region of labelled DNA is moved to a different region, three signals will be seen. A third method is the use of *in situ* PCR. This involves performing a PCR reaction on a section or smear and morphological localization of the products in the cell containing the relevant sequences. The disadvantage of this method is that it can only be applied to translocations that can normally be demonstrated by DNA PCR (Figure 2.19).

Comparative genomic hybridization offers a way of detecting amplification and deletion of regions of the genome without the need to obtain metaphase spreads

In comparative genomic hybridization fluorescently labelled tumour DNA is mixed with normal DNA labelled using a different fluorochrome and

Table 2.4 Chromosomal translocations detectable by PCR and RT–PCR in the lymphoproliferative disorders

Lymphoblastic disease	Non-Hodgkin's lymphoma
t(9;22)	t(2;5)
t(1;19)	t(14;18)
t(4;11)	t(11;14)
t(12;21)	
TAL1 deletions	

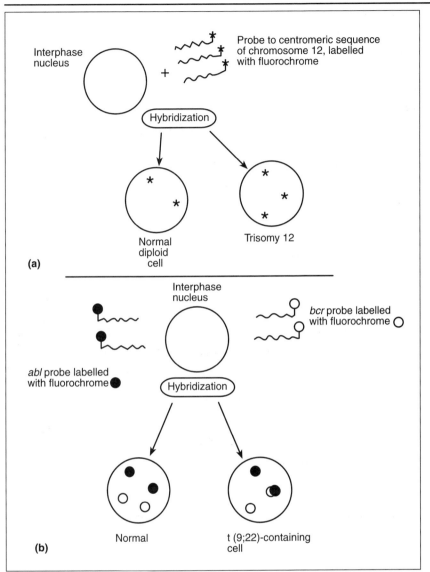

(a)

(b)

Figure 2.19 Fluorescence *in situ* hybridization (FISH). FISH can be used to detect numerical chromosomal abnormalities **(a)** or translocations **(b)**. The resolution of the technique is being improved by sensitive cameras and image processing, which allows the use of small DNA probes

hybridized to a preparation of normal metaphase chromosomes, preferably batched and stored to ensure consistency. Colour imaging techniques are used to assess the relative concentrations of tumour and control DNA bound along the length of individual chromosomes, an excess of either colour indicating either an amplification or deletion. This method is capable of resolving amplified or deleted regions of around 1 Mb and is a useful tool for screening the entire genome. Part of its attraction is that it is not necessary to obtain metaphase preparations of tumour material. Unfortunately at present it will not detect structural abnormalities such as trans-

Figure 2.20 Comparative genomic hybridization. This is a method of detecting deletion or amplification of chromosomal segments. DNA samples from tumour cells and normal cells are labelled with different fluorescent dyes. A mixture of the two labelled samples is hybridized to a metaphase chromosome preparation of normal cell. Image analysis techniques are then used to measure the ratio of the fluorescent dye bound along the length of individual chromosomes. Divergence of this ratio from 1.0 indicates deletion or amplification of the chromosome at that point.

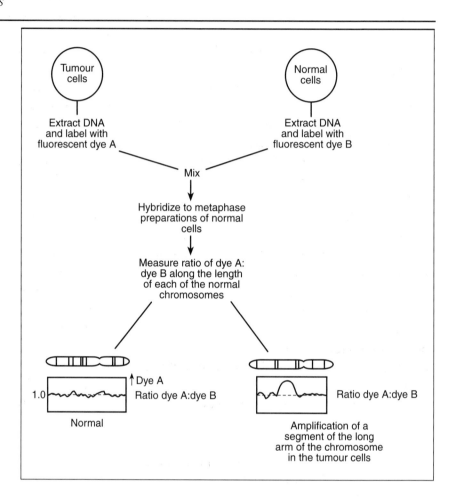

locations. Interestingly, amplifications in lymphoid tumours were thought to be very rare compared to epithelial malignancies, but preliminary results from CGH suggest that they can be seen in 10% of cases (Figure 2.20).

Smaller areas of deletion and amplification can also be detected by PCR amplification of microsatellites close to the area of interest. The highly polymorphic nature of many microsatellite loci means that this technique can also be used to differentiate host and donor cells after allogeneic bone marrow transplants (Figure 2.17).

The detection of residual disease

PCR methods can be used to monitor therapy and detect minimal residual disease

Depending on the disease type, the majority of patients achieve complete clinical remission. Unfortunately, relapse from these remissions is common implying that there is residual tumour below the level of what is detectable by clinical examination. Once no longer detectable clinically, there are a number of potential fates for cells belonging to the malignant clone: they could continue to decline steeply and be eradicated completely or they may persist longer before eventually dying out. Alternatively they may persist at very low but constant subclinical levels or they may gradually increase in number, a course of events that will eventually lead to relapse. An alternative to this pathway to relapse is that the cells are stable at low levels but something acts to destabilize this state and relapse ensues rapidly.

When malignant cells are present at the level of approximately 10% of the bone marrow cells, they can be detected by light microscopy of a bone marrow aspirate. At this level there is persistence of a very large tumour burden, about 10^{10} malignant cells. When bone marrow biopsies are examined, lower levels of marrow infiltration can be detected, though this still represents a high tumour burden. Sensitivity can be further improved by the use of flow cytometry, which can under appropriate circumstances detect one tumour cell in 10^3–10^4 normal cells. However, the detection of clonal populations by PCR can increase the sensitivity to around one clonal cell per million (equivalent to about 10^8 residual tumour cells), which is currently the maximum level of sensitivity that can be obtained (Table 2.5).

Table 2.5 Sensitivity of methods for the detection of residual disease

Morphology	10%
Cytogenetics	10%
Southern blotting	5–10%
IgH-PCR	0.0001%
Clonospecific PCR	0.000001%

Even using the PCR, a range of sensitivities can be obtained and using current approaches most analyses do not reach this theoretical level of sensitivity. The sensitivity for each reaction needs to be determined, as it will depend upon primers and reaction conditions within the reaction tube. These features must always be borne in mind when interpreting published results of minimal disease detection. Another important issue to be considered is that the sensitivity for detecting residual disease in peripheral blood and bone marrow will differ, often markedly.

The PCR can be used to amplify a number of targets that are suitable for residual disease monitoring. The best are tumour-specific chromosomal translocations but these are not present in the majority of cases. In these instances the IgH and TCR gene rearrangements provide more generally applicable targets. Using ethidium bromide visualization of the products of one of these reactions, a sensitivity of 1–10% of a polyclonal lymphoid population can be obtained. In a bone-marrow background the sensitivity is higher and, if combined with incorporation of a radiolabel, sensitivities of up to one abnormal cell in 10^3 normal cells are obtained. This may be improved further by the use of fluorescently labelled primers and an appropriate visualization system. As discussed above, the test detects clonality by identifying the size of the product only; however, a truly clonospecific test can be designed using this system by obtaining the sequence of the N regions inserted by Tdt. This can either be used to design a clone-specific primer for a PCR reaction or be used as a probe for sequences amplified by the consensus primers. This is a widely used technique but is open to large variations in sensitivity due to the primers used.

Some patients appear to have stable long-term persistence of a low level of residual disease detectable by PCR and a single positive test is not predictive of imminent relapse. Ideally a quantitative test should be used to monitor changes in the level of residual disease. At present this is difficult to achieve because of the large number of variables involved in DNA extraction and in the PCR reaction. The use of internal standards in the form of competitor substrates may go some way towards controlling interassay variation.

Similar techniques are used to monitor peripheral blood stem cell or bone marrow harvest specimens for the presence of contaminating tumour cells and to assess the efficacy of purification or purging procedures. Preliminary evidence suggests that the use of stem cells free of neoplastic cells or a post-treatment bone marrow that is free of tumour may be associated with an improved prognosis due to reduced risk of relapse.

2.4 Key references

Barclay, N. A., Birkeland, M. L., Brown, M. H. (1993) *The Leucocyte Antigen Factbook*, Academic Press, London.
Beesley, J. E. (1993) *Immunocytochemistry*, IRL Press, London.

Darzynkiewicz, Z., Robinson, J. P. and Crissman, H. A. (1994) *Flow Cytometry,* Academic Press, San Diego, CA.

Kendrew, J. (1994) *The Encyclopedia of Molecular Biology,* Blackwell Science, Oxford.

Schwartz, L. M. and Osbourne, L. M. (1995) *Cell Death,* Academic Press, London.

Wilkinson, D. G. (1993) *In Situ Hybridisation: A Practical Approach,* IRL Press, London.

3

Staging and imaging of lymphoproliferative diseases

3.1 Introduction

Staging is used to determine the extent of disease prior to treatment

Staging involves the measurement of the bulk of a tumour and its distribution. Staging using agreed criteria is essential for the proper analysis of clinical trials in which treatments are being compared. In the individual patient the stage may be a powerful prognostic factor for some types of tumour and patients with early-stage disease may be selected for local rather than systemic therapy.

For most common types of epithelial malignancy a TNM staging system is used, which takes account of the size and extent of local invasion of the primary tumour (T), the presence of metastatic deposits in draining nodes (N) and spread to distant organs (M). Unfortunately, with the exception of some extranodal lymphomas, such as mycosis fungoides, which have a predictable pattern of spread analogous to carcinomas, this type of staging cannot be readily applied to lymphoproliferative disorders. Among nodal lymphomas Hodgkin's disease has the most predictable pattern of dissemination, beginning in most cases in the thorax or neck and spreading contiguously to adjacent nodal groups. This allows 'anatomical' staging, based on the groups of nodes involved; marrow and extranodal spread being relatively rare late events. In contrast, the pattern of spread of diffuse large B-cell lymphoma is much less constant. In the case of follicle centre lymphomas almost all patients have disseminated disease at presentation and only a small minority will be found to have localized disease. Chronic lymphocytic leukaemia and mantle cell lymphoma typically involve nodes, blood and marrow at presentation but the extent of involvement of these components varies widely between patients at presentation and each may respond differently to therapy. For this reason staging systems for lymphoproliferative disorders need to be appropriate for individual tumour types and these are discussed further in the relevant chapters. The main reasons for staging are listed in Table 3.1.

Measurement of tumour-associated serum proteins may also be helpful in assessing tumour load, notably paraproteins, as in myeloma. In the case of beta-2-microglobulin the value of such measurement is more empirically based.

The examination of the bone marrow is an important part of staging of all lymphoproliferative disorders. As well as providing evidence of the extent of spread of the tumour, the extent of marrow infiltration and bone marrow reserve may affect the delivery of treatment. There are a number of problems in interpreting staging bone marrow specimens which are common to all lymphoproliferative disorders. Firstly, it is essential that a trephine biopsy and aspirate are examined in every case as the use of aspirates alone will result in a considerable underdiagnosis of marrow disease, especially where this is focal or associated with fibrosis. Secondly, it is difficult to quantify the extent of marrow disease. Differential cell counts on a aspirate sample are of dubious validity as they depend on both the number of tumour cells and the overall marrow cellularity. There is no simple method of carrying out absolute cell counts on marrow aspirate specimens, which are variably diluted with blood. Morphometric counting on a trephine biopsy is very time-consuming and may not be valid in populations that have non-random spatial distribution. In some cases marrow infiltration progresses through well defined stages and these may be used as crude estimates of the volume of marrow replaced.

Table 3.1 The purpose of staging

- To determine the extent of disease in a standard, reproducible manner
- To guide therapeutic decision making, for instance, appropriate choice of radiotherapy/chemotherapy
- To stratify patients for therapeutic trials
- To enable comparison of response rates between groups of comparable stage
- To provide a prognostic parameter

The remainder of this chapter will consider the principles of radiology that apply to the anatomical staging and management of lymphoproliferative disorders. The detailed criteria used in staging individual tumours are discussed in later chapters.

3.2 Radiological techniques

The number of imaging options has increased markedly in recent years

The advent of cross-sectional imaging has radically altered the management of patients with lymphoproliferative disorders, and such imaging is now a fundamental component of the diagnostic process and the monitoring of response to treatment. This has led to the gradual replacement of some conventional radiological techniques in lymphoma staging and the need for surgical staging has been largely eliminated.

Conventional radiology has a limited role in staging but can still provide valuable information

The chest radiograph remains a simple and valuable technique for the initial assessment and follow-up of patients with thoracic lymphoma and its complications. Although it cannot compete with the overall thoracic assessment offered by axial CT or multiplanar MR, the chest X-ray allows some assessment of the hilar and mediastinal anatomy, provides a means of reviewing the pulmonary parenchyma for evidence of lymphomatous involvement or infective complications, and gives a rudimentary impression of the structures of the chest wall and pleura.

Full radiological skeletal surveys (involving the production of a large number of conventional radiographs from skull to femora) are now rarely requested as part of the routine baseline investigations in lymphoma. While both the osteolytic and osteoblastic manifestations of skeletal lymphoma may be observed in plain radiographs, CT and isotope scintigraphy are more sensitive and will give more accurate information concerning the extent of skeletal involvement. Conventional X-ray evidence of bone involvement occurs relatively late in the disease process and relies on the detection of cortical bone destruction. Trabecular bone destruction is identifiable on CT images and increased osteoblastic activity will result in a positive bone scintiscan. However, in multiple myeloma, where osteoblastic activity is absent, plain radiographs remain of central importance in the detection of the bone lesions. Marrow involvement, which is often the site of earliest change, will only be detected by MR scanning and at present the relevance of this is not fully defined.

Barium contrast studies, intravenous urography and conventional angiography are rarely indicated as part of the initial work-up of patients with lymphoproliferative diseases and are only performed for specific clinical reasons. One of the main benefits of cross-sectional imaging techniques such as CT has been the replacement of multiple conventional contrast studies (which are generally targeted at one anatomical area or a single organ system) by a single technique which encompasses a number of systems – a contrast enhanced abdominal CT study can assess the solid organs such as liver, spleen, pancreas and kidneys, the large and small bowel, the vascular anatomy and related lymph node groups, as well as the peritoneal and retroperitoneal spaces.

Lymphography is useful in identifying involved nodes but is now of largely historical interest

Bipedal lymphography (lymphangiography), first introduced in 1955, is invasive and requires the subcutaneous injection of methylene blue dye into the first and second web spaces to identify the peripheral lymphatic channels. Using a cut-down technique, a single lymphatic is cannulated from each foot and an oily iodinated contrast agent (Lipiodol) is slowly injected using a pressure pump. Conventional X-rays of the pelvis and abdomen are obtained to monitor the contrast column and the injection is stopped when contrast reaches the fourth lumbar vertebral body. Radiographs are repeated after 24 h, usually accompanied by an intravenous urogram. The procedure is uncomfortable for the patient and time-consuming. It is contraindicated in patients with cardiac and pulmonary disease and in those who have had radiotherapy to any part of the lung. Lymphography will identify enlarged lymph nodes and will demonstrate nodes of normal size that display an abnormal internal architecture. However, even when the examination is technically successful, significant groups of lymph nodes are not opacified by the contrast. These include some para-aortic nodes as well as mesenteric, retrocrural, splenic and porta hepatis nodes. Lymphography does not identify hepatic or splenic involvement. Non-opacification of a lymph node group may lead to an underestimation of tumour load. After the initial study, contrast may remain in the lymph node for 12–18 months, allowing follow-up assessment of tumour bulk and distribution as well as response to therapy.

Lymphography provides information about nodal architecture that is not currently available from ultrasound, CT or MR techniques, which rely entirely on nodal size as the arbiter of normality or abnormality. Interpretation of lymphangiographic nodal architecture is, however, very much dependent on the expertise of the reporting radiologist and it is often difficult to differentiate reactive hyperplasia, fatty infiltration and fibrotic changes from tumour deposits. The specificity and sensitivity of lymphography has been reported as 80–95% for para-aortic and pelvic lymph nodes in Hodgkin's disease, which compares with a specificity of 80–90% and a sensitivity of 65–80% for CT. The accuracy of lymphography is appreciably less in non-Hodgkin's lymphoma. A slightly better performance in comparison with CT has to be weighed against the practical difficulties and reduced efficiency of lymphography in NHL.

Diagnostic ultrasound can avoid the need to expose patients to irradiation

Diagnostic ultrasound avoids the use of ionizing radiation and has a wide range of applications. It is readily applicable to the assessment of intra-abdominal and intrapelvic anatomy, testes and thyroid, and by using Doppler techniques can also give an assessment of blood flow in solid organs and the vascular tree. The lack of ionizing radiation makes ultrasound an ideal choice for the assessment of disease in children or in pregnancy as well as providing a means of safe follow-up, notably in young adults of childbearing age, when serial studies are required.

A major disadvantage of ultrasound is its inability to produce good diagnostic images in the presence of intestinal gas in the abdomen or air in the lungs when scanning the chest. A body habitus with excess fat also significantly compromises the use of ultrasound, particularly in investigating deep-seated anatomical structures such as retroperitoneal lymph node groups.

Scintigraphy has only a limited role in lymphoma management

Currently, scintigraphy has a limited role in the routine evaluation of patients with lymphoma, being generally used for problem-solving rather than for routine staging. Bone scintiscanning remains one of the commonest indications, while gallium-67 scintigraphy is establishing a role in the detection of disease activity within areas of residual nodal mass following initial treatment. As with most radiopharmaceuticals, gallium-67 is not tissue-specific and is taken up by most epithelial tumours as well as lymphomas. Isotope lymphography has made no significant impact on lymphoma staging and, like conventional lymphography, is not part of contemporary routine staging protocols in lymphoma.

Computed tomography (CT) has been the major advance for imaging in the lymphomas

Computed tomography uses an X-ray source that rotates through 360°. An array of detectors records the attenuation of the beam at each point as it exits from the patient. The data can then be used to calculate the attenuation of the X-ray beam at each point on the anatomical slice around which the X-ray tube has rotated. These numerical values are used to construct the image. In most cases this image is in the axial plane and is seen as a cross-section of the body. However, the technique of multiplanar reconstruction allows a series of such images to be used to produce sagittal or coronal sections or in some cases three-dimensional reconstructions (Table 3.2).

Helical (also known as spiral or volumetric) CT represents a significant improvement in CT technology. In conventional CT the X-ray source rotates through 360° and a set of data is generated for that plane. The table is then moved a preset distance and the process is repeated. In helical CT the table moves continuously while the X-ray source is stationary. A volume data set is acquired from which the CT software can reconstruct axial slices at any given interval along the Z axis (the direction in which the table moves). By acquiring overlapping slices, e.g. 10 mm slices reconstructed every 5 mm, partial volume averaging is reduced and high-quality multiplanar reformats and 3D reconstructions can be made. For the patient, helical scanners are significantly quicker than conventional

Table 3.2 The contribution of CT in the management of lymphoma

- Full radiological assessment of disease extent
- Documentation of disease-free sites at baseline assessment
- Monitoring response to treatment
- Documentation of complete remission
- Evaluation and monitoring of residual masses
- Early detection and assessment of relapsed disease
- Early detection of the complications of treatment

scanners and, with state-of-the-art systems, a 50–100 cm volume can be acquired at the rate of 1 cm per second. A helical study of 50 cm will therefore take 50 s to complete compared with a theoretical 6 min 30 s to cover the same distance with an average conventional scanner.

In helical CT the pitch refers to the rate of table movement over the slice thickness. Increasing the pitch reduces scanning time and radiation dose and increases anatomical coverage. After an appropriate period of hyper-ventilation, large areas of the body can be imaged during a single breath-hold. Most patients prefer single or multiple prolonged breath-hold techniques to a large number of stop/start images. Although patient throughput in overall terms is not significantly increased with helical scanning, the time a patient spends in the scanner is significantly reduced.

CT is now established as the main imaging tool both for the initial assessment and staging of lymphomas and for monitoring response to treatment. Although the patient receives a radiation dose, the complexity and duration of the CT protocol can be tailored to the level of information required for the stage of the disease process or the treatment regimen. For the patient, the examination can last an hour or more because of the time required to take the oral bowel contrast that is required to opacify the small intestine. Unopacified bowel can give a pseudo-mass appearance and lead to misdiagnosis of lymphadenopathy. Standard protocols include the chest, abdomen and pelvis with expansion into the neck and brain depending on the clinically detected extent of disease. Centres vary as to whether intravenous (IV) contrast is given for each examination and few would give contrast as a matter of routine. IV contrast studies are generally reserved for problem-solving or assessing areas of possible residual disease where contrast enhancement gives improved differentiation between residual nodal disease and vascular structures. Although IV contrast may demonstrate foci of lymphoma in the solid abdominal organs not appreciated on non-contrast images, the demonstration of such disease usually does not significantly alter management.

Magnetic resonance (MR) offers similar cross-sectional imaging to CT scanning but avoids radiation and has additional advantages

Magnetic resonance imaging involves placing the patient in a strong magnetic field, which causes alignment of protons in tissues. A radiofrequency pulse is applied which is absorbed by the protons. When the pulse is switched off the protons return to their original state and in doing so emit a signal which is detected by the receiver coils. These signals are used to create the image. Different tissue characteristics can be demonstrated by varying the sequence of radiofrequency pulses and the time interval between pulses. The water content of a tissue can be demonstrated by comparison of spin-echo sequences. Water has a low signal intensity on a T1 image and a high intensity on a T2 image. Many types of tumour are detected by having a relatively high water content. Unlike CT, MR images can be acquired in any plane but can also be used for multiplanar reformatting (Tables 3.3, 3.4).

MR avoids the use of ionizing radiation and this is a considerable advantage in investigating young children and in the assessment of lymphoma in the pregnant female. MR is generally contraindicated during the first trimester but there are no restrictions to its use throughout the remainder of pregnancy. However, compared with CT, MR studies require the patient to enter a narrow tunnel and, in most cases, remain fully enclosed for a fairly lengthy period. In children this often requires general anaesthesia, which restricts the frequent use of MR in follow-up. About 5% of patients are not able to cooperate, mainly because of claustrophobia. Although the high-contrast resolution provided by MR represents a significant advance on CT, MR still cannot assess the internal nodal architecture and therefore, like CT, remains reliant on lymph node size in the assessment of pathological change.

Table 3.3 The contribution of MR in the management of lymphoma

- Can be used in the second and third trimesters of pregnancy
- Problem solving technique (especially when CT is equivocal)
- Avoidance of iodinated contrast in patients with an allergy/renal dysfunction
- Differentiation of residual lymphoma from fibrotic masses
- Evaluation of thymic rebound
- Assessment of bone marrow pathology
- Assessment of avascular necrosis occurring as a complication of chemotherapy

Table 3.4 Problems in the use of MR in the management of lymphoma

- Lack of general availability and high cost
- Patient intolerance
- Need for anaesthesia in children
- Not useful for general radiological surveys

MR obviates the need to give large volumes of intravenous iodinated contrast (though an injection of gadolinium may sometimes help to assess a specific diagnostic problem). MR represents an excellent diagnostic tool for the assessment of the bone marrow, providing improved sensitivity when compared with CT and scintigraphy. It is playing an ever-increasing role in monitoring residual masses following treatment, and the technique can give some indication as to whether residual active disease or an inactive fibrotic mass is present. Confident discrimination on the basis of a single examination is often difficult because fibrosis appears similar to tumour but a combination of changing size and signal characteristics can be diagnostic. For follow-up studies, MR could replace CT in most situations. However MR does not currently lend itself to the swift body survey role, which is more than adequately provided by CT. Although MR-guided biopsies are technically possible, these are very time-consuming when compared with CT procedures and require non-ferromagnetic needles and, ideally, open magnet technology. The open low field systems being introduced will allow stereotactic and other biopsy techniques to be performed but MR is unlikely to replace ultrasound or CT for biopsy guidance in the near future.

To fully cover the anatomical areas required for lymphoma staging, an MR study will be lengthy when compared with CT. The information obtained is comparable for the major lymph node groups in the thorax, abdomen, and pelvis, although mesenteric disease may be more difficult to evaluate on MR, especially in patients who lack body fat. MR may provide additional information with regard to lymphomatous involvement of the solid organs such as the liver, spleen and kidneys, as well as giving unique information about bone marrow involvement.

3.3 Imaging nodal disease

On CT, lymph nodes display a similar density to muscle. Lymph nodes showing a lower attenuation than normal may be seen with non-Hodgkin's lymphoma and, occasionally, in treated lymphoma. In the undiagnosed patient, low-density nodes may occur with tuberculous lymphadenopathy or metastatic spread from a testicular tumour. Other causes of low density nodes on CT include Whipple's disease and *Mycobacterium avium/intracellulare* infections (Table 3.5).

The larger the node, the more likely it is to be abnormal. False-negative diagnoses arise when tumour is present in normal-sized nodes

Table 3.5 Causes of low density nodes on CT

- Lymphoma
- Treated lymphoma
- Tuberculosis
- Testicular metastases
- Whipple's disease
- *Mycobacterium avium/ intracellulare*

or when an enlarged node is not recognized. False positives can occur when nodal enlargement is due to a benign process or when a soft tissue structure, such as unopacified bowel, is interpreted as a lymph node mass. Early in the disease process tumour is contained within the node, which displays a well defined border. Eventually tumour spreads through the capsule but, in contrast to carcinoma, lymphomatous masses tend to displace rather than invade adjacent structures. Vascular preservation is usual in lymphomas, a finding that can be helpful in making the distinction from other types of tumour in which vascular compromise is more usual (Table 3.6).

Table 3.6 Guidelines in assessing lymphadenopathy

- Mediastinal nodes – normal if less than 1 cm in diameter
- Retroperitoneal and pelvic nodes – normal if less than 1 cm
- Retrocrural nodes – normal if less than 0.6 cm

Although an individual node measuring about 1 cm may be equivocal, a cluster of nodes of this size would be probably abnormal. It is often stated in the older literature that pelvic nodes must be greater than 1.5 cm to call them pathological but it is now clear that normal pelvic nodes should be no larger than 8–10 mm.

On MR, lymphomatous tissue is hypointense with respect to fat and slightly hyperintense with respect to normal muscle on T1-weighted spin-echo images. On T2-weighted spin-echo sequences, lymphomatous tissue is isointense to fat and hyperintense to muscle. Conventional T1- and T2-weighted spin-echo sequences show very little difference in signal intensity between normal and abnormal nodes, with great overlap between benign and malignant tissue. Before treatment the extent of low signal intensity within a mass on a T2-weighted spin-echo sequence reflects the amount of fibrotic tissue within the tumour. Mature fibrosis typically displays low signal intensity on T2-weighted spin-echo images while active lymphoma will show high signal. Early or immature fibrosis may display high signal intensity on T2-weighted spin-echo images and, as such, cannot be differentiated from persisting active disease. Dense fibrosis, displaying high signal intensity on T2-weighted images, occurs more commonly in Hodgkin's disease than in non-Hodgkin's lymphomas.

3.4 Imaging the thorax

The chest CT is often a key investigation in the assessment of Hodgkin's disease

Thoracic involvement will be demonstrated at presentation in 65–85% of patients with Hodgkin's disease and 25–40% with non-Hodgkin's lymphoma. The distribution of lymphoma in Hodgkin's disease follows a fairly predictable pattern, with initial involvement of the mediastinum, then the hila and subsequently the pulmonary parenchyma. In non-Hodgkin's lymphoma the distribution of disease is less predictable and isolated lung involvement with no evidence of hilar or mediastinal disease is not uncommon.

A wide variety of pulmonary parenchymal changes are found in lymphoma patients. The prevalence of lymphomatous involvement of the lung is 12% in Hodgkin's disease and 4% in non-Hodgkin's lymphoma. Pulmonary parenchymal disease is more frequently seen in the context of generalized as opposed to localized disease.

Additional intrathoracic lesions not seen on chest radiograph may be visualized by CT and MRI

Although the chest X-ray remains a useful investigation, CT can demonstrate abnormalities in up to 30% of patients who have a normal chest radiograph. Moreover, CT will reveal additional lesions in 25% of patients whose chest X-ray is abnormal. These additional findings on CT can lead to alteration in stage and therefore, possibly, of treatment in 10–15% of patients with Hodgkin's disease. When retrocrural or peridiaphragmatic lymph nodes are demonstrated on chest CT, there is an increased likelihood of disease being present below the diaphragm.

Pleural effusions are detected in about 7–10% of patients with intrathoracic malignant lymphoma. No more than one-third contain malignant cells and they are not routinely aspirated as part of the staging procedure. The incidence of pleural effusion is significantly higher when there is concomitant pulmonary parenchymal disease. Pleural plaques of solid tumour tissue are usually associated with malignant effusions and tend to be found with recurrent rather than primary disease. Rather less frequently, pericardial effusions may be detected.

Lymphomatous involvement of the chest wall can usually be demonstrated by either CT or MR. Non-Hodgkin's lymphoma more commonly involves the chest wall than Hodgkin's disease and typically occurs by direct extension from internal mammary nodes. Occasionally, direct involvement of the thoracic spine with neurological sequelae may occur by extension from posterior mediastinal nodes.

Imaging the lungs can provide help in diagnosing the infective complications associated with immunosuppression

In Hodgkin's disease at presentation, pulmonary parenchymal changes that are not associated with mediastinal or hilar lymphadenopathy are almost always due to coincident non-lymphomatous pathology. However, this is not the case for patients with non-Hodgkin's lymphoma or recurrent Hodgkin's disease. Non-lymphomatous complications fall into two major categories. Firstly, there is the pulmonary parenchymal response to chemotherapeutic toxicity with acute alveolitis in the early stages, which may lead on to interstitial pulmonary fibrosis and changes following radiotherapy to the mediastinum and adjacent lung, although these rarely have clinical significance. Secondly, pulmonary infection in this immunocompromised population can lead to a wide variety of lung changes, which may closely mimic those due to the lymphomatous process itself. Both pyogenic and fungal infections are frequently encountered. *Aspergillus* infection can display multifocal lung pathology ranging from well defined cannon ball nodules to areas of ill defined consolidation that may or may not cavitate. If initial clinical and bacteriological assessment fails to clearly differentiate infection from lymphoma then fibreoptic bronchoscopy with bronchial washing is indicated and occasionally open lung biopsy may be required.

Primary pulmonary lymphoma generally presents as pulmonary lobar consolidation that fails to respond to standard antibiotic therapy. Chest radiographs, CT and MR typically show no specific features and percutaneous or open lung biopsy is often required to establish the diagnosis. The radiological differential diagnosis would include alveolar cell carcinoma (Tables 3.7, 3.8).

Table 3.7 Pulmonary parenchymal changes associated with lymphomas

- Direct extension from a mediastinal/hilar mass
- Discrete pulmonary nodules of varying definition and size which may or may not display cavitation
- Lobar or segmental collapse from bronchial infiltration
- A disease pattern similar to lymphangitis carcinomatosa

Table 3.8 Pulmonary parenchymal changes associated with the treatment of lymphoma

- Chemotherapy
  - Acute alveolitis
  - Fibrosis
- Radiotherapy
  - Juxtamediastinal parenchymal densities
  - Atelectasis
- Infection
  - Consolidation
  - Cavitation
  - Pleural effusion

The thymus is enlarged in a high proportion of patients with Hodgkin's disease

The thymus is enlarged in some 30–50% of patients with Hodgkin's disease and remains enlarged in approximately one-third of cases, even after successful treatment.

The incidence of a residual thymic bed mass is higher in patients with bulky mediastinal disease at presentation. Some 64–88% of patients with bulky mediastinal Hodgkin's disease will have a residual mass after treatment while only 14–40% of cases with non-Hodgkin's lymphoma will show this. Approximately 50% of patients with residual masses will relapse; the frequency of relapse is twice that in patients without residual masses. The detection of disease activity within residual masses continues to be a challenge for diagnostic imaging. Surgical resection is associated with significant morbidity and the inherently fibrotic nature of the residual mass does not lend itself to percutaneous biopsy techniques. There is also a significant danger associated with percutaneous 'tru-cut' biopsy using spring-loaded devices with masses that are often situated close to major vessels; hence the need for effective non-invasive imaging techniques of residual mediastinal masses.

As CT relies solely on assessing mass size and stability over time, the technique has a limited role in differentiating active from inactive disease. A residual mass that shows no change in size may still retain active foci of disease. MR and gallium-67 scintigraphy are the techniques of choice to differentiate between fibrosis and residual or recurrent disease. In childhood, the thymus generally displays a lower signal intensity on both T1- and T2-weighted spin-echo images than adjacent mediastinal fat. With increasing age, the thymus displays increasing fatty replacement with corresponding changes in signal intensity. In untreated lymphoma, MR displays a typically homogeneous high signal intensity on T2-weighted spin-echo images. The signal intensity of a residual mass relates to the degree of water and protein content. Lymphoma tissue contains a high water content and therefore displays high signal intensity on T2-weighted spin-echo images. Fibrous tissue contains a relative excess of protein and therefore displays lower signal intensity. Following treatment of a mediastinal mass, a heterogeneous pattern of signal intensity may be demonstrated for up to 6 months. This pattern can also be seen in untreated nodular sclerosing Hodgkin's disease. If a homogeneous low signal intensity is demonstrated on T2-weighted spin-echo imaging, this supports a diagnosis of fibrosis if treatment has been successful on other criteria. Foci of fat can lead to false-positive diagnoses so it is important to assess both the T1- and T2-weighted images. In general, if a mass displays low signal intensity on T1- and T2-weighted spin-echo images, then fibrosis is likely. If, on the other hand, a mass displays low signal intensity on T1-weighted images, but high signal intensity on T2-weighted images, active disease is more likely to be present.

MR can be used to monitor residual masses and has been used to detect recurrent active foci in a residual mass several weeks before any overt clinical evidence of disease. An alternative approach to demonstrate residual disease activity within a residual mediastinal masses is the use of gallium-67 scintigraphy, which has been reported as showing a sensitivity and specificity in excess of 80% for assessing the activity of residual mediastinal masses.

Failure to recognize thymic rebound can lead to inappropriate treatment

The phenomenon of thymic enlargement following treatment, known as thymic rebound, may lead to diagnostic difficulties on follow-up CT studies in differentiating pathological thymic enlargement from hyperplasia. MR is proving a useful problem-solving technique in this situation. With rebound, the thymus is generally of smooth contour, with retention of its bilobular appearance, and gives a typically homogeneous signal intensity on spin-echo imaging. If lymphoma is responsible for the thymic enlargement, diffuse and often asymmetrical lobar enlargement is noted; localized contour abnormalities are typically present and a heterogeneous signal intensity is characteristic.

3.5 Imaging the abdomen

Both conventional radiography and cross-sectional imaging should be used to identify involvement of the gastrointestinal tract

The gastrointestinal (GI) tract is the commonest extranodal site in non-Hodgkin's lymphoma. By contrast, gastrointestinal involvement is rare in Hodgkin's disease. Non-Hodgkin's lymphoma frequently arises from mucosa-associated lymphoid tissue as a primary tumour of the stomach, small bowel or colon and accounts for some 2–5% of all gastric tumours. Lymphoma is the commonest primary tumour of the small bowel and is multifocal in some 10% of cases. Primary lymphoma of the large bowel is, by comparison, rare and typically affects the caecum or rectum.

A wide variety of radiological appearances may be seen. Lesions vary from small nodules to bulky masses, which may ulcerate when they outgrow their blood supply. CT is particularly useful in the diagnosis of gastric lymphoma where diffuse or focal wall thickening is found. As with linitis plastica, upper GI endoscopic biopsy may not be diagnostic because of lack of mucosal involvement. GI lymphoma may be multifocal or manifest diffuse or segmental bowel wall thickening. Complications of bowel lymphoma include abscess formation and perforation, while intussusception is a well recognized presentation, particularly in children. Although bowel strictures may occur, they are relatively uncommon because of the relative lack of fibrous tissue reaction in non-Hodgkin's lymphoma. Aneurysmal dilatation of the small bowel may also be found.

Surgery remains the only definitive way of demonstrating splenic lymphoma

At laparotomy some 30–40% of patients with Hodgkin's disease and 10–40% of patients with non-Hodgkin's lymphoma will have splenic involvement but, to date, imaging has proved rather unsuccessful in the confirmation of splenic pathology. Splenic lymphoma is typically diffuse and relatively few cases will have discrete nodules of such a size as to permit identification with conventional imaging.

Splenic size is not the final arbiter of normality, as diffuse infiltration may be present in normal sized spleens. It is accepted that approximately one-third of pathologically involved spleens are of normal size, while one-third of enlarged spleens show no discrete lymphomatous involvement. Mild to moderate reactive splenomegaly can be found in one-third of patients with Hodgkin's disease and two-thirds of patients with non-Hodgkin's lymphoma. When splenomegaly is marked, however, this almost always means lymphomatous infiltration.

It should be remembered that 10% of patients with Hodgkin's disease apparently restricted to the region above the diaphragm will have splenic involvement documented at either post-mortem or laparotomy as the only site of infradiaphragmatic disease. When enlarged nodes are noted at the splenic hilum, splenic involvement can be predicted with some confidence.

Currently, diffuse splenic infiltration cannot be reliably detected by ultrasound, CT or MR, although contrast-enhanced CT and contrast-enhanced MR may demonstrate focal defects not apparent on non-contrast imaging. Developments in MR, using super-paramagnetic iron oxide particles, may well permit the detection of splenic infiltration even in the absence of splenomegaly. These particles are ingested by normal reticuloendothelial cells and result in a significant reduction of splenic parenchymal signal intensity on T1- and T2-weighted images. Foci of splenic pathology can be distinguished, as the abnormal splenic tissue will not contain reticuloendothelial cells and therefore will not take up the contrast.

MRI may offer some improvements over CT scanning for visualization of hepatic lymphoma

Primary lymphoma of liver is very rare, while involvement as part of generalized disease is usually associated with concurrent lymph node disease. As a general rule, the liver is seldom involved in the absence of splenic disease except in AIDS-related lymphoma. Involvement of the liver occurs less frequently than involvement of the spleen – in non-Hodgkin's lymphoma, if hepatomegaly is demonstrated then lymphomatous involvement of the liver is generally present whereas in Hodgkin's disease it is more often a non-specific finding than an indicator of hepatic involvement.

Although focal nodular changes may occur in approximately 10% of patients with liver disease, hepatic involvement is more typically diffuse and, as with splenic disease, imaging is generally inadequate in its detection. Larger focal lesions can be demonstrated with ultrasound, CT or MR. Developments with hepatic-specific MR contrast, such as superparamagnetic agents, are showing promise in the detection of smaller liver lesions than can currently be shown with gadolinium-enhanced MR. Other elements of the hepatobiliary tree may be involved and in AIDS-related lymphoma involvement of the bile duct and gall bladder has been documented. MR cholangiography is becoming more widely available and is predicted to replace diagnostic ERCP in the near future.

3.6 Imaging the genitourinary tract

Genitourinary involvement is only detected in a minority of patients by imaging techniques

Lymphomatous involvement of the genitourinary (GU) tract is generally a late feature of the disease process and is more likely in non-Hodgkin's lymphoma than in Hodgkin's disease. Renal involvement occurs either as a result of haematogenous dissemination, typically multifocal, or by direct spread from adjacent nodal disease, when the kidney is characteristically surrounded by a soft tissue mass invading the renal parenchyma.

Renal lymphoma can be demonstrated by ultrasound, CT and MR. On non-contrast CT, renal lesions can be hypodense or isodense with respect to normal renal tissue and are difficult to identify. After contrast enhancement, lymphomatous deposits show lower attenuation values than normal cortex. Similar appearances will be demonstrated on MR following gadolinium. Although renal lymphoma is found in 33–52% of patients at post-mortem, disease is only detected in 5% of patients on routine staging CT. The disease is often bilateral and is usually associated with other evidence of lymphoma in retroperitoneal lymph nodes and spleen.

Involvement of the adrenal gland is uncommon and, as with renal lymphoma, there is usually associated retroperitoneal lymphadenopathy. Adrenal disease is generally detected during routine staging procedures but it usually has no specific clinical significance and Addison's disease is rare.

CT has virtually no role to play in the direct assessment of testicular disease. Although MR will demonstrate focal masses and suggest diffuse involvement, ultrasound is the technique of choice for demonstrating all testicular tumours. Non-Hodgkin's lymphoma accounts for one-third of all testicular tumours in the over 50s and is bilateral in 10–25% of patients.

3.7 Imaging bone and bone marrow

MRI can be used to demonstrate early marrow involvement

Skeletal radiographs are not routinely indicated in the current staging protocols for lymphoma, but conventional radiographs of a symptomatic area are appropriate if a patient complains of focal bone or joint pain. MR, using T1-weighted spin-echo imaging, can relatively quickly image the dorsolumbar spine, pelvis and upper femora and may provide an early indication of marrow involvement (Table 3.9).

When the marrow is involved by lymphoma, low signal intensity changes on T1-weighted spin-echo imaging and high signal intensity on T2-weighted images are usually found. In nodular sclerosing Hodgkin's disease, very high signal intensity may be seen on T2-weighted images. MR is very sensitive for the detection of marrow changes following radiotherapy. Depending on the degree of fibrosis present, relatively low marrow signal may be shown on T2. Increased fat deposition is reflected by increased signal intensity on T1-weighted images. Postradiotherapy changes characteristically show clear cut-off points at field margins.

In patients with known or suspected bone involvement by lymphoma, scintigraphy is a useful technique to determine the extent of disease. Isotope scanning has a sensitivity and accuracy of 95% in the detection

Table 3.9 The role of MR in bone marrow lymphoma

- To demonstrate the extent of disease
- To identify an optimum site for biopsy
- To evaluate response to treatment
- To detect disease relapse
- To evaluate complications of marrow or bone involvement, e.g. spinal cord compression

of such pathology. Primary bone lymphoma is very rare and typically involves the femur or pelvis. Bone involvement, as part of disseminated disease, more characteristically involves the axial skeleton.

3.8 Imaging the head and neck

CT and MRI scanning have revolutionized the imaging of head and neck lymphomas

Waldeyer's ring is one of the commonest sites for lymphomatous involvement of the head and neck. An assessment of the nasopharyngeal adenoids, oropharyngeal and lingual tonsils should form a routine part of the initial lymphoma assessment. Approximately 20% of all patients with NHL will have a positive nasopharyngeal biopsy in studies where this has been carried out. Lymphomatous involvement of the paranasal sinuses is the next most common tumour after squamous cell carcinoma. Non-Hodgkin's lymphoma is the commonest primary malignancy of the adult orbit and is bilateral in 40% of cases. In patients who demonstrate bulky supraclavicular or bilateral neck lymphadenopathy approximately one-third will have subclinical infradiaphragmatic disease. Full staging procedures should be carried out even when only localized disease, e.g. in the orbit, is apparent clinically. Many such patients will demonstrate generalized disease either at the time of presentation or at a later stage.

Primary central nervous system (CNS) lymphoma accounts for 1–2% of all brain tumours. CNS involvement occurs in 10–15% of patients with disseminated non-Hodgkin's lymphoma but, of those patients who initially present with CNS involvement, 90% have primary brain lymphoma. Routine imaging of the CNS is not performed as part of a lymphoma staging protocol unless neurological signs are present. The majority of lesions are solitary and centrally situated although 30% of patients with primary brain lymphoma will develop multifocal lesions and 10% will demonstrate diffuse CNS involvement. Multifocal disease is more common in immunocompromised patients. On CT, two-thirds of lesions are hyperdense on non-contrast studies and demonstrate uniform enhancement following contrast. Lymphomas typically lack associated oedema and necrosis and this can be a useful differentiating feature from gliomas.

Leptomeningeal involvement may be present in NHL and is best demonstrated on post-gadolinium spin-echo MR images. Similarly, spinal cord involvement is best demonstrated by MR.

3.9 Imaging studies in children

There are some differences of emphasis in imaging childhood lymphoma

Essentially, the imaging of children with lymphoma is the same as in adults, although particular attention needs to be paid to a number of specific sites of disease that are involved more frequently in childhood. Involvement of the ileocaecal junction, pancreas and kidney are more frequently seen in children than in adults. Non-Hodgkin's lymphoma involves the pancreas in less than 2% of patients overall, but pancreatic lymphoma is reported at post-mortem in one-third of children dying of lymphoma. Pancreatic disease is usually associated with retroperitoneal lymphadenopathy, which typically involves the peripancreatic groups. When the kidneys are involved two-thirds of children will have multifocal bilateral disease. Solitary renal masses or diffuse enlargement of a single kidney are rarely found in the paediatric population.

Extranodal sites in the head and neck are more commonly involved in children than adults, tonsillar lymphoma being the commonest site in children compared with lymphoma of the nasopharynx in the adult population. Parotid gland disease is also more frequently seen in children.

The choice of imaging technique will vary with the site and distribution of disease, as will the required frequency for follow-up imaging. Children younger than 8–9 years will find magnetic resonance a distressing experience and will generally require either sedation or a general anaesthetic, depending on local practice. Ultrasound is an excellent means of investigating the abdomen in children and should be used in preference to CT whenever possible. Although MR would be the ideal choice for follow-up in children, the risks of repeated general anaesthesia may be considered greater than the risk of repeated exposure to ionizing radiation.

3.10 The use of imaging-guided percutaneous biopsy

Diagnostic material can be obtained by guided biopsy in lymphoma

Imaging-guided biopsies allow either cytological or histological assessment. The role of fine-needle aspiration biopsy is controversial but developments in immunological markers and cytogenetics may improve the value of this technique, particularly in follow-up of previously diagnosed patients. Using CT guidance, fine-needle aspiration biopsies can be performed with minimal patient risk at almost any anatomical site. The use of coaxial needle systems has significantly reduced the time taken to perform repeat biopsies under CT guidance. While ultrasound is the most appropriate imaging technique for guiding biopsies of the liver, biopsy of the spleen, kidneys, adrenals and other retroperitoneal biopsies is sometimes best performed under CT guidance. Similarly, the assessment of mesenteric disease is best controlled by CT as ultrasound may have difficulty in differentiating tumour masses from bowel loops.

The advent of spring-loaded biopsy devices has led to an increased use of core biopsy techniques in the assessment of lymphoma. These devices allow a 'tru-cut'-type core to be obtained. The automatic nature of the biopsy device significantly reduces the shearing artefact and other problems that arise with conventional hand held 'tru-cut' biopsy techniques. It is still the case that a full surgical biopsy remains the optimum procedure for obtaining tissue for the accurate diagnosis and characterization of lymphoma.

3.11 Imaging studies following therapy

CT remains the best single technique for the assessment of response to treatment, the follow-up of residual masses, and the early detection of relapse and treatment-related complications. The frequency of follow-up CT will vary from centre to centre but generally CT is carried out following the first two or three cycles of chemotherapy and the result is used to direct further treatment. A CT to confirm complete remission and help determine the total length of treatment is also usual. Subsequently, it is largely a clinical decision as to how often further CT studies are performed, assuming that other indicators of disease suggest continuing remission. Some centres advocate 6-monthly follow-up studies for a period of at least 3 years. However, the clinical value of such frequent investigation is questionable in the absence of clinical signs indicating relapse. In younger patients there is a role for replacing CT with MR in order to avoid repeated doses of ionizing radiation.

3.12 Key references

Elkowitz, S. S., Leonidas, J. C., Lopez, M. *et al.* (1993) Comparison of CT and MRI in the evaluation of therapeutic response in thoracic Hodgkin disease. *Pediatric Radiology,* **23**, 301–304.

Front, D., Ben-Haim, S., Israel, O. *et al.* (1992) Lymphoma: predictive value of Ga-67 scintigraphy after treatment. *Radiology,* **182**, 359–363.

Hoane, B. R., Shields, A. F., Porter, B. A. and Borrow, J. W. (1994) Comparison of initial lymphoma staging using computed tomography (CT) and magnetic resonance (MR) imaging. *American Journal of Hematology,* **47**, 100–105.

Libson, E., Polliack, A. and Bloom, R. A. (1994) Value of lymphangiography in the staging of Hodgkin lymphoma. *Radiology,* **193**, 757–759.

Munker, R., Stengel, A., Stabler, A. *et al.* (1995) Diagnostic accuracy of ultrasound and computed tomography in the staging of Hodgkin's disease. Verification by laparotomy in 100 cases. *Cancer,* **76**, 1460–1466.

Stomper, P. C., Cholewinski, S. P., Park, J. *et al.* (1993) Abdominal staging of thoracic Hodgkin disease: CT-lymphangiography-Ga-67 scanning correlation. *Radiology,* **187**, 381–386.

Tecce, P. M., Fishman, E. K. and Kuhlman, J. E. (1994) CT evaluation of the anterior mediastinum: spectrum of disease. *Radiographics,* **14**, 973–990.

4 Principles of therapy of lymphoproliferative disorders

At present lymphoproliferative disorders are treated using a variety of types of cytotoxic chemotherapy and radiotherapy but there is considerable variation between tumour types in their response to therapy. In childhood acute lymphoblastic leukaemia and Hodgkin's disease, both previously fatal conditions, there is now an expectation that most patients will be cured by current therapy. In contrast to children, most adults with lymphoblastic disease have a poor prognosis despite very intensive therapy. In diffuse large B-cell lymphoma, around one-half of patients will enter a long-term remission with expectation of cure, which contrasts with indolent lymphoproliferative disorders such as follicle centre lymphoma, chronic lymphocytic leukaemia and multiple myeloma; these are not curable by chemotherapy and in most patients the aim of therapy is the control of symptoms. With the increasing knowledge of the regulation and abnormalities of the cell cycle and cell death pathways the reasons why tumours differ in their response to therapy are becoming clearer. A much better understanding of the effects of treatment will also be gained by future clinical trials based on clearly defined disease entities rather than on tumour grade.

Lymphoproliferative disorders are due to multiple genetic abnormalities in the cell-cycle and cell-death pathways

A cell may exist in one of three states. It may be in cycle and continuously dividing, have temporarily exited from the cell cycle in G_0 phase, or it may have permanently lost the capacity for division as a terminally differentiated cell. To these three options must be added programmed cell death (apoptosis). The movement of a cell between these possible states is determined by the integration of a large number of internal and external factors.

A critical regulatory step in the cell cycle is the checkpoint which governs the progression of a cell from G_1 phase in the case of continuously cycling cells and G_0 in the case of resting cells to S phase and hence to cell division. Passage through this checkpoint depends upon appropriate signals from the external environment and on the integrity of genomic DNA (Figures 4.1, 4.2).

External signals such as growth factors or adhesion molecules act through cell surface receptors and are integrated by the cell signalling pathway. The final stage in this signalling process is the induction of members of the cyclin D and E families, which activate cyclin dependent kinases (cdk) in the nucleus. These enzymes phosphorylate the retinoblastoma (Rb) protein, causing release of bound E2F, a transcription factor which forms a heterodimer with non-phosphorylated Rb. E2F is capable of inducing the expression of proteins involved in the replication of DNA and allowing the cell to enter S-phase.

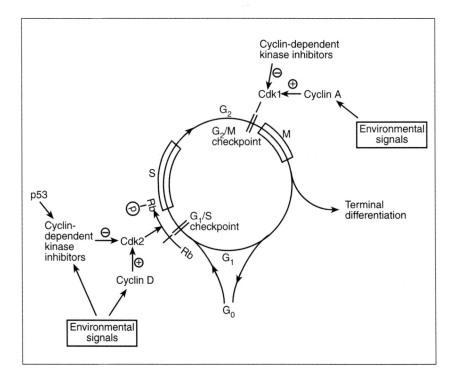

Figure 4.1 The cell cycle. The cell cycle is regulated by a series of checkpoints, which the cell can pass through only in the presence of appropriate environmental signals and the absence of DNA damage. At the G_1/S checkpoint that precedes DNA replication the activity of Cdk-2 is determined by the levels of cyclins and cyclin-dependent kinase inhibitors, each of which in turn are determined by multiple external and internal signals. Cdk-2 phosphorylates the retinoblastoma protein, which in turn results in the activation of the enzymes responsible for DNA replication. A similar system involving Cdk-1 and the cyclin A family regulates the G_2/M checkpoint.

Figure 4.2 The programmed cell death pathway. Most cells contain the enzymes of the cell death pathway in an inactive form. The pathway can be activated by a wide range of internal and external signals. Some of these act by removal of *bcl-2* inhibition of the pathway. Once activated the cell death pathway results in DNA fragmentation, cross linking of the cytoskeleton and membrane changes, resulting in opsonization and rapid phagocytosis.

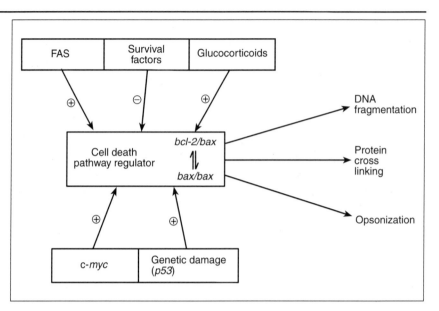

The presence of damaged DNA is a major inhibitor preventing a cell from entering S-phase. DNA damage is detected by an as yet unknown mechanism, which possibly recognizes double-stranded DNA breaks. This signal, which may be transmitted through the product of the ataxia telangiectasia gene, leads to the induction of p53, which prevents a cell with damaged DNA from passing through the G_1/S checkpoint through the induction of cyclin-dependent kinase inhibitors such as p21, which antagonize the effect of the cyclins. In the presence of DNA damage that cannot be repaired the programmed cell death pathway is activated. If the DNA damage is repaired p53 is downregulated and the cell is able to proceed to DNA synthesis.

Later in the cell cycle a similar range of mechanisms act to regulate the cell's passage from the G_2 phase of the cell cycle to mitosis at the G_2/M checkpoint. At this checkpoint members of the cyclin A and B families are the key regulatory molecules.

DNA damage acting through p53 is one of many stimuli that may cause activation of programmed cell death (PCD). Others include activation of *fas* by cytotoxic T-cells, corticosteroids and intracellular calcium. It appears likely that in most cells the enzymes of the PCD pathway are present in inactive forms, the most important of which are proteases of the ICE (interleukin converting enzyme) family. Activation of the pathway results in DNA fragmentation and cross-linking of cytoskeletal proteins, which stabilizes the dying cell. One of the earliest changes appears to be loss of the normal asymmetrical distribution of phospholipids in the plasma membrane. Phagocytosis is promoted by the appearance of phosphotidylserine in the outer layer of the membrane. This process of rapid removal prevents inflammation, a key feature that distinguishes PCD from necrosis.

Lymphoid cells differ from many other types of cell in that they will undergo PCD unless survival signals are present in the environment. Many of these signals act by induction of Bcl-2 or in some cells Bcl-x_L. Both of these molecules form heterodimers with Bax and the relative concentration of Bcl-2/Bax or Bcl-x_L/Bax to Bax/Bax homodimers determines the propensity of the cell to undergo PCD. Removal of the survival factors leads to loss of Bcl-2 and removal of inhibition of the PCD pathway.

There are a number of ways in which these critical pathways may be disrupted by genetic abnormalities found in lymphoproliferative disorders

In mantle cell lymphoma the t(11;14) results in dysregulated production of cyclin D1, a member of the cyclin D family not normally expressed in B-cells, which is likely to destabilize the regulation of the cell cycle, although interestingly the cell-cycle fraction in most mantle cell lymphomas is not particularly high. A small number of diffuse large B-cell lymphomas have deletion of the *Rb* gene with loss of expression of Rb protein, thus removing the key element regulating G_1/S transition. The clinical significance of this abnormality has not been fully evaluated. A more common abnormality in large B-cell lymphomas is inactivation of p53 by mutation or deletion which would normally arrest the cell cycle of genetically damaged cells. Regulation of the cell cycle may also be disrupted by overexpression of the nuclear transcription factor c-Myc, which occurs as a result of the t(8;14). This results not only in continuously cycling cells but also increased levels of cell death.

Failure of the control of terminal differentiation is a feature of many types of lymphoproliferative disorder. For example, surviving germinal centre cells would be expected to become plasma cells and memory B-cells but this occurs to only a minor degree in follicle centre lymphoma. In multiple myeloma the neoplastic clone continues to produce plasma cells while inhibiting the differentiation of normal B-cells. The molecular regulation of the process of terminal differentiation in lymphoid cells is not well understood and few genetic abnormalities have been described which appear to directly affect this process. One possibility is the *bcl-6* gene, which may be involved in the differentiation of germinal centre cells and is deregulated by translocation into chromosome 3q27 in some diffuse large cell lymphomas (Figures 4.3, 4.4).

Evidence from genetically manipulated mice and from cell culture suggests that single genetic abnormalities are rarely sufficient to cause tumour formation. The probability of a single cell acquiring the multiple abnormalities required to undergo neoplastic transformation will be greatly increased if the removal of genetically damaged cells by programmed cell death is disrupted. This is a key factor in the pathogenesis of a number of types of lymphoma. The best described abnormality affecting PCD is t(14;18), which deregulates expression of Bcl-2 and enhances cell survival in the absence of survival signals. A cell containing this abnormality would then accumulate random

Figure 4.3 The action of p53. p53 is produced in response to DNA damage. It is a transcription factor able to activate a wide range of genes. These include the cyclin-dependent kinase inhibitor p21, which can arrest the cell cycle in G_1, allowing time for DNA repair. If this is not competed the cell death programme is activated. p53 also induces the production of MDM2, which can bind to and inactivate p53.

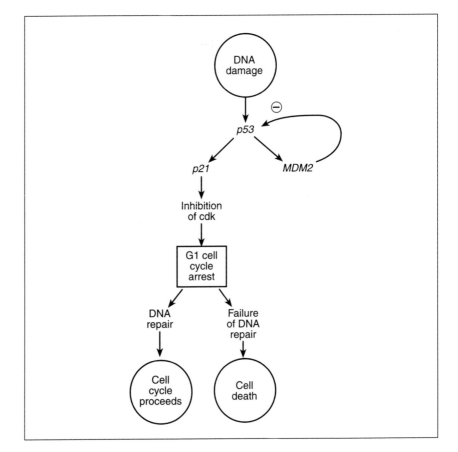

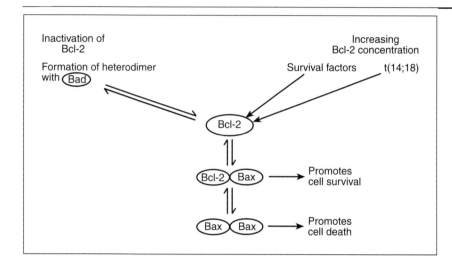

Figure 4.4 Regulation of programmed cell death. The propensity of a cell to enter programmed cell death is dependent on the ratio of Bcl-2/Bax and Bax/Bax dimers. The effective concentration of Bcl-2 available to form dimers depends on its production and by inactivation through dimer formation with Bad.

genetic damage, which eventually in some cells may affect critical genes regulating cell growth or differentiation and lead to the formation of a tumour. It would be expected that this process would be further accelerated if *p53* is also inactivated by deletion or mutation, which is a feature of many transformed lymphoproliferative disorders (Figure 4.5).

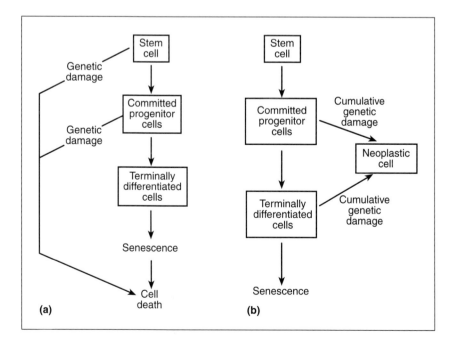

Figure 4.5 Inhibition of cell death and the risk of malignancy. Programmed cell death removes senescent cells and those with damaged DNA. In normal cells there is a steady state between the populations of stem cells, committed progenitors and terminally differentiated cells **(a)**. Inhibition of programmed cell death may lead to expanded populations of cells at risk of transformation and loss of the ability to remove genetically damaged cells **(b)**. Both these factors increase the probability that random genetic damage may affect key regulatory genes in a cell, leading to neoplastic transformation.

4.2 Chemotherapeutic approaches in the treatment of lymphoproliferative disorders

Cytotoxic drugs induce the PCD pathway through a wide variety of mechanisms

The majority of cytotoxic drugs act by causing damage to DNA and activation of PCD. The largest group of drugs in this category act as alkylating agents whereby an alkyl group becomes covalently attached to a DNA base, guanine being the most susceptible. Some drugs have two reactive groups and are therefore capable of cross-linking the DNA strands by reacting with bases on each strand. Alkylating agents include a number of drugs that are effective in the treatment of lymphoproliferative disorders, notably chlorambucil, cyclophosphamide, ifosamide and melphalan (Figure 4.6).

A second major mechanism of DNA damage involves inhibition of topoisomerase activity. Topoisomerase I and II are enzyme systems capable of forming protein–DNA complexes that produce strand nicks, allowing changes in the conformation of DNA and releasing tension

Figure 4.6 Mechanism of action of cytotoxic drugs and radiation. Cytotoxic drugs can be classified into several broad groups according to their mode of action. Together with radiotherapy almost all drugs appear to act by disruption of DNA and activation of programmed cell death by induction of p53. High levels of corticosteroids act on lymphoid cells through specific receptors. It should, however, be noted that the action of many drugs is complex and may not fit readily into a single category.

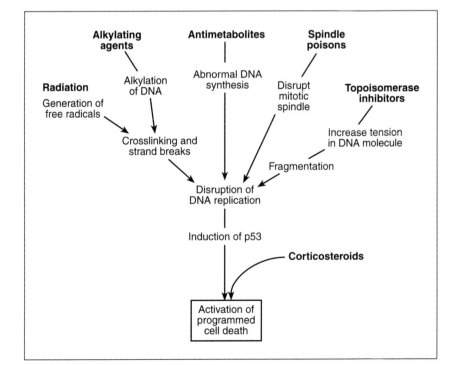

caused by strand separation during DNA replication. This is vital for replication. Inhibitors of both types of topoisomerase are described but most of the drugs used in clinical practice, e.g. etoposides, interact with topoisomerase-II–DNA complexes. The nature of this interaction is complex but the effect appears to be the production of double-stranded DNA breaks and fragmentation (Figure 4.7).

A third general mechanism of DNA damage is interference in the metabolism of DNA bases by antimetabolites. The prototypic member of this group is methotrexate, which is a powerful inhibitor of dihydrofolate reductase. Inhibition of this enzyme arrests the production of tetra-hydrofolate, which is involved in the transfer of single carbon moieties necessary for the synthesis of purines and pyrimidines. This results in impairment of DNA synthesis and repair. A variety of pyrimidine and purine analogues are in routine use for the treatment of haematological malignancies. The mechanism of action of these drugs is complex and each may act through several pathways to cause DNA damage. Cytosine arabinoside, an analogue of deoxycytidine, may act both by inhibition of DNA polymerase and by substituting for cytosine in newly synthesized DNA. The more recently introduced purine analogues, fludarabine, 2-chlorodeoxyadenosine (2-CDA) and 2-deoxycoformycin (DCF), were

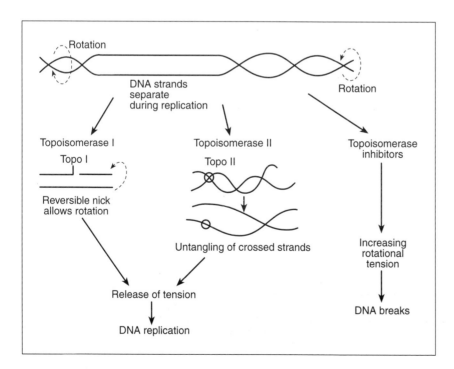

Figure 4.7 Topoisomerases and DNA replication. Chromosomal DNA consists of very long molecules. Separation of the strands of the double helix to allow DNA replication causes rotational stress in the molecule. This stress is relieved by topoisomerase enzymes, which create transient strand nicks to allow rotation to occur or form reversible complexes with DNA, allowing untangling of strands. Drugs that block topoisomerase activity result in DNA strand breaks and disruption of chromosomes.

initially investigated as inhibitors of the enzyme adenosine deaminase (ADA), which is involved in the degradation of adenosine. The accumulation of adenine metabolites inhibits DNA synthesis. However, fludarabine in particular appears to a have a more direct inhibitory effect on DNA polymerase and incorporation into a growing DNA strand results in chain termination. It is likely that these drugs exert a combined effect of producing strand breaks and inhibiting DNA repair.

The effect of all these drugs is to produce DNA strand breaks, base substitutions and failure of DNA synthesis, which lead to the induction of programmed cell death by a p53-dependent mechanism.

However, not all cytotoxic drugs act by causing damage to DNA. Corticosteroids are potent inducers of p53-independent apoptosis in both normal and neoplastic lymphoid cells. This may be mediated by interaction with steroid hormone receptors or by causing a rise in intracellular calcium, which can directly or indirectly activate enzymes involved in the triggering of the PCD pathway. The vinca alkaloids, which are of major importance in the treatment of lymphomas, act by binding to tubulin, which is the major component of microtubules. At low doses the continual cycle of polymerization and depolymerization vital to the function of microtubules is inhibited. At higher doses there is disruption of microtubules and the formation of tubulin crystals. The key cytotoxic effect of the vinca alkaloids is probably to block the mitotic spindle and prevent mitosis.

4.3 Drug resistance and treatment failure

To be effective the drug must be present in sufficient concentration within the tissue containing the tumour cells

The concentration of drugs within the tumour can be affected by a variety of pharmacokinetic factors, which may vary between patients. The presence of sanctuary sites in the CNS and testis caused by blood–tissue barriers is well recognized. The effective concentration of a drug within the cell is also affected by a range of other factors. The membrane pump mdr-1 (P-glycoprotein) is capable of expelling a wide range of cytotoxic drugs, including anthracyclines and vinca alkaloids from cells, reducing their effective concentration. Increased levels of expression of mdr-1 may be present in a number of types of leukaemia or lymphoma at presentation and rather more frequently at relapse. The importance of this mechanism as a cause of treatment resistance *in vivo* remains unclear. Attempts to reverse such resistance with drugs such as verapamil and cyclosporin A have, as yet, shown no clear benefit (Table 4.1).

Intracellular metabolism may also affect the concentration of active drug within the cell. The activity of enzymes such as cytP450 and glutathionine-S-transferase can significantly affect the amount of active cytotoxic agent in the cell by affecting its activation and deactivation. Polymorphisms that affect the activities of these enzymes are relatively common in the population. In some cells there may be failure of intracellular transport of anthracyclines and possibly other drugs from the cytoplasm to the nucleus, which may reduce the effective concentration of the drug at the target site. The effectiveness of particular cytotoxic drugs may be affected by concentrations of *in vitro* target molecules. For example, methotrexate resistance may occur as a result of amplification and overexpression of the gene for dihydrofolate reductase, though this is of limited importance *in vivo*.

Genetic damage with the PCD pathway may also lead to treatment resistance. For example, mutation and inactivation of *p53* may lead to failure of cell-cycle arrest or PCD in response to drug-induced genetic damage. Not only does the presence of these abnormalities allow cells to survive drug toxicity but the mutagenic effects of many drugs may even lead to the accumulation of further genetic defects and accelerated tumour progression. Induction of drug-induced PCD will also be inhibited by increased levels of Bcl-2/Bax or Bcl-x_L/Bax heterodimers.

Table 4.1 Variables affecting the efficacy of cytotoxic drugs

Drug action	Affected by
Drug delivery to tumour cell	Hepatic metabolism Renal function Tumour vascularity
Intracellular concentration	Level of membrane P-glycoprotein (MDR1)
Intracellular activation	Induction and polymorphism of cyt P450 Glutathione-S-transferase
Binding to molecular target	Gene amplification and induction
Damage to DNA	{ Impaired DNA repair { Mutation or deletion of *p53*
Induction of programmed cell death	Bcl-2 and Bax expression

4.4 The development of chemotherapeutic strategies

Despite the increasing understanding of the mechanisms of chemotherapy, many of the drugs in routine use were developed as a result of chance observations. Studies of the toxic effects of mustard gas, as used in the First World War, on bone marrow and lymphoid tissue led to the use of nitrogen mustard in animal models and subsequently in humans with lymphomas. This agent, mechlorethamine, was the prototype for several alkylating agents, including cyclophosphamide, which were often given singly to patients with Hodgkin's disease and other lymphoproliferative diseases. The folate antagonists, notably methotrexate, the corticosteroids and, somewhat later, drugs being investigated as possible antibiotics – daunorubicin and doxorubicin – were also found to have therapeutic activity and were, consequently, applied in treatment. A further agent, synthesized as a potential monoamine oxidase inhibitor but with activity in lymphoma, was procarbazine.

Combination chemotherapy represented a major advance

An era of generally unsatisfactory chemotherapy, mainly with single agents and often in the setting of very advanced disease, came to an end with the combination of four agents with individual activity in the treatment of Hodgkin's disease into a multi-agent regime. The MOPP regimen (mechlorethamine, vincristine ('Oncovin'), procarbazine and prednisolone) was the model for subsequent combination chemotherapy. In essence, the intention was to enhance antitumour effectiveness without producing unacceptable toxicity. The CHOP regimen (cyclophosphamide, hydroxydaunorubicin (doxorubicin) vincristine and prednisolone) subsequently became the standard treatment of the more aggressive, advanced non-Hodgkin's lymphomas. These more intensive, and therefore more myelosuppressive, regimens were given cyclically with intervals between treatment to allow bone marrow recovery.

The basis of many regimens is largely empirical rather than closely related to cell kinetics

Concepts of differential drug efficacy during specific phases of the life cycle of the proliferating malignant cell were suggested as a possible basis for developing chemotherapy schedules. Drugs were identified as phase-specific or phase-non-specific. Tumours with low proliferative activity were considered less likely to respond to agents most effective during S phase than, for example, the alkylating agents, which interact directly with DNA independently of the phase of the cell cycle. More recently, the importance of the programmed cell death pathway as a mode of action of cytotoxic drugs has been recognized. It is clear that, despite this theoretical approach, the evolution of chemotherapy schedules and particular combinations has owed more to empiricism and serendipity than the application of cytokinetic and pharmacokinetic principles.

4.5 Management of therapy-induced cytopenia

Dose-related cytopenias are an inevitable consequence of cytotoxic chemotherapy

Chemotherapy regimens such as CHOP induce predictable neutropenia, which is usually maximal between days 10 and 14 post-chemotherapy, with recovery of normal counts by day 21 when the next cycle of chemotherapy is due. The nadir neutrophil count would be expected to be in the range $0.5-1.5 \times 10^9/l$. There is, however, considerable individual variation, younger patients generally being able to tolerate higher doses of chemotherapy. In principle, it is important to ensure that the chemotherapy is given on schedule in full doses to obtain the best treatment responses. In the event of infection or if the neutrophil count is below $1 \times 10^9/l$ at the time of the next cycle of chemotherapy, it is conventional to delay treatment by a week until the count recovers. Dose reductions are often applied in specific regimens and these may become increasingly necessary with successive cycles of treatment.

Neutropenic sepsis can be a rapidly fatal complication of chemotherapy

Sepsis, particularly when caused by Gram-negative bacteria (GNB), can be rapidly fatal. For this reason it is imperative that antimicrobial therapy is commenced as soon as sepsis is suspected without awaiting the results of microbiological investigations. Empirical therapy is directed against GNB, including *Pseudomonas aeruginosa*, and typically comprises an antipseudomonal penicillin, such as piperacillin, combined with an aminoglycoside, e.g. gentamicin. Such combinations are preferred on the theoretical grounds of synergy, but many institutions claim that monotherapy with an antipseudomonal cephalosporin (such as ceftazidime) or a carbapenem is of equivalent efficacy.

In recent years Gram-positive bacteria have replaced GNB as the most frequent blood culture isolates, reflecting the marked increase in the use of indwelling vascular access lines. Excepting *Staphylococcus aureus*, the organisms most commonly encountered in this setting – the coagulase-negative staphylococci and 'diphtheroids' – can, in most circumstances, be regarded as low-grade pathogens and it is not necessary to include specific agents against these bacteria in the initial empirical regime.

The response to empirical antimicrobial therapy needs to be carefully monitored

Antimicrobials are often reviewed 48 h after commencing empirical therapy in the context of the results of microbiological investigations. However, management is often problematical when the results of these are negative and the patient remains pyrexial. Other clinical and laboratory parameters should be reviewed (e.g. C-reactive protein levels), as 35–50% of patients who ultimately respond to empirical therapy take 4 days or more to defervesce, particularly if there is a pulmonary focus of sepsis. Non-infectious causes of fever should also be considered. If, however, a change of therapy is deemed necessary, then the addition of a glycopeptide (e.g. vancomycin) with activity against Gram-positive bacteria would be an appropriate step. Continuing non-response of the pyrexia following this should heighten suspicion of fungal sepsis and the empirical use of a broad-spectrum antifungal agent, such as amphotericin B, should be considered, particularly in patients who have received chemotherapy over a long period (Figure 4.8).

Antimicrobial prophylaxis may prevent opportunistic infection

Many episodes of septicaemia caused by GNB are a result of the entry of these bacteria into the bloodstream *via* the gut wall, particularly against a background of chemotherapy-associated changes in the gut mucosa. Selective decontamination regimens were developed in an attempt to prevent this by the eradication of aerobic GNB in the colon while preserving anaerobic flora that may protect against gut colonization by new coliforms, including hospital-acquired strains. Problems with patient compliance and a lack of demonstrable efficacy with early strategies, which used non-absorbable oral agents such as neomycin, led to the development of other regimens, most commonly those which employ quinolones (e.g. ciprofloxacin). The efficacy of such approaches is not clearly established or universally agreed. Many institutions using this quinolone prophylaxis report an increased incidence of serious Gram-positive infections.

Prevention of oral candidiasis can be attempted using non-absorbable compounds, such as nystatin; however, more recently, systemically absorbed drugs, e.g. fluconazole, have been used with success, although claims that these agents may also prevent deep fungal infections remain the subject of debate.

Infections due to the Herpesviruses are associated with significant morbidity and occasionally mortality in patients undergoing treatment for lymphoproliferative diseases. Reactivation of Herpes simplex virus infections can be prevented by acyclovir. Higher doses may also prevent the reactivation of Varicella zoster virus.

Previously considered as a protozoan parasite, but now regarded as a fungus, *Pneumocystis carinii* may cause a severe pneumonic illness in this patient group. A number of agents have been used prophylactically but the combination of sulphamethoxazole and trimethoprim (co-trimoxazole) remains the regimen of choice in this setting.

Growth factors can minimize chemotherapy-induced neutropenia

G-CSF (granulocyte colony stimulating factor) can be used to shorten the period of chemotherapy-induced neutropenia. Given as a subcutaneous

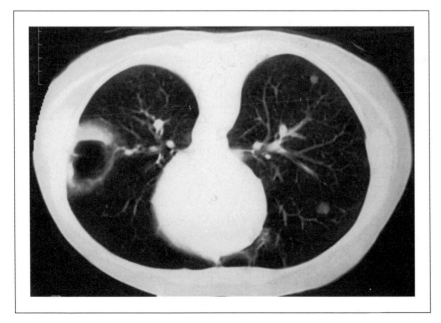

Figure 4.8 Pulmonary fungal infection – CT scan. This scan shows a large cavitating lesion in the left lung which developed in a neutropenic patient. Several other smaller lesions were seen. This was found to be due to *Aspergillus* infection.

injection daily, following the discontinuation of chemotherapy, it is possible to minimize or prevent the period of neutropenia associated with chemotherapy. The optimum time to commence the administration following discontinuation of chemotherapy is not clear and it is variably started immediately or after 5–7 days. Surprisingly, although the period of neutropenia can be shown to be reduced by G-CSF, the clinical benefit in terms of reduced episodes of infection has not clearly been demonstrated.

An alternative approach to using these growth factors is only to treat neutropenic patients who are septic and not responding to appropriate antibiotics. In this instance the clinical benefit of the more rapid regeneration of neutrophils is clear. Another potential use of G-CSF is to use it to increase the dose intensity of standard chemotherapy, such as CHOP, by decreasing the period of time between courses. This approach is limited by non-haemopoietic toxicities (notably mucositis) and improved outcomes have yet to be demonstrated.

Thrombocytopenia is not frequently seen with outpatient chemotherapy but is a significant problem after intensive treatment

Thrombocytopenia following treatment may be reflected in clinical signs such as petechial haemorrhages, mucosal haemorrhage and purpura. Following intensive regimens there is a significant chance of bleeding and platelet transfusions may be required. Platelet transfusions are often given to maintain platelets at levels above $20 \times 10^9/l$, although in the absence of overt bleeding, many centres do not give platelet support until the count falls below $10 \times 10^9/l$. Despite this, in the presence of an infection or pyrexia the count needs to be maintained at higher levels, in order to prevent clinically significant haemorrhage. Regular fundoscopy is important in the presence of thrombocytopenia and the detection of retinal haemorrhage would be an indication to maintain higher platelet counts. The platelet growth factor thrombopoietin, TPO, has now been cloned and its use in the clinical setting is being investigated.

Anaemia is also an inevitable consequence of intensive treatment that is not regularly seen after outpatient chemotherapy

Anaemia may occur towards the end of CHOP-type regimens but is mainly a consideration in the elderly. Full blood counts should be monitored and packed red cell transfusions should be initiated in the presence of significant anaemia (haemoglobin less than 10 g/dl) and/or the presence of symptoms such as breathlessness or heart failure. Anaemia is an inevitable consequence of intensive treatment and the haemoglobin level is usually maintained above 10 g/dl by regular transfusion. There is a general consensus that for the transfusion of Hodgkin's disease irradiated blood should be used to prevent engraftment of donor lymphocytes and graft *versus* host disease (GvHD). The need for irradiated blood for transfusion during the treatment of other lymphoproliferative disorders is less clear, although treatment with fludarabine is an indication. Following autologous transplantation significant rates of GvHD can occur and irradiated blood products are therefore required. In young patients with long-term transfusion requirements consideration should be given to the use of erythropoietin, EPO. This may avoid some of the hazards of long-term transfusion such as iron deposition and exposure to viruses.

4.6 Stem cell therapy

The use of stem cells allows chemotherapy to be given in supralethal doses

Dose escalation is one way of increasing the effective intracellular level of cytotoxic agent, but a limiting factor with this approach is the risk of irreversible myelosuppression. This can be avoided by the reinfusion of stored autologous stem cells not exposed to treatment. The clinical indications for such a strategy are in the process of being established but patients who may benefit include some large cell lymphomas at presentation, relapsed large cell lymphomas, myeloma and relapsed Hodgkin's disease with poor prognostic features. In most of these indications the use of peripheral blood stem cells is increasingly preferred to marrow because of the more rapid engraftment and reduced morbidity.

Peripheral stem cells are obtained in most patients by induction of neutropenia using a dose of cyclophosphamide ($2-4 \text{ g/m}^2$) followed by daily subcutaneous injections of G-CSF. This results in a rapidly rising white cell count at around day 10 when the harvests are performed using a continuous flow cell separator. This separates and collects the

Figure 4.9 Mobilization of stem cells into the peripheral blood. Progenitor cells capable of bone marrow reconstitution can be mobilized into the peripheral blood by two main methods. **(a)** Most commonly, G-CSF is given by daily injection after a single dose of a myelotoxic agent. The cells are harvested during white cell count recovery after day 10. **(b)** An alternative method for use in those who do not have malignant disease, e.g. bone marrow donors, is to administer daily doses of G-CSF and harvest around day 4, by which time the donor will have a very high white cell count.

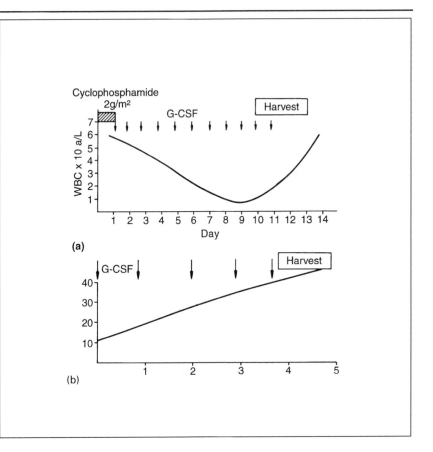

mononuclear-cell-rich fraction and returns the remainder to the patient (Figure 4.9).

There are two methods in common use to assess the number of stem cells in the harvest. A sample of cells can be plated in semi-solid medium and the number of CFU-GM colonies counted. These are cumbersome to perform and poorly reproducible. More commonly the number of CD34 positive cells in the harvest are counted by flow cytometry (Figure 4.10).

This fraction includes pluripotent stem cells as well as lineage-committed cells. Although both the above tests provide reassuring information, they do not directly measure stem cells and, in general, if an adequate number of mononuclear cells is obtained during the time of a rapidly rising white cell count there will be sufficient stem cells for engraftment. The usual reasons for an inadequate harvest are age and heavy pretreatment with alkylating agents.

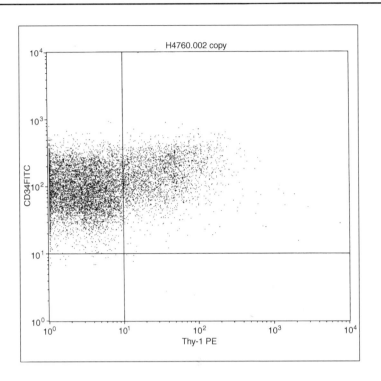

Figure 4.10 Flow cytometric analysis of CD34⁺ cells. This is the product from a CD34-selected peripheral blood stem cell harvest in which the cells are labelled with anti-CD34 and anti-Thy-1. The CD34 Thy-1-positive population appears to contain the true pluripotent stem cells.

There are a number of potential advances in stem cell technology

Many harvests contain contaminating tumour cells. These can now be removed by positive selection for CD34-expressing cells and negative selection of contaminating tumour cells using antibodies directed against cell surface proteins known to be present on the tumour cells. Improved methods of detecting subpopulations of stem cells in the CD34⁺ fraction could result in the production of stem cell products that contain a balance of pluripotent and committed progenitors cells, which would combine the shortest possible cytopenic phase with the certainty of long-term marrow repopulation. The techniques of gene transfer are now well established in experimental systems and one possible clinical application of gene transfer is to transfect harvested stem cells with genes that can confer drug resistance. This would allow further relatively intensive therapy to be given after a stem cell autograft. Finally, greater understanding of the processes of stem cell mobilization may allow more effective harvesting of cells in patients where this is currently difficult or impossible (Figure 4.11).

Figure 4.11 CD34 selection of peripheral blood stem cells. This is a method of specifically selecting stem cells and progenitor cells which constitute only a small proportion of harvested mononuclear cells based on the expression of CD34. The major application of this method is in the removal of contaminating tumour cells, which do not express CD34. The method may be combined with further selection aimed specifically at killing or removing neoplastic cells.

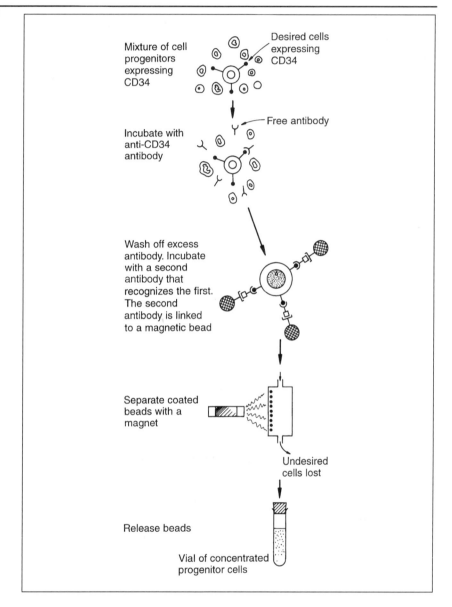

4.7 Radiotherapeutic approaches in the treatment of lymphoproliferative disorders

Radiotherapy kills cells by the generation of electrons in target tissues

Radiation is a means of delivering energy to a tissue so as to generate electrons, causing ionization and the formation of free radicals; this leads to cellular damage and ultimately cell death. The amount of energy absorbed by the tissue depends on the energy of the incident radiation beam and the atomic number of the atom absorbing the photon of radiation. In general, the absorbed dose falls exponentially with its path length within the tissue. The energy absorbed is measured in grays (Gy); 1 Gy = 1 J/kg (Figure 4.12, Table 4.2).

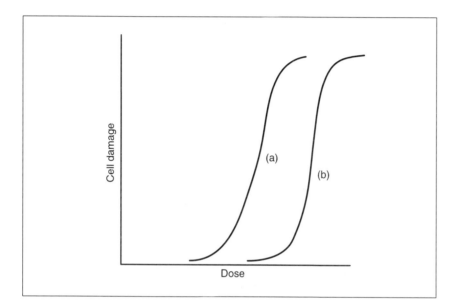

Figure 4.12 Typical radiotherapy dose–response curve. If radiotherapy is to be curative, curve **(a)** must apply to the tumour tissue and curve **(b)** to the normal tissue so that a tumoricidal dose can be given with minimum risk of damage to normal tissue.

Table 4.2 Radiotherapy dose limits for normal tissue (based on daily 2 Gy fractions – the tolerance depends on the volume treated and may be reduced by previous treatment and coexisting disease)

Tissue type	Maximum dose
Whole lung	20 Gy
Spinal cord	
< 10 cm	50 Gy
10–20 cm	40 Gy
Whole	30 Gy
Heart	40 Gy
Kidney	20 Gy
Liver	25 Gy
Small intestine (part)	45 Gy
Testis	1 Gy
Ovary	2–3 Gy
Lens	5 Gy
Salivary gland	30 Gy
Thyroid	<4–5 Gy

High-energy or megavoltage photons produced by linear accelerators are most commonly used to treat deep-seated tumours. When irradiating deep structures more than one beam of megavoltage radiation is often required to produce a homogeneous therapeutic dose within the target tissue while reducing the dose to surrounding normal tissues. Linear accelerators also have the facility to produce high energy (megavoltage) electrons. These are less penetrating than megavoltage photons and deliver 90% of their dose within a few centimetres of the skin surface. These are useful in treating superficial tumours, e.g. skin tumours.

The potential for radiation therapy to cure a tumour is determined by the ability to achieve local control of the tumour and the natural history of the disease

To obtain local control of a tumour it must be possible to deliver a lethal dose of irradiation to the malignant cells without producing functional failure of the surrounding normal tissue. This is dependent on the normal tissue having a greater capacity to repair radiation damage than the tumour and/or being able to limit the volume of normal tissue treated so that the non-irradiated normal tissue can compensate for that damaged by radiotherapy (Figure 4.13, Table 4.3).

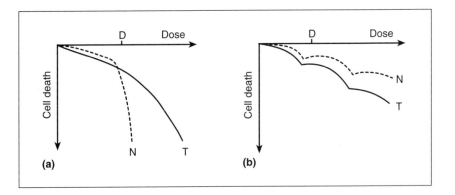

Figure 4.13 (a, b) Single and fractionated radiotherapy dose–response curves. Tissues can be classified into early- or late-responding depending on the shape of the dose–response curve. Radiosensitive tumours have early-responding characteristics and most normal cells are late responders. When radiation is given as a single fraction there is a dose D at which the dose–response curves cross and above which larger numbers of normal cells will be killed. If fractions, each less than D, are given then the favourable differential between normal and tumour cells can be maintained at higher total dose levels.

Table 4.3 Key factors in achieving local control

- Radiosensitivity of the tumour
- Size of tumour
- Radiosensitivity of surrounding normal tissue

Lymphomas are relatively radiosensitive tumours although there is variation between tumour types. In Hodgkin's disease, 35 Gy is usually sufficient to control subclinical disease and 40 Gy to control clinically involved lymph nodes. In indolent lymphomas, 35 Gy will control 93% of tumours but in aggressive lymphomas a plateau is seen in the dose–response curve at between 40 and 50 Gy, with control being achieved in only about 75–80% of cases. The reasons for these differences are not well understood, but some of the factors that interfere with chemotherapy-induced apoptosis, such as *p53* mutations, may also be important.

In general, it is more difficult to eradicate larger tumours, where cellular hypoxia may have a protective effect. A further problem with more infiltrative tumours is minimizing damage to surrounding tissues: the tissue adjacent to the tumour is sometimes more sensitive to irradiation than the tumour. This can be the limiting factor in determining the given dose of radiation. In sensitive tissues, such as the spinal cord, dose fractionation can allow an increase in the total dose given. Both tumour size and radiosensitivity of adjacent tissues influence the decision to give chemotherapy rather than radiotherapy to patients with Hodgkin's disease who have mediastinal lymph node masses more than 10 cm in diameter.

Radiotherapy is relatively efficient in obtaining local control of lymphomas within the irradiated area. In Hodgkin's disease, where the pattern of spread tends to be predictable and contiguous, using extended-field techniques to irradiate lymph node groups adjacent to the tumour will improve the chance of cure. In non-Hodgkin's lymphomas, which are usually systemic diseases with a less predictable pattern of spread, extended-field techniques are of no benefit. Local radiotherapy will cure patients with truly localized disease and will reduce local relapse in patients previously treated with chemotherapy.

There are some well-defined radiotherapy techniques adopted in the treatment of lymphomas

4.7.1 Involved field radiotherapy
This treats involved nodes with a margin of 5 cm in the line of lymphatic drainage and 2 cm laterally. The side effects are those due to local tissue damage.

4.7.2 Mantle radiotherapy
The aim of treatment is to irradiate all of the major supradiaphragmatic lymph node groups in continuity from the mandible to the lower

Figure 4.14 Radiotherapy fields. The field covered by mantle irradiation is shown in **(a)** and inverted Y in **(b)**. The hatched areas are shielded by individually made lead equivalent blocks.

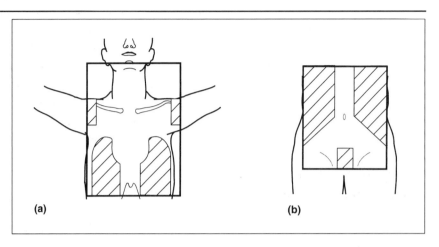

border of T10 and laterally into the axillae. Lead shielding is used for all the treatment to protect lungs and heart and for part of the treatment to protect spinal cord, as far as is compatible with achieving the objective of treatment. The acute side effects of mantle radiotherapy include skin reactions, local hair loss, sore throat and dysphagia. Radiation pneumonitis may produce a dry cough and dyspnoea in the weeks after radiotherapy. These symptoms are self-limiting but can be controlled by steroid therapy. This is not indicative by itself of developing symptomatic chronic lung damage. The major late effects of mantle radiotherapy are pulmonary fibrosis and an increased risk of ischaemic heart disease, depending on the extent of the irradiated area and dose delivered (Figure 4.14).

4.7.3 Inverted Y radiotherapy

This is a method of irradiating the para-aortic, iliac, inguinal and femoral nodes in continuity. The field extends from the lower border of D10 to the lower extent of the femoral nodes in continuity. Individualized shielding must be produced to cover the abdomen lateral to the para-aortic nodes and the central pelvis including the bladder and rectum. In men, the testicular dose is measured and, if it exceeds tolerance, additional lead shielding is used to protect against scattered irradiation. Irradiation of the testis beyond a tolerance dose will lead to loss of sperm production, although hormonal failure is rare. In women, however, retention of ovarian endocrine and reproductive function requires orchidopexy to remove the ovaries from the treatment field.

Acute gastrointestinal side effects in the form of nausea, vomiting and diarrhoea are common during treatment with inverted Y radiotherapy.

These can be managed with standard antiemetic and/or antidiarrhoeal therapy. Skin reactions may occur, especially in the groin, and can be treated with simple cleaning and application of moisturizing cream. The commonest long-term complication is peptic ulceration. There is a small risk of avascular necrosis of the femoral head, which is increased in patients also receiving steroids. Early recognition of the complication may allow treatment by decompression of the femoral head.

4.7.4 Total nodal irradiation

This technique is a combination of mantle and inverted Y radiotherapy. The components are given sequentially to reduce acute morbidity, often with a 1 month rest interval. As radiotherapy fields diverge, it is essential to accurately calculate a gap between the fields to avoid overdosage of the spinal cord and at the same time to ensure an adequate dose to the nodes at the junction of the fields.

4.7.5 Electron beam therapy for skin lymphoma

Megavoltage electrons are used to treat skin lesions. The effective treatment depth increases with the energy of the electrons used. The dose/fractionation schedule required depends on the type of tumour. For solitary skin lymphomas doses of 30–40 Gy in 10–15 fractions will usually produce long-term local control. For patients requiring palliative treatment a single fraction of 6–8 Gy will often suffice.

The use of electron beam therapy for the treatment of cutaneous T-cell lymphomas have excited much interest. Localized lesions requiring treatment may be treated as above. For more widespread disease total skin electron therapy is used. This is a specialized technique only available in some centres. The aim is to irradiate the whole of skin surface to a depth of about 6 mm. If the head is not involved it should be shielded to avoid alopecia; the nails are shielded to prevent loss and the eyes to avoid cataracts. The precise radiotherapy technique and dose fractionation regimen varies from centre to centre.

4.7.6 Cranial prophylaxis of ALL

This reduces the risk of CSF relapse. The whole brain and meninges are irradiated, including the cord adjacent to the upper two cervical vertebrae and the optic nerve. A Perspex immobilization mask is made for the patient's head to allow accurate reproduction of the treatment. Shielding blocks are made to protect the areas of the head outside the treatment volume. Dose/fractionation regimens vary but, for adults, 24 Gy in 12 fractions is often used.

The treatment is usually well tolerated. Occasionally patients may develop a somnolence syndrome in the weeks following treatment. This is self-limiting and does not imply any long-term damage. Neuropsychiatric damage after cranial radiotherapy in children is well documented.

In patients with CSF involvement, craniospinal radiotherapy can be used to irradiate the whole of the meninges and may be used in addition to intrathecal chemotherapy.

4.7.7 Total body irradiation

This technique is usually used in conjunction with high-dose therapy prior to bone marrow or peripheral blood stem cell transplantation. The aim of treatment is to deliver a homogeneous dose of radiotherapy to the whole body. Various techniques are employed but they all involve treating the patient at an increased distance from the radiotherapy machine (usually 3–4 m) to produce a beam large enough to cover the patient. This reduces incident dose rate and increases the treatment time. The treatment is usually given in several fractions, often treating twice a day, for example 14.4 Gy in eight fractions over 4 days. Since the advent of $5\text{-}HT_3$ antagonists, the treatment seldom produces any immediate side effects. In the short term, mucositis is common. In the longer term, pneumonitis has been a problem but current dose/fractionation schemes seem to be safer. The incidence of cataracts after TBI increases with time.

4.7.8 Palliative radiotherapy

The aim of palliative radiotherapy is to produce symptomatic relief for the patient for the remainder of his or her life with the minimum of side effects and inconvenience. This can often be achieved by either a single fraction or a short course of radiotherapy to the relevant area.

4.8 Cytokine and immunological therapy

Cytokines and cytokine inhibitors can be used to manipulate the tumour cells

The growth and differentiation of normal and neoplastic lymphoid cells is, at least in part, regulated by cytokines, most of which act through a superfamily of cell surface receptors that in turn activate a number of intracellular signalling pathways (Figure 4.15).

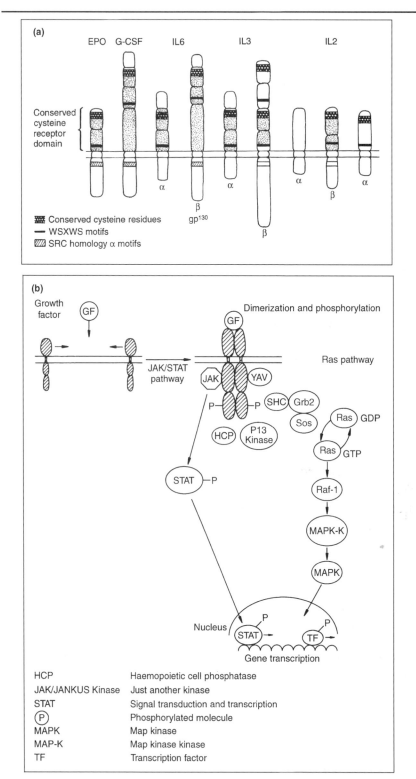

Figure 4.15 Intracellular signalling by cytokines. Many cytokines that regulate the growth and differentiation of haematopoietic cells act through a superfamily of cell surface receptors (a). Cytokine binding leads to dimerization of its specific receptor and to activation by phosphorylation of members of the JAK kinase family which in turn phosphorylate STAT transcription factors, leading to dimerization and transport to the nucleus, where they activate transcription of specific genes. Cytokine receptors may also act through a second signalling pathway in which the dimerized receptor binds Grb-2 and Sos leading to the activation of Ras by exchange of GDP and GTP. GTP-Ras initiates a kinase cascade, which leads to the activation of MAP-kinases. These enzymes are transported to the nucleus, where they phosphorylate and activate a range of transcription factors (b).

The use of cytokines or cytokine inhibitors should, in principle, be a valid approach to the treatment of lymphoproliferative disorders. Alpha interferon has a well established role in the treatment of hairy cell leukaemia but its effectiveness in other disorders remains to be clearly established. IL6 inhibitors may soon be entering preliminary clinical trials in myeloma. Increasing understanding of the cellular action of individual cytokines may lead to a more rational basis for therapy.

Attempts to modulate the immune response have been tried for many years

A persistent strand in oncological research for almost 30 years has been the idea that the immune response may be important in the treatment of tumours, but the evidence for a host response to most human tumours is very sparse. However, a special case where lymphocytes do have potent antitumour activity is in the context of allografting for chronic myeloid leukaemia. The antileukaemic effect of lymphocytes is clearly illustrated in the increased relapse rate of patients who received T-cell-depleted marrow. This graft *versus* leukaemia phenomenon is now being manipulated by using donor lymphocytes to induce remission in patients who have relapsed after non-T-cell-depleted grafts. Whether this effect is mediated by tumour specific antigens or is an antihistocompatibility antigen response is not known, although the close relationship with graft *versus* host reactions suggests that the latter is at least partly responsible. A similar graft antitumour response may occur in some other haematological malignancies treated by allogeneic bone marrow transplantation. The utility of this technique may be increased in the future by genetic manipulation of T-cells to allow them to be readily destroyed if a significant graft *versus* host reaction develops.

Another example of the important role of T-cell-mediated immunity comes from the study of lymphomas that arise in immunosuppressed individuals. In these cases failure of anti-EBV-related immunity appears to be a major factor in pathogenesis. Some of these tumours can be treated by reducing the level of immunosuppression but it is also possible to induce remissions by the use of cloned donor anti-EBV lymphocytes.

Unlike most human tumours, the majority of lymphomas have a tumour-specific antigen in the form of idiotypical determinants of immunoglobulin or T-cell receptors. There is still continuing debate about the role of anti-idiotype responses in regulating the normal immune system, but whether or not this is the case, the use of antitumour idiotype monoclonal antibodies or T-cells offers an opportunity for highly specific antilymphoma therapy. The realization of the potential has been hindered by the impracticality of producing anti-idiotype monoclonal antibodies or specifically primed T-cells except in the occasional patient.

Monoclonal antibody therapy may also be directed against lymphocyte cell surface proteins other than the idiotypical determinants of immunoglobulin or the T-cell receptor, e.g. humanized CD20 or CAMPATH-1H (CD52). Such reagents will kill normal lymphocytes but should cause minimal damage to non-lymphoid tissues. Therapeutic monoclonal antibodies may be conjugated to toxin or rely on fixation of complement or antibody-dependent cell killing for their effect. *In vitro* many monoclonal antibodies can alter the behaviour of cells by cross-linking their target molecule and substituting for the effect of the natural ligand and this may also be a useful property that can be applied to therapy.

4.9 Gene transfer and antisense therapy

The activity of aberrantly expressed genes may be modified using antisense oligonucleotides

The rapid growth in understanding the pathogenesis of lymphomas at a cellular and molecular level raises the prospect of therapy aimed specifically at neutralizing the effects of particular molecular abnormalities. An attractive prospect is to use antisense oligonucleotides, which complex with mRNA and block translation of a particular gene. Various chemical modifications allow the production of antisense agents that are relatively stable within the cell and therefore have the potential to function as active agents. However, the investigation of the value of antisense therapy is greatly complicated by the finding that the nucleic acids used often have effects on protein function that are not mediated by sequence-specific binding to mRNA. The second major barrier to the use of antisense therapy is the problem of targeted drug delivery to the tumour cells. Perhaps the best hope for the manipulation of oncogenes lies with small peptide molecules which will penetrate cells more easily.

Gene transfer therapy may be used to modify the tumour or the host response

Gene therapy represents a novel option for the treatment of lymphoproliferative diseases, although at present this is far from being a clinical reality. The principle of gene therapy is modification of the behaviour of cells by the introduction and stable expression of novel genetic material. The technique may be used to cause the production of proteins that are not normally found in a particular type of cell or the modification or replacement of defective genes. There are three main types of strategy under current investigation.

4.9.1 Gene addition

This involves the use of gene transfer to add a gene not normally expressed in the cell concerned. This can be used in a number of ways in the context of lymphoproliferative diseases. If a system could be designed that delivered a gene only to the tumour cells it would be possible to deliver a gene that conferred sensitivity to a chemotherapeutic agent that was not otherwise cytotoxic. This approach has some merit but relies on the use of vector systems that work *in vivo* and recognize only the tumour cells, a difficult goal to achieve. Additionally, they should recognize and modify all the tumour cells, otherwise unmodified cells will remain after treatment, a situation reminiscent of chemotherapy.

The other approach using the concept of gene addition is to directly modify the normal haemopoietic stem cells. It is possible, by expressing a gene that makes these cells more resistant to chemotherapy, to increase the dose of standard chemotherapy or to use agents that previously gave unacceptable myelotoxicity. In these circumstances other non-haemopoietic toxicity becomes dose-limiting. This approach is now a clinical reality using retroviral vectors to deliver either the multidrug resistance (*mdr*) gene or the alkyl transferase gene to haemopoietic stem cells.

The other potential application of gene addition is to deliver exogenous genes to the tumour cells that modify the host response to the tumour. These have been tried with some limited success clinically and have concentrated mainly on delivering and overexpressing cytokine genes in the tumour cells such as IL2 and GM-CSF. Rather more elegant approaches have tried to break the immune tolerance to the tumour cells by delivering extra copies of immune accessory molecules such as B7.1 (CD28).

A further variant of this technique is to attempt to vaccinate the patient against a tumour-specific molecule such as a mutated *ras* protein by overexpression of the antigen in muscle cells. There is some evidence to suggest that this can be achieved, at least against some viral proteins, by direct intramuscular injection of naked DNA coding for the antigen, which is taken up and expressed by the skeletal muscle cells.

4.9.2. Gene replacement

This approach would seek to add back to a malignant cell normal copies of an abnormal gene critical to the malignant process. An example of this would be adding normal copies of *p53* to cells which were abnormal because of a mutated *p53*. There is, however, a catalogue of difficulties to overcome before this would be expected to work:

1. All the tumour cells need to be corrected or the modified cells will be selectively lost by overgrowth of the unmodified cells.
2. Once in the cell the exogenous gene needs to be regulated appropriately.
3. The added gene should restore the normal function of the gene.
4. The corrected gene should be crucial to the malignant behaviour of the cell and, in the context of multistep carcinogenesis, replacing the lost function should return the cell to a premalignant state if not to normal.

4.9.3 Gene modification

This approach would seek to achieve the same end results as those brought about by gene replacement, but rather more elegantly. It relies upon using techniques such as homologous recombination to modify the regulatory sequences of a gene to alter the pattern of its expression. Oncogenes could be downregulated and tumour-suppressor genes upregulated with the aim of restoring normal cellular function. This approach is the most appealing but the least close to clinical use.

A major problem in all types of gene therapy is the efficient introduction of the novel DNA into specific target cells

There are many approaches that have been used to insert DNA into cells, including liposomally coated DNA particles, colloidal gold coated with DNA shot at high pressure at the target cells and a variety of viral vectors, but all have suffered from a lack of efficiency and have been unable to target cells present in low numbers and to maintain continued expression within these cells. At present the preferred clinical system is retroviral gene transfer and current vectors are based on the Moloney murine leukaemia virus,

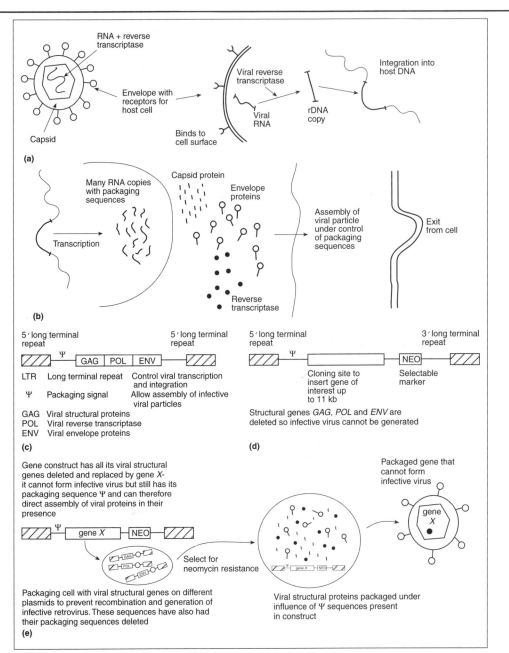

Figure 4.16 The use of retroviral vectors in gene therapy. Retroviruses can be used to integrate novel genetic material into cells. A normal retrovirus (a) attaches to a cell through specific receptors, a property that can be exploited for targeting gene therapy, and after reverse transcription the viral genome becomes integrated into a host chromosome. Given the appropriate signal, intact viruses may produce large numbers of RNA copies (b) which are packaged in protein and bud from the cell surface as infective particles. In the production of a gene therapy vector (c–d), the genetic material to be transferred and a selectable marker replaces the genes coding for the viral structural proteins (c) making the spontaneous production of infective virus impossible (d). Viral particles for use in therapy are prepared in a packaging cell that contain plasmids coding for the missing viral genes (e). This is designed to minimize the risk of recombination, which could result in novel types of infective retrovirus.

modified so that it is no longer able to complete an infective life cycle. High-titre virus can be generated, which gives the efficiency required to transfect small numbers of target cells such as haemopoietic stem cells. Major drawbacks of these vectors are the limited amount of DNA (9–12 kb) that can be packaged and transferred by the virus, targeting the vector to specific cells and safety considerations. Despite using non-replication-competent retrovirus, it is theoretically possible that infective retrovirus will be generated by recombination with endogenous human retroviral sequences and generate a transmissible disease. A further potential hazard is integration of the retrovirus next to an endogenous oncogene, which can lead to its deregulation (Figure 4.16).

4.10 Problems of therapy for lymphoproliferative disorders in children

In addition to the usual complications seen in all patients, the use of chemotherapy and radiotherapy in children may result in impairment of normal physical and intellectual development. The long life expectancy of many children also means a much greater cumulative risk of long-term complications

Cranial prophylaxis for children with ALL is associated with a range of complications

Early studies of treatment and prophylaxis for CNS disease in acute lymphoblastic leukaemia and lymphoma involved cranial irradiation, including spinal irradiation and occasionally intrathecal methotrexate. Spinal irradiation was found to cause myelosuppression, immunosuppression and growth retardation and is no longer routinely used. It is also now recognized that cranial irradiation is associated with cranial calcification, particularly of the basal ganglia, ventricular dilatation and white matter damage described as leukoencephalopathy. Late sequelae of cranial irradiation are related to the dose of radiotherapy and to the age of the child at treatment. Younger children have greater late effects. Growth retardation occurs secondary to damage to the hypothalamic-pituitary axis. There is a suggestion that therapy may impair the IQ of children, although there is a lack of consensus on the appropriate methods of sequential measurement. Again this is age- and dose-related. This effect is said to be most noticeable in the area of mathematics.

Cranial irradiation is now used solely in children with high count ($> 50 \times 10^9$/l) ALL, CNS disease at presentation and in relapsed ALL (when cranial irradiation is given in combination with total body irradiation for BMT conditions). A randomization is under way within the auspices of an MRC trial (UKALL XI) between continuing intrathecal methotrexate alone *versus* high-dose intravenous methotrexate with intrathecal MTX in low-count ALL and high-dose intravenous MTX with intrathecal MTX *versus* 18 Gy cranial irradiation for high-count ALL. The benefits of HDMTX with respect to reduction of CNS relapse (and potentially bone marrow and other site relapse) will be evaluated. Importantly, whether high-dose MTX will result in less long-term morbidity (compared with cranial irradiation) is being monitored. Secondary tumours in children following treatment for ALL have an estimated cumulative risk of 2.5% at 15 years. CNS neoplasms are among the commonest tumour and seem to occur only in children who have been irradiated. Age is an important consideration for the delivery of cranial prophylaxis as all complications of CNS-directed therapy are believed to be worse in young children under the age of 3 and particularly 2. None of the secondary CNS tumours arose in children irradiated over the age of 5.

Secondary malignant neoplasms are an important consideration in selecting chemotherapeutic agents for use in children

Secondary malignancy is recognized to occur in patients being treated with chemotherapy. It is clearly highly desirable to reduce this risk in children who have a high chance (60%) for being cured of their disease and may have a long life expectancy. Alkylating agents, such as cyclophosphamide, have been known for some time to be associated with a small risk of secondary malignancy, particularly acute myeloid leukaemia. Topoisomerase II inhibitors are particularly associated with the risk of secondary AML with abnormalities at 11q23. Combinations of drugs may potentiate the risk, which is further increased when chemotherapy is administered in association with radiotherapy. There is a cumulative risk for second malignant neoplasms following treatment for Hodgkin's disease in young people below the age of 24 (8.2% after 15 years follow-up). The major predisposing factor is having treatment with combined chemoradiotherapy.

Infertility is becoming more amenable to treatment

Infertility with complete azoospermia is almost invariably seen after treatment with combination chemotherapy in boys. Girls do not commonly become infertile but are likely to have an early menopause. Prior to starting therapy sperm storage can be undertaken in postpubertal boys, although many of them are oligospermic or azoospermic at presentation. Recently, techniques have been described for ovarian slicing with salvage and long-term storage of eggs in girls. This can be undertaken in girls prior to puberty.

Cardiac toxicity is specifically associated with anthracyclines

Anthracyclines have long been recognized to be associated with cardiotoxicity. In a small percentage of children this may result in severe cardiac failure. There are established guidelines on cumulative dose of anthracyclines but there is wide variability in individual susceptibility.

Radiotherapy to the chest may also result in cardiac dysfunction as well as radiation pneumonitis.

4.11 Key references

4.11.1 The cell cycle and cellular effects of chemotherapy

Begleiter, A., Lee, K., Israels, L. G. *et al.* (1994) Chlorambucil induced apoptosis in chronic lymphocytic leukemia (CLL) and its relationship to clinical efficacy. *Leukemia*, **8**(Suppl. 1), S103–S106.

Boise, L. H., Gottschalk, A. R., Quintans, J. and Thompson, C. B. (1995) Bcl-2 and Bcl-2-related proteins in apoptosis regulation. *Current Topics in Microbiology and Immunology*, **200**, 107–121.

Chilosi, M., Doglioni, C., Magalini, A. *et al.* (1996) p21/WAF cyclin-kinase inhibitor in non-Hodgkin's lymphomas: a potential marker of p53 tumour-suppressor gene function. *Blood*, **88**, 4012–4020.

Cordon-Cardo, C. (1995) Mutations of cell cycle regulators. Biological and clinical implications for human neoplasia. *American Journal of Pathology*, **147**, 545–560.

Ewen, M. E. (1994) The cell cycle and the retinoblastoma protein family. *Cancer and Metastasis Reviews*, **13**, 45–66.

Goldstein, L. J. (1995) Clinical reversal of drug resistance. *Current Problems in Cancer*, **19**, 65–124.

Hainaut, P. (1995) The tumor suppressor protein p53: a receptor to genotoxic stress that controls cell growth and survival. *Current Opinion in Oncology*, **7**, 76–82.

Hannun, Y. A. (1997) Apoptosis and the dilemma of cancer chemotherapy. *Blood*, **89**, 1845–1853.

Imamura, J., Miyoshi, I. and Koeffler, H. P. (1994) p53 in hematologic malignancies. *Blood*, **84**, 2412–2421.

Kang, Y. K., Zhan, Z., Regis, J. *et al.* (1995) Expression of *mdr-1* in refractory lymphoma: quantitation by polymerase chain reaction and validation of the assay. *Blood*, **86**, 1515–1524.

Lane, D. P., Midgley, C. A., Hupp, T. R. *et al.* (1995) On the regulation of the p53 tumour suppressor, and its role in the cellular response to DNA damage. *Philosophical Transactions of the Royal Society of London – Series B: Biological Sciences*, **347**, 83–87.

Lee, W. P., Lee, C. L. and Lin, H. C. (1996) Glutathione S-transferase and glutathione peroxidase are essential in the early stage of Adriamycin resistance before P-glycoprotein overexpression in HOB1 lymphoma cells. *Cancer Chemotherapy and Pharmacology*, **38**, 45–51.

Mancini, M. A., Shan, B., Nickerson, J. A. *et al.* (1994) The retinoblastoma gene product is a cell cycle-dependent, nuclear matrix-associated protein. *Proceedings of the National Academy of Sciences of the United States of America*, **91**, 418–422.

Milner, J. (1994) Forms and functions of p53. *Seminars in Cancer Biology*, **5**, 211–219.

Payne, C. M., Bernstein, C. and Bernstein, H. (1995) Apoptosis overview emphasizing the role of oxidative stress, DNA damage and signal-transduction pathways. *Leukemia and Lymphoma*, **19**, 43–93.

Russo, D., Marie, J. P., Zhou, D. C. *et al.* (1994) Evaluation of the clinical relevance of the anionic glutathione-S-transferase (*GST pi*) and multidrug resistance (*mdr-1*) gene coexpression in leukemias and lymphomas. *Leukemia and Lymphoma*, **15**, 453–468.

Yang, E. and Korsmeyer, S. J. (1996) Molecular thanotopsis. *Blood*, **88**, 386–401.

Zwall, F. A. and Schroit, A. J. (1997) Pathophysiological implications of membrane phospholipid asymmetry in blood cells. *Blood*, **89**, 1121–1132.

4.11.2 Stem cell transplantation

Bensinger, W., Appelbaum, F., Rowley, S. *et al.* (1995) Factors that influence collection and engraftment of autologous peripheral-blood stem cells. *Journal of Clinical Oncology*, **13**, 2547–2555.

Demuynck, H., Delforge, M., Verhoef, G. *et al.* (1995) Comparative study of peripheral blood progenitor cell collection in patients with multiple myeloma after single-dose cyclophosphamide combined with rhGM-CSF or rhG-CSF. *British Journal of Haematology*, **90**, 384–392.

Fruehauf, S., Haas, R., Conradt, C. *et al.* (1995) Peripheral blood progenitor cell (PBPC) counts during steady-state hematopoiesis allow to estimate the yield of mobilized PBPC after filgrastim (R-metHuG-CSF)-supported cytotoxic chemotherapy. *Blood*, **85**, 2619–2626.

4.11.3 Genetic and immunotherapy

Friedmann, T. (1997) Making gene therapy work. *Scientific American*, **276**, 79–103.

Johnston, J. V., Malacko, A. R., Mizuno, M. T. *et al.* (1996) B7-CD28 costimulation unveils the hierarchy of tumor epitopes recognized by major histocompatibility complex class I-restricted CD8[+] cytolytic T lymphocytes. *Journal of Experimental Medicine*, **183**, 791–800.

Lacerda, J. F., Ladanyi, M., Louie, D. C. *et al.* (1996) Human Epstein–Barr virus (EBV)-specific cytotoxic T lymphocytes home preferentially to and induce selective regressions of autologous EBV-induced B cell lymphoproliferations in xenografted C.B-17 scid/scid mice. *Journal of Experimental Medicine*, **183**, 1215–1228.

Syrengelas, A. D., Chan, T. T. and Levy, R. (1996) DNA immunisation induces protective immunity against B-cell lymphoma. *Nature Medicine*, **2**, 1038–1041.

5 The development of classifications of lymphoproliferative disorders

Classifications of tumours are essentially tools to facilitate the understanding of particular aspects of the disease process and it is possible that a classification useful in predicting the response of a tumour to chemotherapy may be less valuable as a tool to investigate the cause of the tumour. In comparing classifications it is necessary to consider the classification in the context of the techniques and concepts that were current at the time the classification was devised and the purpose for which it was intended.

5.1 Hodgkin's disease

Modern classification begins with the definition of Hodgkin's disease as a separate type of tumour

The origin of lymphoma classification was the description by Thomas Hodgkin in 1832 of a distinctive tumour that affected lymph nodes and spleen. Hodgkin was effectively proposing that the pattern of spread of a tumour is an important characteristic that can be used to distinguish one type of tumour from another. It is important to realize that in Hodgkin's time the term 'tumour' carried its literal meaning of a swelling rather than that of a neoplasm and that the modern concept of neoplasia was not clearly formulated until much later. Microscopy was beginning to be used in medical diagnosis but the lack of adequate techniques of section preparation and staining did not permit histological studies to be performed at that time. A more detailed description of the disease was published in 1856 by William Wilks. In his paper 'Cases of Lardaceous Disease and Some Allied Affections' Wilks gave an accurate description of the contiguous pattern of spread that remains one of the key features of Hodgkin's disease. He also generously proposed the name 'Hodgkin's disease'.

Towards the end of the 19th century, when cell theory and histological techniques were becoming established, Greenfield and other contemporaries recognized that histology could be used to separate Hodgkin's disease from leukaemic infiltration of lymph nodes. At this time the cell that was to become known as the Reed–Sternberg cell was first recognized. Sternberg's description appeared in 1899 but the definitive paper is probably that published by Reed in the *Johns Hopkins Hospital Reports* in 1902. In this paper Reed reviewed a chaotic literature on the subject and posed the fundamental question as to relationship between Hodgkin's disease and infection, in particular tuberculosis. Reed correctly concluded that the strong relationship between Hodgkin's disease and TB was due to the increased susceptibility of patients to infection. She proposed that Hodgkin's disease should be defined histologically and gave a modern description of the basic histological features of the disease. It is remarkable that a disease entity that predated a clear understanding of the nature of neoplasia should have survived to the present day.

During the next 50–60 years a plethora of terms were applied in the classification of lymphomas. An important contribution was the work of Jackson and Parker, published mainly in the mid-1940s which subdivided Hodgkin's disease into paragranuloma, granuloma and sarcoma. However, modern classifications of Hodgkin's disease (HD) stem from the studies of Lukes and Butler published in the 1960s. They recognized that patients with HD had differing rates of disease progression and sought to identify the histological features predictive of prognosis while emphasizing the need for a coherent and uniform terminology. The Lukes–Butler classification was based on the observation that the number of lymphocytes varied inversely with the number of Reed–Sternberg cells and that this correlated with prognosis. In addition to the cellular content, fibrosis in the node was also an important feature, based on the finding that patients with fibrosis appeared to respond better to radiotherapy. There was also the suggestion, based on the degree of morphological atypia, that Reed–Sternberg cells might exist in benign and malignant forms. The Lukes–Butler classification included six subtypes, which were amalgamated into the familiar four types of the Rye classification (Tables 5.1, 5.2).

In the mid to late 1960s cellular immunology was becoming established and the four categories of the Rye classification were meant to

Table 5.1 Lukes and Butler classification of Hodgkin's disease

- Lymphocytic and histiocytic
  - Nodular
  - Diffuse
- Nodular sclerosis
- Mixed cellularity
- Lymphocyte depleted
  - Diffuse fibrosis
  - Reticular

Table 5.2 Rye classification of Hodgkin's disease

- Lymphocyte-predominant
- Nodular sclerosing
- Mixed cellularity
- Lymphocyte-depleted

reflect the 'dynamic state of the host response to the tumour'. Inherent in the concept is that progression to a more malignant histological type with far fewer lymphocytes could occur if the host response diminished in the course of the disease. It is of interest that in the Rye classification the category of nodular lymphocytic and histiocytic HD was lost despite the fact that the publications of Lukes and Butler had shown that this type had a strikingly more favourable prognosis than any other type of Hodgkin's disease.

In recent years the increased understanding of cellular and molecular pathology of lymphocytes has emphasized the relationship between Hodgkin's disease and other types of lymphoma at a cellular level. Hodgkin's disease itself is no longer seen as a single entity but rather as two distinctive clinical syndromes – lymphocyte-predominant nodular Hodgkin's disease and classical Hodgkin's disease.

5.2 Non-Hodgkin's lymphoma

Modern concepts of non-Hodgkin's lymphomas (NHL) began around 1950 with the work of Rappaport

In the early 20th century it was apparent that there was a group of primary disorders of lymph nodes that could be separated from

Hodgkin's disease, metastatic tumours, leukaemia and specific infections such as TB and syphilis. It was recognized that there was a wide variation in clinical behaviour and a number of classifications were proposed, the best known being that of Gall and Mallory. From the mid-1950s Rappaport in the United States began the process that led to the present systems of classification of NHL. In order to understand the classifications being proposed at that time it is important to remember that until the mid-1960s the development and function of the lymphocyte was not understood. As late as 1961 it was being suggested that the lymphocyte acted as a mobile source of energy for cells involved in inflammation.

In the 1950s there remained considerable difficulties in reliably separating follicular lymphoma and reactive follicular hyperplasia. In part this was due to the lack of a clear concept of the fundamental difference between these conditions. Rappaport and others evaluated and clarified the histological criteria for making this distinction and correlated these with clinical outcome. As a result the use of highly ambiguous terms such as 'Brill–Symmers disease' and 'giant follicular hyperplasia' fell into disuse. Rappaport recognized that the morphological features of the cell in follicular lymphoma were the same as those in diffuse lymphomas and he proposed that lymphomas should be classified according to the types of cell present and whether the growth pattern was diffuse or nodular, both of which correlated with clinical outcome. This evolved into the definitive versions of the Rappaport classification. It is of interest that the earliest versions included a Hodgkin's variant as a subtype of follicular lymphoma, possibly representing lymphocyte-predominant nodular Hodgkin's disease. The Rappaport classification, which is based purely on morphological description, was used as a tool for predicting the clinical outcome of patients with lymphoma and to some extent is still successful for this purpose.

The Lukes–Collins and Kiel classifications are based on comparison between tumour cells and the stages of normal lymphocyte development

In the late 1960s the functions of the lymphocyte in the immune response were being elucidated. *In vitro* studies showed that when lymphocytes were activated they progressed through a number of stages of maturation. The separate development and functions of T- and B-cells were described and the first immunological methods became available to distinguish lymphocyte subsets. These observations led to the proposal of a radically new type of classification of NHL by Lennert in Germany and Lukes and

Collins in the United States. The basic concept was that lymphomas were populations of defective lymphocytes that were arrested at one of the intermediate stages of differentiation. Lukes and Collins suggested that this process was in some way analogous to the cellular defects seen in congenital immunodeficiency disorders, where a block in normal maturation led to impaired immune function. It was soon recognized that a considerable proportion of tumours contained cells of the type found in germinal centres and that most lymphomas were of B-cell type. The importance of these classifications was that, although they were still dependent on the morphological examination of the cells, it was recognized that the tumours could be classified within a framework based on abnormalities of the normal processes of cellular differentiation rather than by arbitrary features such as cell size and shape. It was also recognized that new techniques would develop to make this process more effective. In comparison with the Lukes–Collins classification, the Kiel classification was more morphologically orientated and placed considerable emphasis on tumour grade. The definition of grade in the Kiel classification is the size of cells in a given tumour; low-grade tumours have small cells and high-grade tumours have large cells. These pathological grades rapidly became linked to two broad clinical lymphoma syndromes: low-grade, corresponding to indolent chemoresistant tumours with a low growth fraction, and high-grade, corresponding to aggressive, rapidly dividing chemosensitive tumours (Table 5.3).

The International Working Formulation was devised to allow translation of data between different systems of classification

In the late 1970s there were six lymphoma classifications with a significant following in different parts of the world, which created a major problem in the comparison of data. In order to address this problem, the National Cancer Institute commissioned a study to compare the clinical value of these classifications; this was published in 1982. The study found that the degree of reproducibility and their ability to predict prognosis was similar for all the classifications. To allow data from trials that used any of these classifications to be compared, a Working Formulation was proposed that would act as a translation device. The ten main categories in the working formulation are based on pure morphology and are heavily influenced by the Rappaport classification. A further proposal was that these categories could be split into three clinical grades – high, intermediate and low – based on patient outcome data generated by the NCI study. This is conceptually very

Table 5.3 The Kiel classification

B-cell	T-cell
Low grade lymphoma	
Lymphocytic	Lymphocytic
CLL	CLL
PLL	PLL
Hairy cell	
	Small cell
	Mycosis fungoides and Sézary
Lymphoplasmacytic/-cytoid	Lymphoepithelioid
Plasmacytic	Angioimmunoblastic
Centroblastic–centrocytic	T-zone
Follicular ± diffuse	
Diffuse	
Centrocytic (mantle cell)	Pleomorphic, small cell (HTLV1)
Monocytoid/marginal zone	
High-grade lymphoma	
Centroblastic	Pleomorphic medium and large cell
Immunoblastic	Immunoblastic
Burkitt's lymphoma	
Large cell anaplastic	Large cell anaplastic
Lymphoblastic	Lymphoblastic

different from the grades proposed in the Kiel classification, which are based on cell size.

The grades used in the Working Formulation are problematical in two respects. Firstly, the criteria used to separate tumours that differ in grade is in some cases poorly defined or difficult to apply. Secondly, basing the definition of these grades on survival data ensures obsolescence as treatment improves with time. Despite the stated aims of its authors, the Working Formulation has evolved into a major classification and is widely used clinically and in reporting the results of clinical trials. As a tool for studying the cellular pathology or cause of lymphomas or developing new treatment strategies it has little value (Table 5.4).

For largely historical reasons lymphoid leukaemias have been classified separately

The concept of leukaemia as an abnormal expansion of white blood cells has existed for over a century and as described above it was soon

Table 5.4 National Cancer Institute Working Formulation for clinical usage

Low-grade

A. Malignant Lymphoma Small Lymphocytic
   Consistent with CLL
   Plasmacytoid

B. Malignant Lymphoma Follicular, predominantly small cleaved cell
   Diffuse areas
   Sclerosis

C. Malignant Lymphoma Follicular, mixed, small cleaved and large cell
   Diffuse areas
   Sclerosis

Intermediate grade

D. Malignant Lymphoma Follicular, predominantly large cell
   Diffuse areas
   Sclerosis

E. Malignant Lymphoma Diffuse, small cleaved cell
   Sclerosis

F. Malignant Lymphoma Diffuse, mixed small and large cell
   Sclerosis
   Epithelioid component

G. Malignant Lymphoma Diffuse, Large cell
   Cleaved cell
   Non-cleaved cell
   Sclerosis

High-grade

H. Malignant Lymphoma Large cell Immunoblastic
   Plasmacytoid
   Clear cell
   Polymorphous
   Epithelioid cell component

I. Malignant Lymphoma Lymphoblastic
   Convoluted cell
   Non-convoluted

J. Malignant Lymphoma Small Non-Cleaved Cell
   Burkitt's
   Follicular areas

Miscellaneous
   Composite
   Mycosis fungoides
   Histiocytic
   Extramedullary plasmacytoma

recognized that leukaemia could infiltrate and cause enlargement of lymph nodes and other organs. The key concepts that were used to subclassify leukaemias were the distinction between myeloid and lymphoid cells and the subdivision into acute progressive disease, where primitive blast cells predominate, and chronic indolent disease, in which the majority of cells are similar to their normal peripheral blood counterparts. This approach to classification was used in the morphologically based FAB (French, American, British) system first published in 1976. In the FAB classification acute leukaemias were further divided, in the case of acute lymphoblastic leukaemia by basic cellular characteristics such as nuclear shape and morphology. Acute myeloid leukaemia was subdivided by lineage and degree of development. Classification by this method has been a central element in almost all modern therapeutic trials.

The introduction of antibody-based cell markers greatly improved the reliability by which acute lymphoblastic and myeloblastic leukaemia could be distinguished and most individual subtypes of leukaemia within the FAB classification are now defined by cell marker and cytogenetic as well as morphological criteria. However, the increasing use of cell markers and understanding of the normal immune system has also clearly demonstrated the relationship at a cellular level between many of the common types of leukaemia and lymphoma and the largely artificial nature of a distinction that is essentially based on the pattern of spread of the tumour In the majority of cases of acute lymphoblastic leukaemia/lymphoma and chronic lymphocytic leukaemia/B-lymphocytic lymphoma there is involvement of blood, bone marrow and nodal tissues although the relative proportions of each may vary widely between patients.

5.3 New classifications

The REAL classification is based on the recognition of clinico-pathological entities

The Kiel classification in its revised form is widely used in Europe and has been clinically useful but a number of its features have been criticized. These include the classification of peripheral T-cell lymphomas which is seen as poorly reproducible and of doubtful clinical value. Equally, similar problems arise in the subdivision of large B-cell lymphomas into a number of categories based on arbitrary histological criteria. There is also some confusion in the phenotypic and clinical relationships between various types of low-grade B-cell lymphoma. These problems have been addressed in the Revised European American Lymphoma (REAL) classification, published in 1994 (Table 5.5). In many respects this is a direct descendent of the Kiel classification but it has a number of distinctive features. Firstly, the classification includes both Hodgkin's disease and non-Hodgkin's lymphoma. Secondly, much greater emphasis is placed on the integration of clinical and pathological features. The original rather general concept of arrested normal maturation is gradually being refined by the growing understanding of the detailed molecular pathogenesis of lymphoproliferative disorders. Some of the categories in the REAL classification correspond closely with key molecular abnormalities such as the t(14;18) or t(11;14). A further advantage is that, unlike many of its predecessors, the REAL classification is likely to prove more adaptable to the introduction of new developments in cellular and molecular pathology. The recognition of a single group of diffuse large cell lymphoma, for example, is a basis on which future molecular or immunophenotypic subdivisions can be built to replace morphological categories that are poorly reproducible and of doubtful clinical value.

Figure 5.1 The standardized annual incidence of lymphoproliferative disorders in adults living in West and North Yorkshire in 1991.

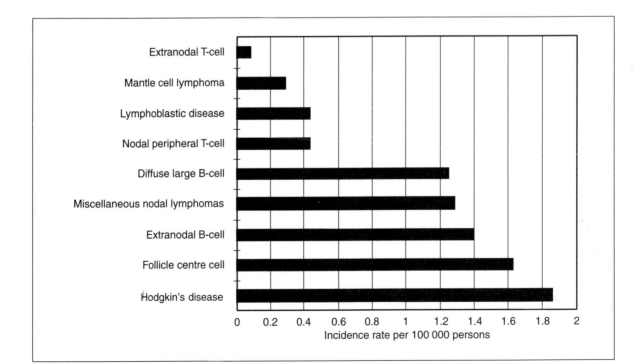

Table 5.5 Revised European–American classification of lymphoid neoplasms

B-cell neoplasms

Precursor B-cell neoplasms
Precursor B-lymphoblastic leukaemia/lymphoma

Peripheral B-cell neoplasms
B-cell chronic lymphocytic leukaemia/lymphocytic lymphoma/B-prolymphocytic
    leukaemia
Lymphoplasmacytoid lymphoma/immunocytoma
Mantle cell lymphoma
Follicle centre lymphoma
Marginal zone lymphoma
   Nodal
   Extranodal (low-grade MALToma)
Hairy cell leukaemia
Plasmacytoma/multiple myeloma
Diffuse large cell lymphoma
Primary mediastinal (thymic) large B-cell lymphoma
Burkitt's lymphoma
Provisional entities
   Splenic marginal zone lymphoma/SLVL
   High-grade B-cell lymphoma – Burkitt-like

T-cell and NK cell neoplasms

Precursor T-cell neoplasms
Precursor T-lymphoblastic lymphoma/leukaemia

Peripheral T-cell neoplasms
T-cell chronic lymphocytic leukaemia/prolymphocytic leukaemia
Large granular lymphocyte leukaemia
   T-cell
   NK-type
Mycosis fungoides/Sézary syndrome
Peripheral T-cell lymphoma, unspecified
Angioimmunoblastic T-cell lymphoma
Angiocentric lymphoma
Intestinal T-cell lymphoma
Adult T-cell lymphoma/leukaemia (HTLV-1)
Anaplastic large cell lymphoma (CD30$^+$)
   T-cell
   Null

Hodgkin's disease

Lymphocyte predominance (paragranuloma)
Classical Hodgkin's disease
   Nodular sclerosis
   Mixed cellularity
   Lymphocyte depletion
Provisional entities
   Lymphocyte-rich classical Hodgkin's disease
   Anaplastic large cell lymphoma – Hodgkin's-like

The next major development in this field is likely to be the introduction of the WHO classification of haematological malignancies. In draft form the section on lymphoproliferative disorders is broadly similar to the REAL classification with only a few relatively minor modifications. Unlike the REAL classification the proposed WHO classification will include myeloproliferative disorders and histiocytosis.

In the chapters that follow emphasis is placed on describing the lymphoproliferative disorders as syndromes encompassing morphological, immunophenotypical, molecular genetic and clinical features. Each of these tumour entities presents distinctive clinical problems and attempting to group disparate tumour types together into high, low and intermediate grade for the purpose of treatment selection may be an obstacle to further progress. For this reason the use of these terms has been avoided (Table 5.5, Figure 5.1).

5.4 Key references

Bain, B. J. (1990) *Leukaemia Diagnosis: A Guide to the FAB Classification.* Gower Medical, London.

Hodgkin, T. (1832) On some morbid experiences of the absorbent glands and spleen. *Medico-Chirurgical Transactions*, **17**, 68–97.

International Lymphoma Study Group (1994) A revised European–American classification of lymphoid neoplasms: a proposal from the International Lymphoma Study Group. *Blood*, **84**, 1361–1392.

Jaffe, E. S. (1997) Introduction to the WHO classification. *American Journal of Surgical Pathology*, **21**, 114–121.

Lennert, K. and Feller, A. C. (1990) *Histopathology of Non-Hodgkin's Lymphomas.* Springer-Verlag, Berlin.

Lennert, K., Mohri, N., Stein, H. and Kaiserling, E. (1975) The histopathology of malignant lymphoma. *British Journal of Haematology*, **31**(Suppl.), 193–203.

Lukes, R. J. and Butler, J. J. (1966) The pathology and nomenclature of Hodgkin's disease. *Cancer Research*, **26**, 1063–1081.

Lukes, R. J. and Collins, R. D. (1975) New approaches to the classification of the lymphomata. *British Journal of Cancer*, **31**(Suppl.), 1–26.

National Cancer Institute (1982) Sponsored study of the classification of non-Hodgkin's lymphomas. *Cancer*, **49**, 2112–2135.

Rappaport, H., Winter, W. J. and Hicks, E. B. (1956) Follicular lymphoma. *Cancer*, **9**, 792–821.

Reed, D. (1902) On the pathological changes of Hodgkin's disease with especial reference to its relation to tuberculosis. *Johns Hopkins Hospital Reports*, **10**, 133–196.

Part Two

The Lymphoproliferative Disorders

Precursor cell lymphoproliferative disorders

6

6.1 Introduction

Precursor cell lymphoproliferative disorders are tumours derived from B and T lineage lymphocytes early in their development when they are in the process of rearranging their immunoglobulin and T-cell receptor genes. This category includes most acute lymphoblastic leukaemias, as defined by FAB criteria, and lymphoblastic lymphomas. Lymphoblastic leukaemia and lymphoma are sometimes separated in clinical trial protocols but, given that the distinction is usually based only on an arbitrary percentage of blast cell in the bone marrow rather than on fundamental cellular differences, the justification for this seems doubtful. In this chapter precursor cell leukaemia and lymphoma will be considered as aspects of the same disease composed of the same cell type and differentiated only by differences in the pattern of spread.

In a proportion of acute lymphoid leukaemias in both adults and children the neoplastic cells are immunocompetent rather than precursor lymphocytes. Morphologically this includes many cases in the FAB L3 category of acute lymphoblastic leukaemia. This type of leukaemia is part of a spectrum of disease that includes Burkitt's lymphoma and related solid tumours; it is discussed in more detail in Chapter 8. In this book the term 'acute lymphoblastic leukaemia' (ALL) is the preferred term and is used solely to describe precursor cell lymphoproliferative disorders.

The cells found in precursor cell lymphoproliferative disorders show morphological, phenotypical and immunogenetic features similar to those found in normal lymphocytes during the precursor cell stage of their life cycle. All lymphocytes are derived from pluripotent bone marrow stem cells. The progeny of stem cells that are committed to becoming B-cells remain in the bone marrow; the critical developmental event for these cells is the rearrangement of the immunoglobulin genes to produce a functional immunoglobulin molecule, which is expressed on the surface of the mature immunocompetent B-cell as part of the B-cell antigen receptor complex. The rearrangement of the immunoglobulin genes proceeds in a predictable sequence. The immunoglobulin heavy chain is rearranged with the coupling of a VDJ region to the Cμ constant region. This is followed by kappa light chain gene rearrangement and, if this is unsuccessful, the lambda light chain is rearranged. T-cell maturation is different, with bone marrow stem cells migrating to the thymus where they become committed T-cell progenitors and begin the process of T-cell receptor (TCR) rearrangement. The gamma and delta genes rearrange to produce a TCR1 (gamma/delta) receptor, which is expressed with CD3 on the cell surface. In most T-cells further rearrangement of the alpha and beta genes occurs with partial deletion of the delta gene. The TCR2 receptor produced is expressed with CD3 and CD4 or CD8. This process is considered in more detail in Chapter 1.

6.2 *Clinical features of acute lymphoblastic leukaemia (ALL)*

The pattern of incidence of ALL differs from other lymphoproliferative disorders

The overall incidence of ALL is around 1–2 cases per 100 000 per year, with a male predominance. Although lymphoblastic disease can occur at any age, the distinctive feature is a peak of incidence in children which may reflect an increased turnover of lymphoid cell precursors present in this age group. Between the ages of 2 and 4 years the age-specific incidence is around 8/100 000, which is about 15 times greater than in adults over 20 years. If the cases are separated according to lineage, 10–25% of cases are of T-cell lineage with almost all of the remainder showing some evidence of B-cell lineage differentiation.

Acute lymphoblastic leukaemia is the commonest type of paediatric malignancy in developed countries. Although it is a heterogeneous disease and the cause is unknown, recent epidemiological research has focused attention on the probable role of immune stimulation due to infection. In developed countries the age at which children are exposed to common infections, may be later than in Third World countries. Differences in the response to these infections may be a factor predisposing to the development of leukaemia. This hypothesis is supported by incidence data from Third World countries, in which the high peak incidence of childhood acute lymphoblastic leukaemia at 2–5 years typical of Europe, USA and Japan is strikingly absent.

Most cases of ALL present with the features of bone marrow involvement, but more generalized disease is often present

In most cases of ALL there is dense marrow infiltration by lymphoblasts with resulting pancytopenia, which may be accompanied by large numbers of circulating blast cells. However, a proportion of cases present with a normal or low white cell counts and few detectable circulating blast cells. Patients present with symptoms of bone marrow failure, with anaemia, bleeding and infection. In children in particular, bone or joint pain causing difficulty in walking can be the presenting feature. Bone destruction of sufficient severity to cause pathological fracture may occur but is exceedingly rare.

Some degree of lymphadenopathy is almost always present in lymphoblastic disease; significant enlargement of the liver and spleen is more likely to be present in children. In T-cell lymphoblastic disease involvement of the thymus and mediastinal nodes is very common and in some cases associated respiratory symptoms or superior vena caval obstruction may be the initial presenting feature. Presentation with such masses is much less common in B-cell tumours. A few patients with ALL present with skin infiltration, although this is more typical of AML. Almost all cases of lymphoblastic disease have evidence of bone marrow infiltration at some stage of the clinical course. In children suspected of having ALL a node or tissue biopsy should only be carried out when investigation of marrow and blood has been shown to be negative by morphological and immunophenotypical examination (Figure 6.1).

The tendency for ALL to relapse in the CNS, with meningeal infiltration, or in the testis is well known. However, it is rare for patients to present with symptoms mainly localized to these sites, though all patients should be screened for CSF involvement at presentation. In patients who die of fulminant disease at presentation, or relapse, infiltration may be present at almost any site, including heart, lung, brain and gastrointestinal tract.

Figure 6.1 T-ALL mediastinal mass – CT scan. **(a)** This adult patient presented with a mediastinal mass which was found to be due to T-ALL. **(b)** After initial induction therapy the mass was no longer detectable.

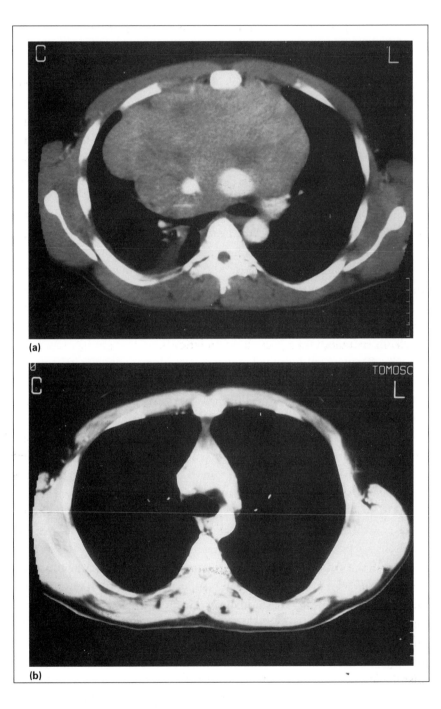

The blast cell morphology does not correlate with cell lineage

The FAB classification is a morphological classification of lymphoid blasts seen by light microscopy. It was developed in the 1970s and predates detailed understanding of lymphoid immunophenotyping. It remains the definitive guide to the cellular morphology of lymphoblastic disease. Three categories are recognized. In L1 the blasts are relatively small and may be only a little larger than a normal lymphocyte. They have regular round nuclei with one, often indistinct, nucleolus, and the cytoplasm constitutes less than 10% of the surface area. In L2 the blast cells are larger, with more cytoplasm and irregular nuclei, with more distinct nucleoli. Both forms may have granular or blocks of PAS positivity in the cytoplasm, though this is now of little value as a diagnostic test. As described above, the FAB L3 category corresponds mainly to the leukaemic phase of Burkitt's-like and related forms of B-cell lymphoma, but precursor cell neoplasms may sometimes have these morphological features. L3 blasts can be distinguished from the other forms of ALL morphologically by the presence of deeply basophilic cytoplasm, a stippled chromatin pattern and multiple nucleoli; frequently cytoplasmic vacuolation may be seen but this is not specific (Figure 6.2).

These morphological descriptions illustrate the range of cytological appearance likely to be encountered in blood and marrow films. However, in most laboratories classification is now based on cell marker studies and increasingly on cytogenetic abnormalities. There is a poor correlation between L1 and L2 morphologies and cell lineage although T-cell tumours are more likely to have L2 features. It should also be noted that variation in blast morphology may be seen at different sites. Bone marrow blasts are often more pleomorphic than those in the peripheral blood and this is often more evident in a trephine biopsy.

Lymphoblastic disease is rarely diagnosed on a solid tissue biopsy and only about 1% of diagnoses are made on node biopsy. The node and often the surrounding perinodal tissues are diffusely infiltrated by a monomorphic population of cells that correspond to the descriptions of L1 and L2 ALL. As with aspirate samples it is not possible to distinguish morphologically between T- and B-cell lineage on routine histological examination. One problem that can arise in older patients is that when the size of the blast cells approaches that of a small lymphocyte such cases are occasionally misdiagnosed as CLL or other types of lymphoma, especially if the histological material is suboptimal.

Figure 6.2 (a, b) B-lineage ALL – bone marrow aspirate. Typical blast cells in cALL. The cells are of intermediate size with a granular nuclear chromatin pattern and small nucleoli. Some of the cells have a moderate amount of cytoplasm.

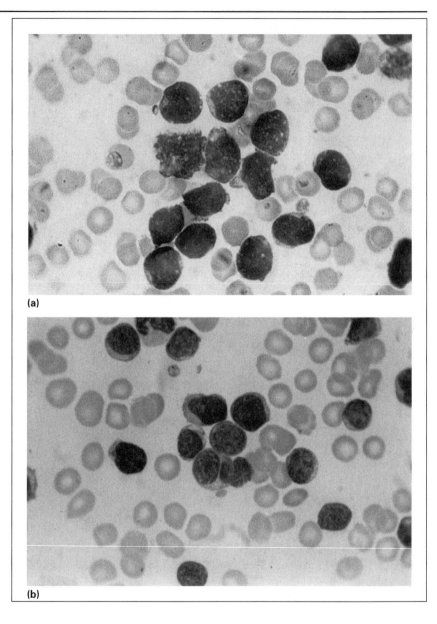

(a)

(b)

It is therefore important that the diagnosis of lymphoblastic disease is always confirmed by marker studies (Figure 6.3).

The defining feature of B-lineage lymphoblastic leukaemia is the demonstration that the cells are in the process of rearranging their immunoglobulin genes

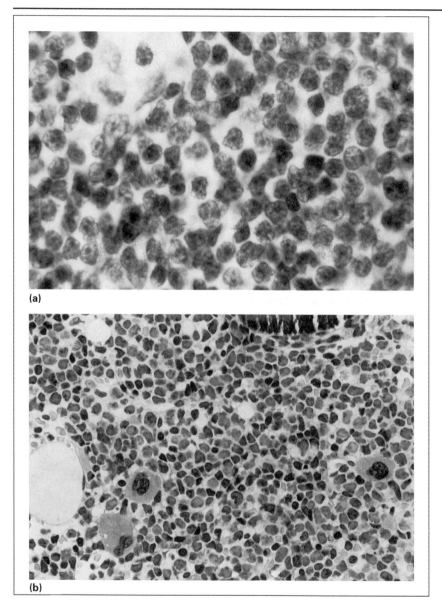

(a)

(b)

Figure 6.3 ALL – lymph node and bone marrow. In this case the patient presented with bulky nodal disease, which was biopsied. The lymph node was diffusely replaced by lymphoblasts **(a)**. The bone marrow biopsy **(b)** showed extensive infiltration by blasts of similar morphology with replacement of normal marrow elements but with sparing of megakaryocytes.

The precursor nature of the cells is routinely shown in two ways. Firstly, surface immunoglobulin expression is not detectable, although in a proportion of cases cytoplasmic μ heavy chain may be seen. Secondly, all cases have detectable Tdt in the nucleus, although this may not be present in all cells. Tdt is involved in the random addition and excision of nucleotides at the junctions between the rearranging immunoglobulin or

Figure 6.4
Immunophenotypical analysis of cALL. This set of flow cytometric histograms shows features of a typical case of cALL. The positively stained cells are within the M2 region of the histogram. There is strong CD19, CD10 and CD34 expression and lack of CD20, CD45 and cell surface CD79.

T-cell receptor genes and is hence an integral part of the process of generation of antibody diversity. (These phenotypic features contrast with the presence of sIg and lack of Tdt in immunocompetent B-cells, Burkitt's-like lymphoma and most acute leukaemias with L3 morphology.) The precursor nature of the cells in B-lineage ALL is also shown by the expression of the stem-cell-related marker CD34 and by the presence in the cytoplasm of CD22 and CD79b, which are normally found on the

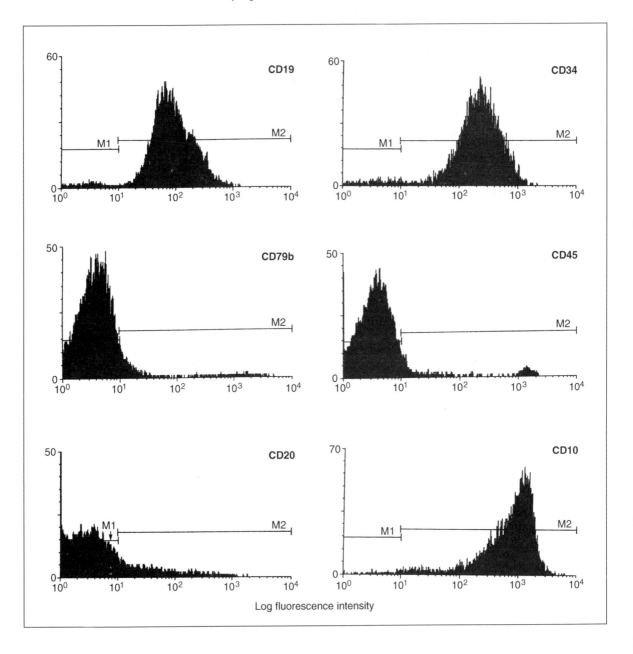

cell membrane of immunocompetent peripheral B-cells (Figure 6.4, Table 6.1).

After the precursor nature of the blast cells has been established using these markers, subclassification is then based on the degree of differentiation of the blast cells, beginning with the earliest identifiable B-cell precursor and ending at the stage before they become immunocompetent peripheral B-cells. The defining immunophenotypical features of cells belonging to the B-cell lineage is the expression of CD19, part of a B-cell-specific signalling pathway together with class II MHC, usually detected using anti-HLA-DR antibodies. Precursor B-ALL is usually subdivided into pre-pre-B-ALL, common ALL and pre-B-ALL. These stages are differentiated by expression of CD10, a membrane aminopeptidase, in c-ALL and pre-B-ALL and then by the expression of cytoplasmic mu heavy chain in pre-B-ALL. It must be emphasized that these categories are defined according to arbitrary criteria, for example the diagnosis of cALL requires more than 20% of CD10-expressing cells and the proportion of CD10-expressing cells may differ in samples taken from different sites in the same patient. It should also be noted that these apparent differentiation stages seen in ALL may not correspond exactly to normal B-cell development.

The approach used for the diagnosis and classification of B-lineage ALL can be used for T-cell ALL

The precursor nature of the cells is demonstrated by the fact that they are rearranging their T-cell receptor genes. As with B-cells they express

Table 6.1 Lymphoblastic disease – B-cell lineage

- **Morphology**: Variable – subdivided in FAB classification into L1 (monomorphic blast with minimal cytoplasm) and L2 (larger blasts with more irregular nuclei and abundant cytoplasm).
- **Immunophenotype**: Shows feature of precursor lymphocytes with expression of Tdt ± CD34. B-cell lineage markers CD19, cytoplasmic CD22 and CD79. Subdivided into pre-pre B, cALL and pre-B by CD10 and cytoplasmic mu heavy chain expression.
- **Cytogenetics**: t(9;22) is commonest in adults. t(12;21) is commonest abnormality in children.
- **Pattern of disease**: Acute leukaemia with variable nodal disease; rare cases may present with nodal disease alone. Meningeal and testicular infiltration.

Tdt and lack cell surface expression of the T-cell antigen receptor (TCR). CD3 is part of the antigen receptor complex, which is common to cells expressing either the gamma/delta receptor or the alpha/beta T-cell receptor, and in cases of T-lineage ALL, CD3 is found in the cytoplasm rather than on the cell surface. The rearrangement of the TCR-delta and gamma genes occurs early in the commitment of precursor cells to the T-cell lineage and, as would be expected, most cases of T-lineage ALL have a detectable TCR-gamma rearrangement. A much smaller number of cases have a rearrangement of the TCR-beta genes (Figure 6.5, Table 6.2).

Table 6.2 Lymphoblastic disease – T-cell lineage

- **Morphology:** Blast cells are likely to have L2 morphology but the correlation between morphology and lineage is relatively poor.
- **Immunophenotype:** Shows features of precursor lymphocytes with Tdt and sometimes CD34 expression. Some cases express the common thymocyte marker CD1. T-cell lineage is shown by CD7 and cytoplasmic CD3 and variable expression of other pan-T-cell markers.
- **Cytogenetics:** Deletion affecting the *TAL1* gene on chromosome 1 is the commonest abnormality.
- **Pattern of disease:** Acute leukaemia. Presentation with mediastinal or other tissue mass is commoner than B-lineage disease. Meningeal infiltration.

Figure 6.5 T-lineage ALL. This patient presented with a mediastinal mass, which was biopsied **(a)**.

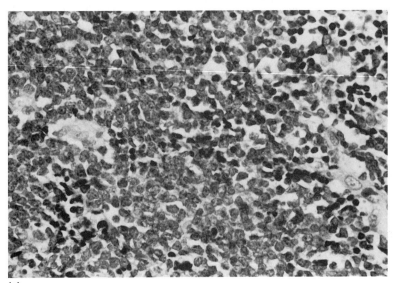

(a)

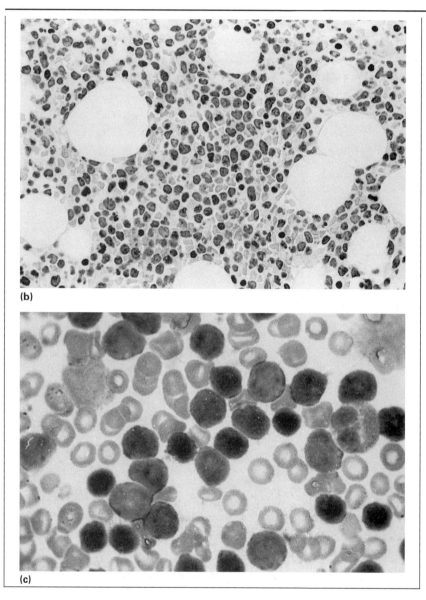

(b)

(c)

Figure 6.5 The staging bone marrow was heavily infiltrated. The tumour consisted of intermediate sized blast cells, many of which appeared highly convoluted on the trephine biopsy **(b)** although this was less obvious on the marrow aspirate **(c)**.

Again, as with B-lineage ALL, CD34 may be detected but only in the small proportion of cases that have a phenotype corresponding to a very early stage in T-cell development. In such cases CD7 and cytoplasmic CD3 may be the only features indicative of T-cell differentiation. (It should be noted that CD7 by itself is not lineage specific.) Blast cells with a more mature phenotype have CD2 and CD5 with coexpression of CD4 and CD8. When CD1 is expressed this corresponds to the phenotype of the normal common thymocyte (Figure 6.6).

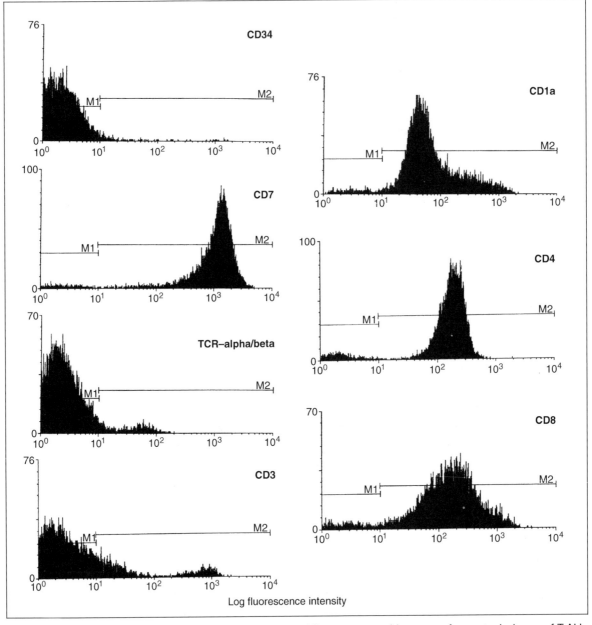

Figure 6.6 Immunophenotypical analysis of T-ALL. This set of flow cytometry histograms form a typical case of T-ALL. There is expression of CD1a, CD2 and CD7 and coexpression of CD4 and CD8. There is no cell-surface CD3 or TCR expression, although cytoplasmic CD3 was present on APAAP staining.

Rearrangement of immunoglobulin and T-cell receptor genes cannot be used to assign B- and T-cell lineage

Cells at the lymphoblastic stage of development continue to express genes responsible for the process of recombination at the immunoglobulin and T-cell receptor loci. Probably because of this activity cross-lineage rearrangements can easily be demonstrated. It is for these reasons that molecular detection of Ig or TCR rearrangement cannot be used to assign lineage.

The distinction between lymphoblastic disease and acute myeloid leukaemia can be difficult

Prior to the widespread use of flow cytometry and molecular biological techniques, there were a significant number of cases of acute leukaemia that could not be assigned to myeloid or lymphoid lineage by morphology and cytochemistry. A proportion of cases in which a morphological diagnosis is made will be reassigned to another group when marker studies are carried out. Unfortunately, a number of areas of ambiguity remain. Around 10% of cases of otherwise typical ALL will express the myeloid markers CD13 and CD33 and some cases will express CD14, CD11b or CD11c. In a very few cases myeloperoxidase will be detected by immunocytochemistry, although cytochemical reactivity is very rare. Conversely, it is relatively common to find CD7 or Tdt expressed on cells otherwise typical of acute myeloid leukaemia, with other lymphoid markers such as CD5 or CD10 being much less commonly found. One way to overcome these problems is to establish a hierarchy of markers depending on their lineage specificity – CD79a, CD22, cIg, CD3 and myeloperoxidase are considered the most lineage-specific. Although c-*kit* (CD117) is expressed on normal stem cells, and in AML, it is rarely found in ALL. Using these markers it is then possible to assign almost all cases to one of five groups – ALL, ALL with atypical myeloid markers, AML, AML with atypical lymphoid markers and a small residual group of true acute biphenotypic leukaemia where there is expression of myeloid and lymphoid lineage-specific markers. Around 2–3% of cases of morphologically typical AML have rearrangement of T-cell receptors of immunoglobulin genes but when one or more lymphoid markers are present this proportion is higher and rearrangement is present in around half of true biphenotypic leukaemia.

6.3 *Chromosomal abnormalities in ALL*

Aneuploidy is common in patients with lymphoblastic leukaemia

Abnormal numbers of chromosomes can be detected in leukaemic blast cells by cytogenetic analysis and by DNA flow cytometry. Around one-third of adult patients and about half of children with ALL will show an abnormal chromosome number. These abnormalities are subclassified according to whether chromosomes have been gained or lost by the leukaemic cells. Hyperdiploid cells have between 47 and 57 chromosomes, and more rarely near-triploid (58–80) and near-tetraploid (83–103) cells have been identified. This is a near random process but chromosomes 8, 16, 18, 21, and 22 are more commonly involved than other chromosomes. When chromosome loss has occurred cells are classified as hypodiploid (35–45) or near haploid (< 27).

Calculating the DNA index is a method of describing the nuclear DNA content that can be readily measured by flow cytometry. Haploid cells have a DNA index of 1.0. Cells with increased chromosomes will have a DNA index of more than 1.0, and fewer than 46 of less than 1.0 (Figure 6.7).

About 20% of children with ALL have hyperdiploidy. This is most common in younger children who have cALL and a low blast count ($< 10 \times 10^9$/l). This group has the best prognosis of all types of ALL. Hyperdiploidy with low blast count is much rarer in adult patients. Little is known as to why a gross cellular abnormality such as hyperploidy should correlate with a favourable prognosis. In contrast, ALL with a near-haploid chromosome count is very rare and has a very poor prognosis (Table 6.3).

The t(9;22) is the commonest genetic abnormality in adult B-lineage ALL

The t(9;22) was first described in chronic myeloid leukaemia, where it is the defining abnormality of the disease. The translocation results in the fusion of 5′ sequences from the *bcr* gene on chromosome 9 with 3′ sequences of the *abl* gene on chromosome 22. This translocation can be routinely detected using RT-PCR. With PCR techniques the t(9;22) is subclassified according to which exons of *bcr* are involved. In almost every case *abl* exon 2 is the site of gene fusion, but this can join with exon 1 or exons b2 or b3 of the major breakpoint cluster region of the *bcr* gene; these translocations are denoted as E1A2, B2A2 and B3A2. When this

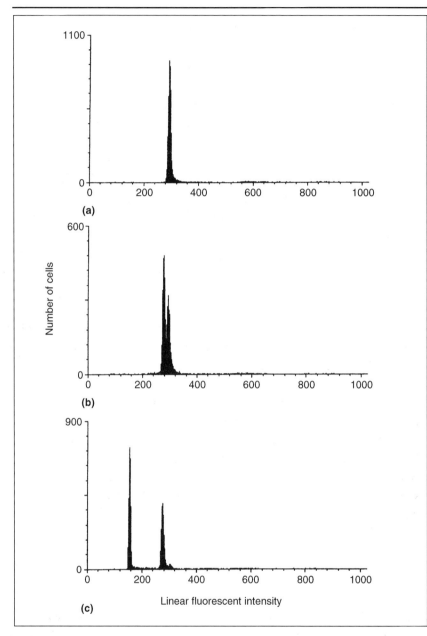

Figure 6.7 Ploidy in B-lineage ALL. These DNA histograms show a tumour with a normal DNA content **(a)**, one with a hyperdiploid clone **(b)** and a case where the predominant population is hypodiploid **(c)**. In this case the peak at around 280 is the diploid population.

abnormal gene is transcribed a fusion protein of 190 kDa is produced by the E1A2 translocation and a 210 kDa protein by the others. These fusion proteins have elevated tyrosine kinase activity. The *bcr–abl* gene product has many functions within the cell, including an antiapoptotic effect, and it has been suggested that the 190 kDa protein is more actively transforming (Figure 6.8).

Table 6.3 Main cytogenetic abnormalities in ALL

- t(9;22)
- t(1;19)
- t(4;11)
- t(12;21)
- 9p–
- 12p–
- Hyperdiploidy
- Hypodiploidy
- *TAL1* deletions

Figure 6.8 The Philadelphia chromosome – t(9;22). The t(9;22) is the commonest chromosomal abnormality in adult ALL. As a result of this translocation the *abl* gene (ch9) is translocated to the *bcr* gene on ch22. The result of this is a fusion protein with tyrosine kinase activity, which can be of one of three types depending on the site of *bcr* breakpoints. In CML the breaks occur in the M-*bcr* region and give rise to two products depending on the presence of the *bcr* B3 exon. In ALL a 190 kDa protein is found where the *bcr* e1 exon is fused to the *abl* a2 exon. The presence of t(9;22) in ALL appears to indicate a very poor prognosis.

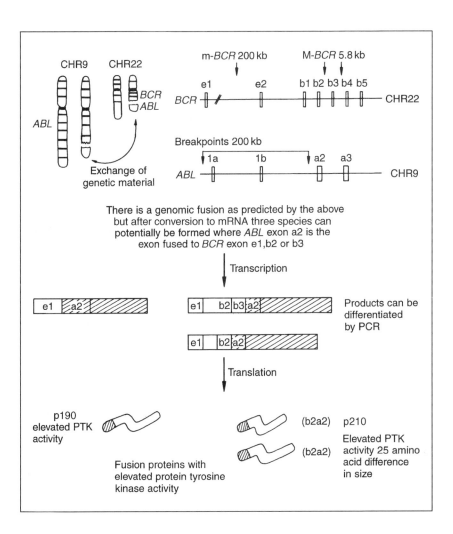

Almost all cases of CML have the B2A2 and B3A2 translocations but all three variants are found in ALL, which may have either the 190 or 210 kDa fusion protein. It has been postulated that cases with 210 kDa proteins represent lymphoid blast transformation of CML whereas those with p190 are *de novo* ALL. The incidence of the t(9;22) increases with increasing age and irrespective of the fusion protein produced the presence of t(9;22) indicates a very poor prognosis in all age groups. Induction of remission is normal, but the relapse rate is higher and very few patients are long-term survivors.

The (12;21) translocation is the commonest translocation in paediatric ALL

Characterization of this translocation revealed the involvement in ALL of two genes previously known to be involved in AML. A fusion gene results, consisting of the *TEL* gene from chromosome 12 and the *AML1* gene from chromosome 21. Interestingly, this translocation is only rarely identified by cytogenetics but preliminary studies using PCR suggest that it may be the most common genetic abnormality in ALL. It occurs in approximately 30% of paediatric ALL but is only seldom seen in adult cases, the converse of the situation with the t(9;22). The *AML1* gene is also altered in the t(8;21) seen in myeloid leukaemia. Furthermore, the inv16 of AML M4 works through the same transcription factor pathway with altered function of core binding factor beta, through which *AML1* exerts its effects. This is an interesting link between acute lymphoblastic and acute myeloid leukaemia, the further characterization of which may improve understanding of the mechanisms of lineage commitment within precursor cells. Some reports suggest that the t(12;21) is a favourable prognostic factor (Figure 6.9).

Other chromosomal abnormalities are much less common but may affect prognosis

About 3–4% of both adult and childhood cases of ALL have a t(1;19), although within the pre-B subgroup with cytoplasmic Ig mu expression the incidence is about 25–30%. The effect of this translocation is to produce a fusion gene, which can be transcribed to produce a novel transcription factor. The fusion gene includes sequences from the *E2A* gene on chromosome 19, which is an immunoglobulin enhancer binding factor and homeobox gene of unknown function on chromosome 1. The breakpoints of this translocation are conserved and so an RT-PCR method

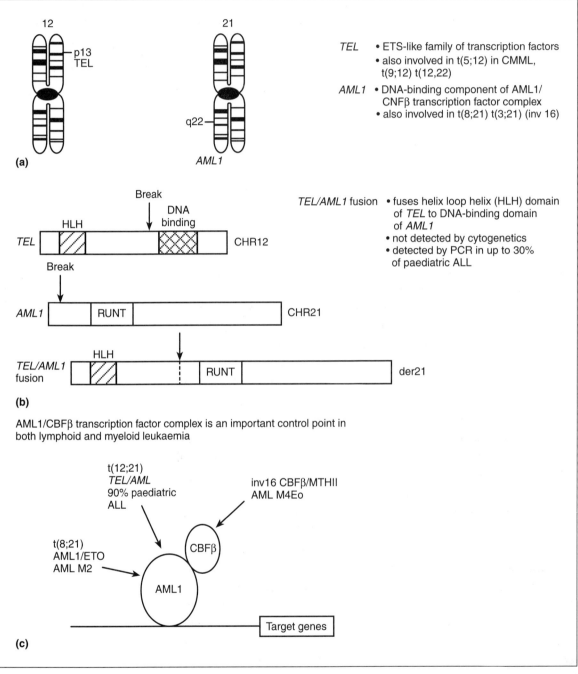

Figure 6.9 The t(12;21) (p13;q22) creates a *TEL/AML1* fusion protein.

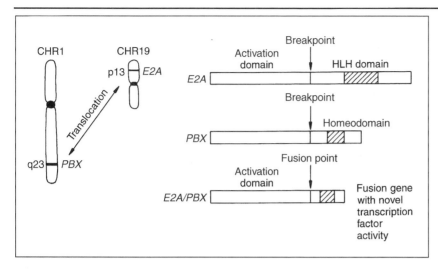

Figure 6.10 The t(1;19). This translocation, which involves the long arm of ch1 and the short arm of ch19, is found in 30% of cases of pre-B ALL. Both partners in the translocation are nuclear transcription factors. The effect is to produce a fusion protein in which the E2A protein is given a novel DNA-binding domain.

can be used to detect the translocation. It has been suggested that this translocation may be an independent prognostic factor (Figure 6.10).

Another abnormal transcription factor is the fusion protein produced by the t(4;11). The gene involved on chromosome 11 is *HRX* (MLL), which is the human homologue of a gene involved in the trithorax homeotic mutation in *Drosophila*, and this fuses with the *AF4* gene on chromosome 4. Less commonly fusion genes are produced between the *HRX* gene and partners on chromosomes 6, 9 or 19. In each a transcription factor is produced with DNA-binding properties not seen in normal lymphoid cells; this in turn may deregulate a range of other genes. The t(4;11) and other *HRX* translocations are associated with a distinctive clinical syndrome. Most cases occur in early infancy and are associated with very high blast cell counts. In most cases the blasts are CD10⁻ and often have one or more myeloid-associated markers. In older children and adults only 2–3% of cases will have this translocation although this may be increased if highly sensitive techniques are used. In all cases the presence of the translocation is associated with a poor prognosis (Figure 6.11).

About 10% of both adult and childhood ALL have deletions in 6q, 9p and 12p. Interestingly these occur in both B- and T-lineage ALL. These deletions raise the possibility of tumour-suppressor genes but as yet none have been identified at these loci. The prognostic significance of these deletions is not yet clear. The most common abnormality in T-ALL is a deletion on the long arm of chromosome 1, which results in the *TAL1* gene coming under the control of the *SCL* gene promoter and subsequent abnormal expression of the *TAL1* transcription factor (Figure 6.12).

Figure 6.11 The t(4;11). This translocation is commonest in young infants with a high blast cell count. In addition to 4q21, 6q27, 9q22 and 19q13 may also form reciprocal translocation with 11q23. The gene at 11q23 (*HRX*) is a homologue of a *Drosophila* homeotic gene. The translocation alters the DNA-binding characteristic of the *HRX* gene and hence its function as a transcription factor. Abnormalities of this type could affect the pattern of expression of a number of genes under the regulatory control of *HRX*.

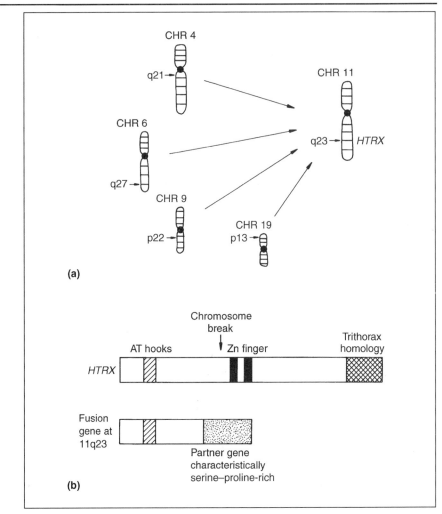

Figure 6.12 *SCL/TAL* deletion. Deletions of chromosome 1 are found in 35% of T-ALL. These result in dysregulation of the *TAL1* gene, which comes under the regulatory control of the *SCL* gene promoter The deletion can be detected by PCR because of the approximation of primer binding sites that are normally separated by a sequence too large to be amplified.

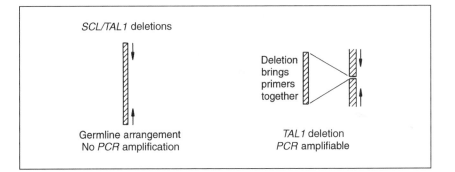

The translocations that deregulate c-*myc* (t(8;14), t(2;8) and t(8;22)) are found in Burkitt's lymphoma and related leukaemia (B-ALL) and are not seen in the tumours of lymphoid precursors that are the subject of this chapter.

6.4 Other prognostic factors in ALL

Age and blast cell count are major prognostic factors in ALL

There are few other malignant diseases in which age of the patient is such a critical prognostic factor as in ALL. The optimum survival after treatment is in children between 1 and 9 years with a slight advantage to those between 2 and 5 years. It is within this age group that favourable prognostic factors such as hyperdiploidy and low blast count are most common. In adolescents, there appears to be a gradual decrease in the 5-year survival and event-free survival over the age of 14 years. In very young infants (< 1 year) the prognosis is very poor. This is a combination of poor tolerance of intensive treatment and the high frequency in this group of very poor prognosis subtypes such as the t(4;11). Within this subgroup of infant ALL, if cases with a t(4;11) are excluded the outcome approaches that seen in older children (Table 6.4).

The prognosis of adult ALL is poor and decreases with age. In clinical trial data with modern intensive treatment about 30% of adults appear to be cured as compared with 70% of children. However, the success rate in treating adults is likely to be overstated. About 20–30% of adults may be too ill to be entered in trials or may fail to achieve remission. Trial data may also be biased towards young adults. When these factors are considered the proportion of adults cured may be as low as 15–20%.

Table 6.4 Poor prognostic features in paediatric ALL

- Less than 1 or greater than 10 years of age
- Mediastinal mass
- Male sex
- CNS disease at presentation
- High white cell count
- t(1;19) t(9;22) t(4;11)
- Hypodiploidy

The blast cell count is a continuous variable affecting survival in both adults and children. Prognosis decreases when presentation blast cell count is above $50 \times 10^9/l$ and falls further when greater than $100 \times 10^9/l$. When the count is greater than $200 \times 10^9/l$ the prognosis becomes very poor.

Males have a worse prognosis, which may be explained by the incidence of testicular relapse (Figure 6.13). The testis is regarded as a sanctuary site where lymphoblasts may survive treatment but the biological basis of this is

Figure 6.13 Testicular relapse of cALL. This testicular biopsy shows heavy infiltration by cALL blasts although there is relative sparing of seminiferous tubules (a). Most of the cells express nuclear Tdt (b).

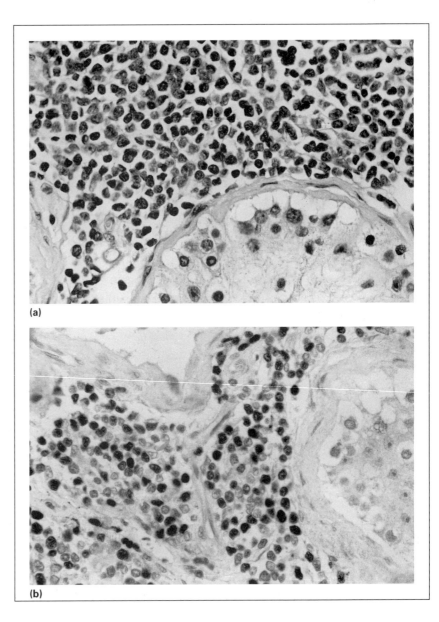

(a)

(b)

not well explained. However testicular relapse does not account for sufficient cases to be the only reason for poorer prognosis in boys. There may be biological differences between the sexes with respect to intracellular handling of 6-mercaptopurine so that boys functionally have a less effective intracellular level of the same treatment dose. Difference in survival between the sexes is seen more than 1 year into treatment.

The difference between T-cell and the subtypes of B-lineage ALL are slight and are tending to disappear due to improvement in therapy. Morphological subtypes are poorly reproducible and do not have independent prognostic significance.

6.5 Treatment of ALL

Current protocols for the treatment of ALL have evolved from previous experience in national and international trials. Although there are some differences between the schedules used, the principles of treatment are similar worldwide. It was recognized early on that remissions could be induced relatively easily using a combination of vincristine and glucocorticoids, which continue to be important drugs in combination with anthracyclines for the induction of remission. These remissions are then consolidated with blocks of chemotherapy, using multiple chemotherapeutic agents with different mechanisms of action and side effects. The blocks of treatment are usually called intensification and consolidation (Figure 6.14).

The propensity for relapse in the CNS prompted specific prophylaxis in the form of intrathecal methotrexate (MTX) and craniospinal radiotherapy (Figure 6.16). In children in particular this has been associated with some degree of intellectual impairment and, with the advent of high-dose methotrexate (HD-MTX), which crosses the blood–brain barrier, there has been a re-evaluation of prophylactic measures. Cranial irradiation remains the 'gold standard' and is still used in adults but in children it is now usually reserved for high count ALL ($> 50 \times 10^9$/l) and randomized against HD-MTX in the trial setting; low-count ALL children receiving continuing intrathecal MTX or HD-MTX. The testis in boys is a common site of relapse, but no specific treatment is given to this region (unless testicular disease is present at diagnosis) in first remission.

A further treatment approach peculiar to the treatment of ALL is the use of maintenance chemotherapy. This takes the form of pulses of vincristine and prednisolone at monthly intervals, with daily 6-mercap-

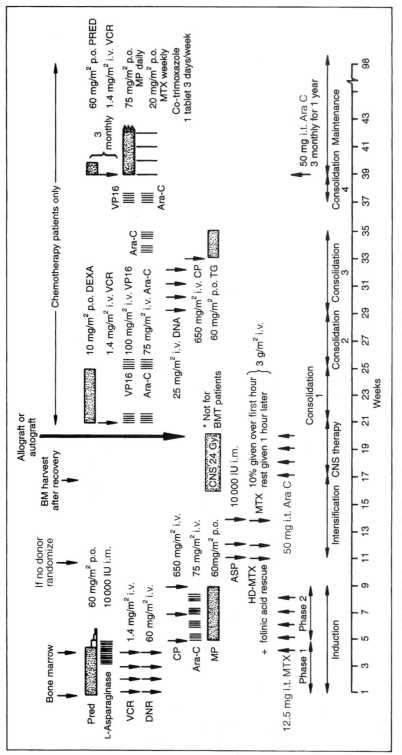

Figure 6.14 Treatment of ALL. This is a typical scheme for treatment of adult ALL (MRC UKALL XII).

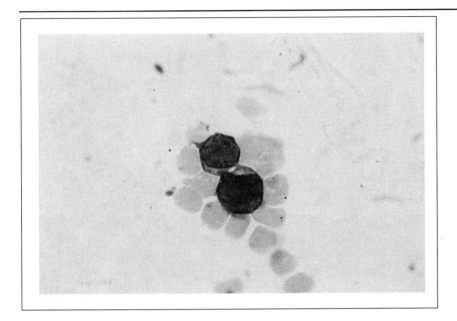

Figure 6.15 cALL – cerebrospinal fluid. This patient with cALL was found to have lymphoblasts present on routine examination of the cerebrospinal fluid.

topurine and weekly methotrexate, and is continued for a 2-year period.

Continued escalation of the intensity of treatment in children has led to excellent long-term survival, in the order of 75% for standard-risk disease. The success of these regimens, exemplified best by the German BFM protocols, was not without cost in terms of growth retardation and mental impairment. The realization of the impaired quality of life for these children and that some long-term survivors were maintained with vincristine and prednisolone alone has led to a critical re-evaluation of these regimens. Current trials are therefore directed towards identifying good-risk patients who will have excellent long-term survival in whom dose intensity can be reduced.

The treatment of adult ALL has lagged behind that of children. However, very intensive treatment based on the successful paediatric regimens are now in use. Unfortunately, despite using very similar regimens, outcome in adults is much less successful than in paediatric cases, with only 15–25% long-term survivors.

It is important to consider why there is such a major difference in outcome between paediatric and adult ALL. It is generally felt that this difference is due to sensitivity of the immortalized cell to chemotherapy. In paediatric cases the cell is more likely to be a lymphoid precursor, which is very sensitive to the induction of apoptosis as a consequence of its level of differentiation. In adults, however, the tumour is more likely to include a proportion of pluripotent stem cells with capacity for both myeloid and lymphoid differentiation. Pluripotent stem cells of this type may have a higher threshold for the induction of apoptosis by chemotherapy than committed lymphoid progenitors. Poor-risk paediatric cases will have molecular features similar to these in adult cases. For example the t(9;22) conveys a resistance to apoptosis but additionally is often present in cells with stem cell features. Mutations within *p53* will also confer a resistance to apoptosis. Tumours with a t(4;11) also show features consistent with the immortalization of a cell with a stem cell phenotype.

Detection of relapse is an important part of the management of ALL

Overall about 30% of children will relapse. This may present as a bone-marrow relapse, but despite CNS-directed therapy children also often relapse in the CNS (Figure 6.15). This may occur even with the marrow in remission but is treated as a herald of marrow relapse and salvage therapy is directed systemically as well as at the CNS. In boys testicular relapse may be isolated but again is regarded as a herald of more widespread disease relapse. Occasionally, relapse may manifest at other sites (Figure 6.16). Children relapsing can still achieve remission and long-term survival although the chances of this are certainly reduced compared to those of long-term survival in first remission. Chances of survival are to a large degree related to the time of relapse. Children who relapse on therapy or within 6 months of stopping treatment have a much reduced chance of long-term remission. Bone marrow transplantation may be considered in these groups of children.

The PCR can be used to monitor residual disease following treatment

A proportion of children and the majority of adult patients with ALL will relapse after the completion of therapy. The identification of these patients prior to clinical relapse by evidence of residual disease may in the future allow more effective therapy to be given without exposing other patients to additional chemotherapy. If blast cells can be detected by morphology or by immunophenotypical studies the patient will have a relatively high tumour load and symptomatic relapse is probably

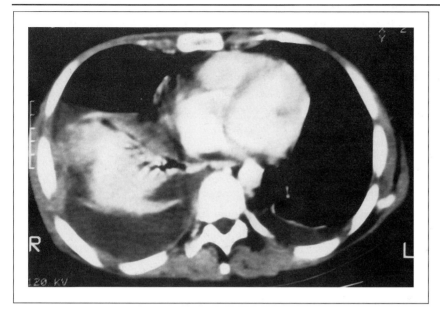

Figure 6.16 cALL: pleural relapse –CT scan. This patient, who was in complete remission following treatment of cALL, developed a massive pleural effusion. The CT scan shows extensive pleural infiltration and relapse was confirmed by pleural aspirate.

inevitable. The use of PCR-based techniques will increase the sensitivity of detection by 100–1000-fold. The most commonly used method is the detection of immunoglobulin heavy chain rearrangement. Almost all cases of B-lineage ALL have a clonal rearrangement of the IgH genes at presentation. The sensitivity of the technique can be further increased by sequencing the PCR product from the presentation sample and preparing patient specific oligonucleotides. The range of suitable targets for monitoring residual disease can be increased by using the various chromosome translocations described above. Additionally T-cell receptor gene rearrangements in B-lineage ALL and immunoglobulin rearrangements in T-lineage ALL may be useful tumour-specific markers. A problem that may arise in some cases is that clonal progression occurs with deletion or modification of the marker being used for follow-up. For this reason negative results need to be treated with caution.

It is very important that the clinical significance of minimal residual disease detected by these methods is established. Results obtained with conventional, fluorescent or ASO PCR are not directly comparable, because of differing sensitivity. At present the clinical significance of a positive PCR result is uncertain, though a positive result at the end of maintenance is thought to be an adverse feature. The significance of positive results before this time are the subject of active investigation.

6.6 Key references

6.6.1 Classification and diagnosis

Anonymous (1993) Collaborative study of karyotypes in childhood acute lymphoblastic leukemias. Groupe Français de Cytogenetique Hematologique. *Leukemia*, 7, 10–19.

Breit, T. M., Wolvers-Tettero, I. L. and van Dongen, J. J. (1994) Phenotypic and genotypic characteristics of human early T-cell differentiation: the T-cell acute lymphoblastic leukaemia model. *Research in Immunology*, 145, 139–143.

Buijs, A., Sherr, S., van Baal, S. *et al.* (1995) Translocation (12;22) (p13;q11) in myeloproliferative disorders results in fusion of the ETS-like TEL gene on 12p13 to the MN1 gene on 22q11. *Oncogene*, 10, 1511–1519.

Clare, N. and Hansen, K. (1994) Cytogenetics in the diagnosis of hematologic malignancies. *Hematology – Oncology Clinics of North America*, 8, 785–807.

Gauwerky, C. E. and Croce, C. M. (1993) Chromosomal translocations in leukaemia. *Seminars in Cancer Biology*, 4, 333–340.

Loffler, H. and Gassmann, W. (1994) Morphology and cytochemistry of acute lymphoblastic leukaemia. *Baillières Clinical Haematology*, 7, 263–272.

Ludwig, W. D., Raghavachar, A. and Thiel, E. (1994) Immunophenotypic classification of acute lymphoblastic leukaemia. *Baillières Clinical Haematology*, 7, 235–262.

Mclean, T., Ringold, S., Neuberg, D. *et al.* (1996) TEL/AML dimerizes and is associated with a favourable outcome in childhood lymphoblastic leukemia. *Blood*, 88, 4252–4258.

Reynolds, T. (1995) Is childhood leukemia the price of modernity? *Journal of the National Cancer Institute*, 87, 560–563.

Sato, Y., Suto, Y., Pietenpol, J. *et al.* (1995) TEL and KIP1 define the smallest region of deletions on 12p13 in hematopoietic malignances. *Blood*, 86, 1525–1533.

6.6.2 Therapy of acute leukaemia

Campana, D. and Pui, C. H. (1995) Detection of minimal residual disease in acute leukemia: methodologic advances and clinical significance *Blood*, 85, 1416–1434.

Copelan, E. A. and McGuire, E. A. (1995) The biology and treatment of acute lymphoblastic leukemia in adults. *Blood*, 85, 1151–1168.

Ochs, J. and Mulhern, R. (1994) Long-term sequelae of therapy for childhood acute lymphoblastic leukaemia. *Baillières Clinical Haematology*, 7, 365–376.

Scheinberg, D. A. (1995) Adult leukaemia in 1995: new directions. *Lancet*, 346, 455–456.

Volm, M. D. and Tallman, M. S. (1995) Developments in the treatment of acute leukemia in adults. *Current Opinion in Oncology*, 7, 28–35.

Hodgkin's disease

7

7.1 Introduction

The nature of Hodgkin's disease has been the subject of debate for over 100 years. From its earliest description there has been discussion as to whether Hodgkin's disease was a true neoplasm or an atypical response to infection. This debate continues, with the discussion of the role of EBV and studies of the clonality of Reed–Sternberg cells. The cell lineage of origin of the Reed–Sternberg (RS) cell has provoked great controversy, with almost every haematolymphoid cell having been proposed as a possible candidate. There is now wide acceptance of the idea that RS cells are abnormal lymphoid cells, in most cases probably of B-cell lineage, which by cytokine secretion or other cellular interactions are able to stimulate an intense reaction involving lymphoid cells, macrophages, granulocytes and connective tissue cells.

Although Hodgkin's disease has distinctive clinical and pathological features it is clear that it is closely related to other lymphoproliferative disorders. In a number of cases the distinction between Hodgkin's disease and other types of lymphoma may be impossible, which is probably a reflection of a continuous spectrum of disease.

Hodgkin's disease has a bimodal age distribution

In the UK the incidence of Hodgkin's disease is about 2/100 000 and there is little if any regional variation. There is an overall male preponderance with a 3:2 male to female ratio. The incidence increases with age continuing into the sixth decade but in addition there is a distinct peak in the 15–34-year age group. In these younger patients the male predominance is less pronounced and almost all cases are of the nodular sclerosing type. Because of this and an apparent seasonal variation in incidence it has been suggested there may be an infective cause, but definitive epidemiological evidence is lacking.

Hodgkin's disease includes two distinctive clinical and pathological entities

The recent clinical and pathological literature on Hodgkin's disease is dominated by the Rye classification, which was first published in 1966, coinciding with the beginnings of effective treatment.

It was a modification of the preceding Lukes–Butler classification, which was based on the idea of varying degrees of host responses to the malignant Reed–Sternberg cell as judged by the number of lymphocytes and other reactive cells. Since 1966 there have been major changes in the diagnosis of Hodgkin's disease, with much stricter adherence to diagnostic criteria and the routine use of immunological marker studies. This has led to a decrease in the number of lymphomas diagnosed as Hodgkin's disease and has affected all the Rye subgroups but especially the lymphocyte-depleted form, which is now very rarely diagnosed. An additional major change has been the rediscovery of the importance of the distinction between lymphocyte-predominant nodular subtype (LPNHD; syn: nodular paragranuloma) and other types of Hodgkin's disease (classical Hodgkin's disease). This distinction was part of the Lukes–Butler classification but was lost when the Rye classification was introduced.

7.2 Lymphocyte-predominant nodular Hodgkin's disease (LPNHD)

The morphological and phenotypic features of LPNHD suggest that it is a disorder of the germinal centre, clearly distinct from other forms of HD

In LPNHD all or most of the lymph node structure is replaced by expanded nodules. These nodules contain a complex mixture of cells including small mantle-zone-type B-cells, T-lymphocytes, germinal centre cells and follicular dendritic cells. T-cells expressing CD57 (a marker of activated cytotoxic T-cells and NK cells) are often a prominent feature of the nodules, which in non-neoplastic lymph nodes tend to be localized to the germinal centre. In most cases moderate numbers of epithelioid histiocytes are also present, sometimes forming microgranulomas. This

Table 7.1 Lymphocyte-predominant nodular Hodgkin's disease

- **Morphology**: Polylobated Reed–Sternberg cells in the context of expanded B-cell nodules containing a mixture of germinal centre B-cell, mantle cells, T-cells and macrophages with follicular dendritic cell networks.
- **Immunophenotype**: CD20$^+$, CD75$^+$, CD45$^+$, CD30$^-$, CD15$^-$; some cases express epithelial membrane antigen or J-chain. Rosettes of CD57$^+$ T-cells often present. May express cytoplasmic kappa light chains.
- **Cytogenetics**: No specific abnormality.
- **Pattern of disease**: Localized nodal enlargement, almost always in neck.

cellular composition is good evidence that the expanded nodules seen in LPNHD are derived from germinal centres. In some cases a rim of compressed normal tissue is seen at one pole of the node.

The features of LPNHD are summarized in Table 7.1.

The Reed–Sternberg cells seen in LPNHD differ in a number of important respects from those seen in the other forms of Hodgkin's disease so that the use of the term Reed–Sternberg cell is itself misleading. At the centre of the expanded nodule described above there are variable numbers of large atypical B-cells, which may have morphological features similar to centroblasts or immunoblasts. The cell type that is the hallmark of LPNHD has a polylobated, folded nucleus, with in most cases relatively small nucleoli (Figure 7.1).

These may be referred to as polylobated RS cells, popcorn cells or L&H cells. Classical or lacunar-type Reed–Sternberg cells are not seen in this condition. The polylobated cells and the mononuclear large B-cells all strongly express CD20, CD45 and CD75, with absence of CD30 and CD15. A population of CD30$^+$ blast cells similar to those seen around the follicle of reactive nodes may be present occasionally in LPNHD and this may lead to difficulty in making the distinction from classical Hodgkin's disease.

In some cases epithelial membrane antigen, a carbohydrate antigen closely related to CD15, or the immunoglobulin J-chain are expressed but both can be absent in otherwise typical cases. The increase in CD57$^+$ T-cells has already been described and it has been suggested that adherence of these cells to the polylobated B-cells is a specific diagnostic feature of LPNHD that is useful in making the distinction from T-cell-rich B-cell lymphoma; again this is not present in every case of LPNHD. Most studies have not been able to demonstrate that the polylobulated cells are a monoclonal population, but some studies have shown that when light chains are expressed these are almost always of kappa type. The reason for this is not understood.

The relationship of LPNHD to the germinal centre is further emphasized by its close similarity to progressive transformation of the germinal centre (PTGC). This is a benign condition in which some of the B-cell follicles in a reactive node expand and then become extensively infiltrated with mantle B-cells and T-cells, producing a nodule similar to that seen in LPNHD, although it lacks polylobated RS cells and usually

Figure 7.1 Lymphocyte-predominant nodular Hodgkin's disease. In LPNHD polylobated-type Reed–Sternberg cells with a B-cell phenotype are found in the context of an expanded nodule, which consists of germinal centre and mantle zone B-cells and reactive T-cells. The polylobated cells (arrow) have multiple often closely packed lobes **(a)**. In some cases these cells show strong expression of epithelial membrane antigen **(b)**.

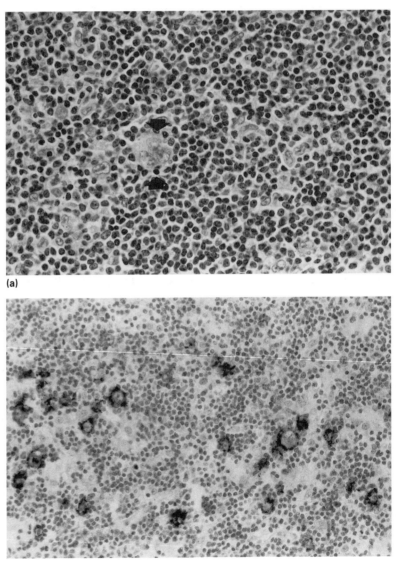

(a)

(b)

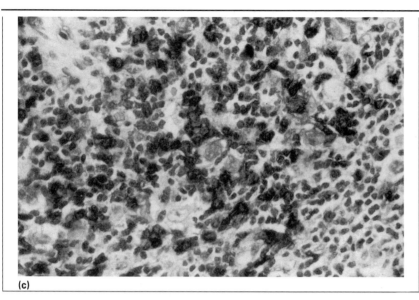

Figure 7.1 **(c)** The T-cells in the normal germinal centre express CD57 and in LPNHD these cells often form rosettes with the polylobated cells **(c)**.

large numbers of epithelioid histiocytes are not seen. PTGC occurs in the context of reactive follicular hyperplasia and could be a normal part of the life cycle of the follicle. Occasional progressively transformed follicles are relatively common in reactive nodes, but only rarely affect the majority of the node. When this is seen there is a small risk that Hodgkin's disease (usually but not always LPNHD) will be present in an adjacent node or will develop subsequently.

Most cases of LPNHD present with cervical lymphadenopathy

LPNHD is a cause of localized, sometimes massive lymphadenopathy. In the vast majority of cases cervical nodes are affected, with the axilla as the second most common site. Mediastinal masses and infradiaphragmatic or intra-abdominal disease are rare, as are B symptoms. Few patients have disease progression beyond stage II and in many cases most of the clinically detectable disease may be removed at the time of lymph node biopsy. If there is evidence of infiltration of the spleen or marrow, the diagnosis should be carefully reviewed, with T-cell-rich B-cell lymphoma being the main differential diagnosis.

Most patients have a good prognosis although some may have a relapsing course

LPNHD may occur at any age although the median age of onset is in the fourth decade, with a small number of cases described in young children.

As in HD in general there appears to be a male predominance. It is a localized condition and most patients are treated with radiotherapy to the involved field. The role of chemotherapy for Stage II disease is uncertain and the extent to which any modality of treatment influences survival is not clear from clinical trial data based on the Rye classification. Whatever the treatment, deaths due directly to LPNHD are very uncommon although there appears to be continued mortality unrelated to relapse, the cause of which is uncertain. In the original data published by Lukes and Butler the survival of patients with LPNHD was much better than those with other types of HD. However, relapse of the condition at the original site of disease may be seen in an as yet ill-defined proportion of patients up to 10 years or more after the original diagnosis. Relapses do not imply refractory or progressive disease and can be retreated as at initial presentation. Given the relationship of LPNHD to reactive hyperplasia and PTGC it should not be assumed that recurrent lymphadenopathy always means relapsed Hodgkin's disease.

LPNHD may transform to diffuse large B-cell lymphoma

LPNHD does not transform into other types of HD as was originally suspected. Instead a proportion of patients, between 2% and 10%, will transform into a diffuse large cell lymphoma of B-cell type. The diagnosis of transformation depends on the demonstration of replacement of part or all of the node by cohesive sheets of large B-cells. These have the same

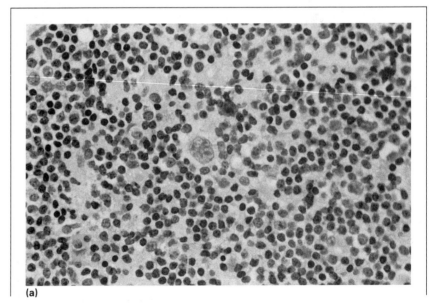

Figure 7.2 Transformed LPNHD. This patient had a solitary enlarged cervical node. Part of the node showed typical LPNHD **(a)**, although some of the polylobated cells had unusually prominent nucleoli.

(a)

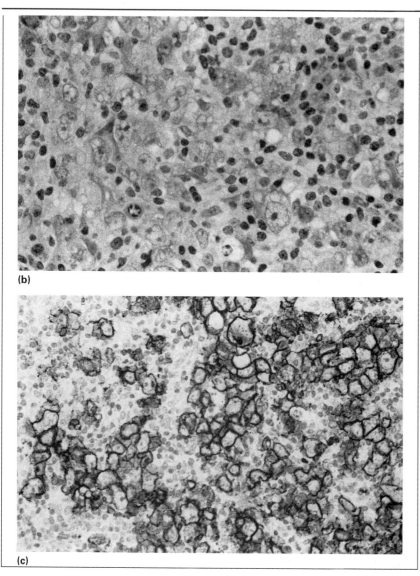

(b)

(c)

Figure 7.2 (b) Other parts of the node had diffuse infiltration by highly pleomorphic large lymphoid cells, which strongly expressed CD20 **(c)**.

phenotype as described above and the link to LPNHD may be further emphasized by the presence of polylobated cells. It can be shown in some cases, using sensitive PCR techniques, that the clone from which the large cell lymphoma arises is present in the underlying LPNHD although the polylobated RS cells may not be monoclonal (Figure 7.2).

In some patients who present with localized diffuse large cell lymphoma in a cervical node there may be some residual evidence to suggest underlying LPNHD although a previous history of HD is lacking. The prognosis for such transformed cases has not been clearly defined but the evidence from a number of small studies suggests that it is better than other transformed lymphomas. In part this may be a reflection of localized early-stage disease.

The relationship of LPNHD to T-cell-rich B-cell lymphoma remains unclear

In a small number of cases many of the cellular features of LPNHD may be present without nodule formation. The classification of such cases and their distinction from T-cell-rich B-cell lymphoma is difficult because of the lack of clearly defined criteria. Indeed it is possible that LPNHD and some cases of T-cell-rich B-cell lymphoma may represent a continuous spectrum of disease (it is unlikely that T-cell-rich B-cell lymphoma represents a unified diagnostic entity). In most of these cases the patient has localized disease but in a small number, advanced-stage aggressive disease is present with spleen and marrow infiltration.

7.3 Classical Hodgkin's disease

Classical HD spreads contiguously to adjacent nodes and usually begins in the neck or mediastinum

Nodular sclerosing and mixed cellularity Hodgkin's disease constitute a distinct clinical entity, which is now called classical-type Hodgkin's disease. In most cases the disease will begin with cervical or mediastinal nodal involvement; mediastinal masses will be present in the majority of cases, especially of the nodular sclerosing subtype. The disease spreads contiguously to adjacent nodes, with late involvement of bone marrow and extranodal sites. Fewer than 10% of patients present with localized Hodgkin's disease below the diaphragm, in intra-abdominal or inguinal lymph nodes. Primary extranodal Hodgkin's disease has been reported but is exceedingly rare.

It is essential that the pattern of disease at presentation is considered together with the biopsy features in making a firm diagnosis. Hodgkin's disease needs to be considered as a syndrome with the distribution of the disease in the patient (contiguous nodal spread) and the cellular characteristics as integral components. When there are atypical clinical or pathological features at diagnosis the clinical course and response to treatment may also be unpredictable. In addition, the diagnosis should be reconsidered if the patient has early-stage nodal disease but evidence of bone marrow, splenic or hepatic infiltration, in which case possibilities such as anaplastic lymphoma or T-cell-rich B-cell lymphoma should be considered.

The diagnosis of classical-type Hodgkin's disease depends on the presence of Reed–Sternberg cells in an appropriate background

The accurate diagnosis of Hodgkin's disease involves demonstrating destruction of the normal nodal architecture by an infiltrate that includes Reed–Sternberg cells in the appropriate cellular background. This definition is constructed to exclude reactive conditions where Reed–Sternberg-like cells may be found in the context of a normal or hyperplastic node.

Two main morphological variants of RS cell are found in nodular sclerosing and mixed-cellularity Hodgkin's disease. The classical RS cell is several times the diameter of a lymphocyte with abundant eosinophilic cytoplasm and the highly characteristic bilobular nucleus with 'mirror image' eosinophilic nucleoli (Figure 7.3).

The lacunar cell typical of NSHD is of similar size but shows artefactual retraction of the cytoplasm and more crowded bi- or multilobular nuclei and smaller nucleoli. In most cases there will be a range of other obviously related cell types, including a variable number of large mononuclear cells in association with classical RS cells. In some

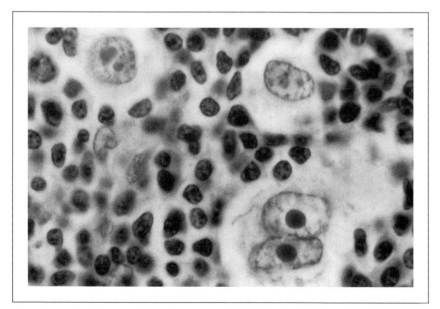

Figure 7.3 Classical-type Reed–Sternberg cell. This figure shows a typical RS cell from a case of mixed cellularity HD. The cell is six to seven times the diameter of the adjacent small lymphocytes and has a bilobular nucleus with large symmetrical nucleoli.

cases of NSHD, in particular, the neoplastic population may be highly pleomorphic and include bizarre multinuclear forms. Compacted, densely staining degenerate RS cells may be numerous and are sometimes known as mummified cells.

The features of classical-type Hodgkin's disease are summarized in Table 7.2.

Immunophenotypical studies are essential for the accurate diagnosis of HD, including the distinction between LPNHD and classical HD. In almost every case the RS cells will express CD30; with modern antigen retrieval techniques only 1–2% of otherwise typical cases of Hodgkin's disease will be negative, although there may be heterogeneity of expression within the tumour. CD30 is a growth factor receptor that has been shown to be a member of the TNF family. The ligand of this receptor has now also been characterized but the effect of CD30 stimulation by its natural ligand is not yet well understood. A smaller percentage of cases will be CD15$^+$. CD15 is a carbohydrate antigen expressed on myeloid cell and various epithelia. Not all anti-CD15 antibodies react equally with RS cells; those that do show a dense area of positivity in the paranuclear region. Membrane staining is less specific and the strength of CD15 reactivity with eosinophils may sometimes cause problems of interpretation. For this reason paraffin or resin section are preferable to frozen sections (Figure 7.4). A further strong immunohistological feature of RS cells is the lack of CD45 expression in fixed tissue by the majority of RS cells. This can be difficult to interpret if, as is often the case, there are mature T-cells close to or adherent to the RS cell membrane.

Evidence of T- or B-cell differentiation is a less constant feature of RS cells. The most consistent finding in over 70% of cases is reactivity with the B-cell/histiocyte marker BLA36, which is part of the CD20 cluster.

Table 7.2 Classical-type Hodgkin's disease

- **Morphology**: Classical- or lacunar-type Reed–Sternberg cell in a background of T- and B-lymphocytes, macrophages and eosinophils. Nodule formation and fibrosis characterizes the nodular sclerosing types.
- **Immunophenotype**: CD30$^+$, CD15$^+$, CD45$^-$, CD3$^-$, BLA-36$^+$. Rosettes of adherent T-cells are often present.
- **Cytogenetic**: No specific abnormality.
- **Pattern of disease**: Contiguous nodal spread beginning in neck or mediastinum.

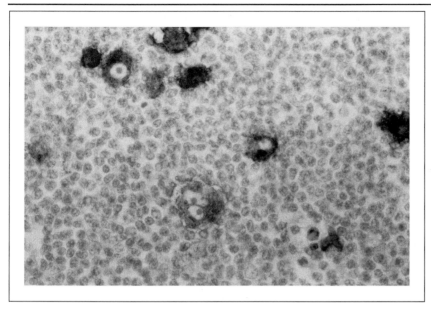

Figure 7.4 Mixed-cellularity Hodgkin's disease – anti-CD15. A key immunophenotypical feature of classical Hodgkin's disease is cytoplasmic staining, often strongest in the paranuclear area, by CD15.

Reactivity with other CD20 antibodies is rarer. A highly distinctive feature is the presence of T-cell rosettes around RS cells (the T-cells are CD57-negative, in contrast to LPNHD). This cell-to-cell adhesion is mediated by CD2-LFA-3 binding and may involve activation of CD40, which is widely expressed by RS cells (Figure 7.5). In B-cells CD40 activation by binding to its ligand expressed by T-cells is a survival

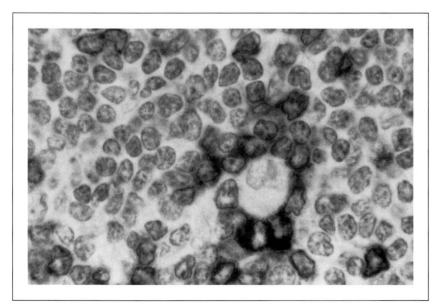

Figure 7.5 Mixed cellularity HD – T-cell rosettes (anti-CD3). In classical HD the Reed–Sternberg cells form rosettes with T-cells. Unlike LPNHD these are CD57⁻. This interaction may be mediated by the adhesive interaction of CD2-LFA-3 and may result in the activation of CD40 on the Reed–Sternberg cells by CD40L on the T-cells.

stimulus leading to *bcl-2* induction, and in RS cells may also lead to cytokine release.

In a very small number of cases with morphological features of Hodgkin's disease RS cells show elements of a cytotoxic T-cell phenotype. The relationship of these cases to T-lineage anaplastic lymphoma and their clinical significance is not yet clear.

About 70% of cases of HD other than LPNHD are of nodular sclerosing type (Figure 7.6).

Figure 7.6 Nodular sclerosing Hodgkin's disease. This is a typical case of type 1 NSHD. One of the key diagnostic features of this condition is the presence of nodules surrounded by fibrous tissue, which contain a mixed population of lymphocytes, macrophages and eosinophils **(a)**. **(b)** Many of the RS cells are lacunar cells and show extensive retraction artefact of the cytoplasm, which is connected by thin strands to the cell membrane (arrow).

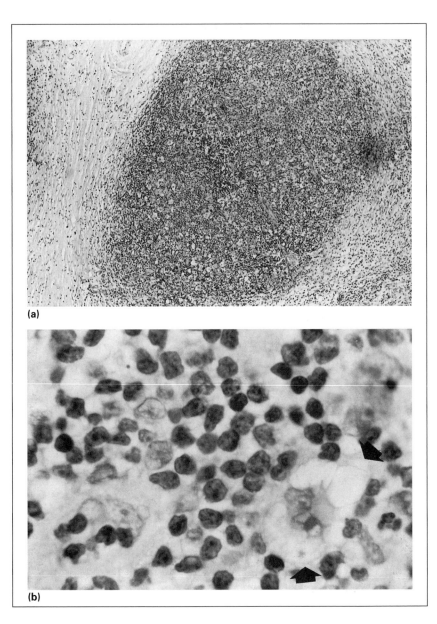

(a)

(b)

This has three essential diagnostic features; a nodular growth pattern, bands of mature fibrous connective tissue and lacunar-type Reed–Sternberg cells. Within this broad definition there may be considerable variation. The nodules may have a mixed cellular background pattern with mature T- and B-cells, macrophages, plasma cells and eosinophils. Even within the same biopsy some nodules may have a lymphocyte-depleted pattern or consist of a mixture of spindle-shaped connective tissue cells and macrophages. These latter patterns are associated with variable amounts of necrosis. The number of lacunar-type RS cells and their morphology also varies. In a minority of cases these may be very sparse, although this is the exception. At the other extreme cohesive sheets of highly pleomorphic lacunar cells may be present that give the appearance of a syncytium (Figure 7.7).

NSHD may be subdivided into type 1 and 2, based on the number of lymphocyte-depleted nodules. The BNLI criteria define the type 2 variant as having more than 25% of nodules with a lymphocyte-depleted pattern, which is characterized by diffuse sheets of large pleomorphic tumour cells. Cases are also included in the type 2 category if more than 50% of the nodules have a fibrohistiocytic background. The association between a type 2 pattern and poor prognosis has been shown in a number of clinical trials. However, many patients with type 2 NSHD have a normal response to therapy and conversely some patients with type 1 disease are refractory to treatment. The classification is not an accurate predictor of

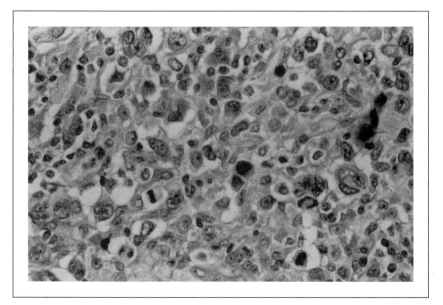

Figure 7.7 Relapsed NS Hodgkin's disease. At presentation this patient had typical type 1 NSHD. The relapse biopsy shows relative lymphocyte depletion with cohesive sheets of highly pleomorphic mononuclear cells that showed a typical Hodgkin's disease immunophenotype.

probable response in the individual patient and if complete remission is achieved with standard therapy there is probably no survival difference between the groups. A further problem with the classification is the accuracy that can be achieved in small biopsy samples, where only a few nodules may be present.

Some biopsy specimens may show lacunar-type RS cells but without nodular fibrosis. This is sometimes classified as cellular-phase NSHD. There is no advantage to recognition of this subtype, which should be included in the mixed cellularity variant.

The term 'mixed-cellularity HD' applies to cases of classical HD that do not meet the strict criteria for NSHD (Figure 7.8).

Most cases of mixed cellularity HD have a mixture of lymphocytes, eosinophils and macrophages with classical-type Reed–Sternberg cells. A small number of cases have a histiocyte- and lymphocyte-predominant background; these are distinguished from LPNHD by the morphology and phenotype of the RS cells. The term lymphocyte-rich classical HD is sometimes used to describe these cases but there seems little reason to consider this group as distinct from MCHD. In a few cases there are areas of lymphocyte depletion that may be associated with either high concentration of RS cells and atypical mononuclear cells or dense diffuse fibrosis.

True cases of pure lymphocyte-depleted Hodgkin's disease are very rare, although this diagnosis was used more commonly in the past. Nodes involved with MCHD sometimes show B-cell hyperplasia either as follicular hyperplasia or as an expansion of monocytoid parafollicular B-cells. This may sometimes appear as the predominant feature of the node, with the presence of HD in the interfollicular areas being overlooked (Figure 7.9). In general MCHD behaves in a similar way to NS1 HD with the majority of patients having a good response to standard treatment.

The distinction between Hodgkin's disease and anaplastic lymphoma may be difficult

The difficulty in distinguishing Hodgkin's disease from anaplastic large cell lymphoma has been recognized in the REAL classification by the suggested term 'Hodgkin's-like anaplastic large cell lymphoma'. This diagnosis recognizes the not uncommon finding in which a tumour may have, at least in part, a nodular sclerosing pattern but the nodules contain sheets of large pleomorphic cells and few or no morphologically typical RS lacunar-type cells. Similar cells may be seen to have a sinusoidal

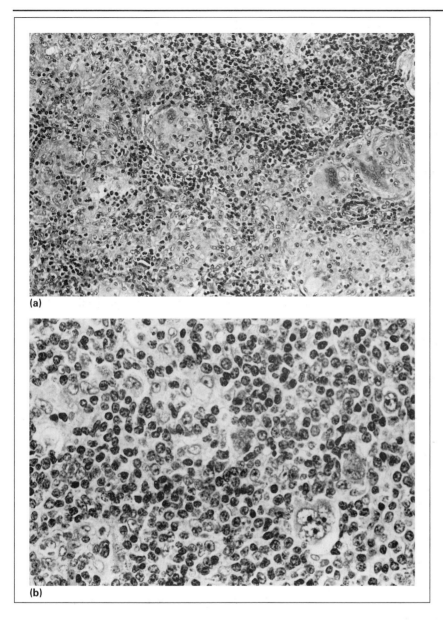

(a)

(b)

Figure 7.8 Granulomatous Hodgkin's disease. In this otherwise typical case of mixed cellularity HD large parts of the lymph node biopsy were replaced by epithelioid cell granulomas **(a)**. A large bizarre Reed–Sternberg cell with a trilobular nucleus is present **(b)**.

pattern of infiltration. There are insufficient published data to comment on whether it is important to separate this type of tumour from type 2 NSHD and definitive diagnostic criteria for making this distinction have not been developed; again this may be a reflection of a continuous spectrum of disease. Other types of ALC lymphoma are distinguished mainly by the pattern of infiltration and by phenotype. Most cases of ALC lymphoma have some evidence of a T-cell phenotype and many have

Figure 7.9 Follicular Hodgkin's disease. This patient, who had typical NSHD, relapsed several years after treatment. The node was replaced by expanded follicles shown on the reticulin stain **(a)**. **(b)** Most of these follicles included reactive germinal centres surrounded by numerous Reed–Sternberg cells (arrows).

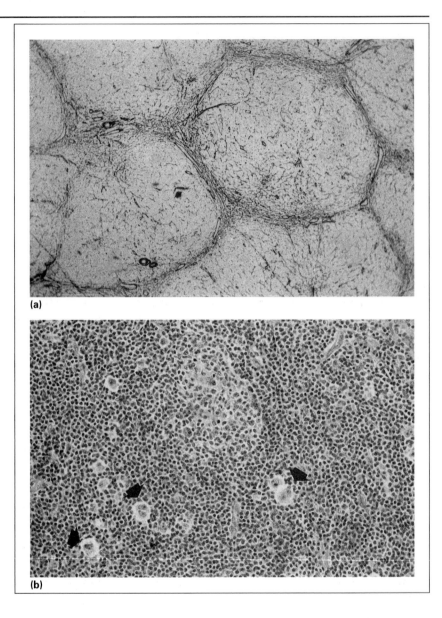

(a)

(b)

distinctive features such as EMA or BNH9 expression or a t(2;5) and associated NPM-ALK expression.

The majority of cases of Hodgkin's disease of NS and MC types are diagnosed without difficulty although there may be some interobserver variation in subclassification. Residual problems occur with T-cell lymphomas, especially angioimmunoblastic and Lennert's type, but in general these can be solved by immunophenotypic and immunogenetic studies.

7.4 The pathogenesis of classical Hodgkin's disease

The aetiology and pathogenesis of Hodgkin's disease is still poorly understood, but considerable advances have been made. The origin of the Reed–Sternberg cell and its interaction with non-neoplastic cells is a subject of considerable contemporary interest. The other main strand of investigation is the part played by EBV and possibly other viruses in the pathogenesis of the disease.

Reed–Sternberg cells in most cases appear to be of B-cell origin

In most cases of classical HD the RS cells express the B-cell marker BLA36 and in a smaller number of cases react with other anti-B-cell antibodies. Using standard Southern blot or IgH PCR techniques a clonal B-cell rearrangement can be detected in about one-third of cases but these studies are clearly limited by the sensitivity of the detection techniques in cases where RS cells may be a small fraction of the total population. More recently, microdissection techniques have been used to isolate and study individual RS cells. These data show that most, if not all, RS cells have rearranged immunoglobulin genes, although sequencing shows that in a few cases the RS cells sampled are not monoclonal. This suggests that the monoclonality of RS cells may develop by clonal evolution during the course of the disease. These studies are not extensive enough for clinical differences between monoclonal and polyclonal HD to have been fully investigated.

A further interesting aspect of this work is the finding that the immunoglobulin genes in many RS cells are hypermutated indicating that they may have been derived from post-germinal centre B-cells. In the small number of cases examined the expression of immunoglobulin genes appears to have be abrogated by mutation at critical sites. This has led to the suggestion that a fundamental element in the pathogenesis of classical HD is the ability of the RS cells to escape apoptosis, the usual fate of abnormal germinal centre cells.

About one-third of cases have a strong association with Epstein–Barr virus

The bimodal age incidence of HD and reports of case clustering have led to intensive investigation of the possibility of an infective cause. Case control studies have identified a past history of infectious mononucleosis as a risk factor. This has led to extensive investigations of the role of EBV and other Herpesviruses in the pathogenesis of HD.

There is no direct evidence for a causative link between Epstein–Barr virus and Hodgkin's disease but in about 40% of cases the presence of virus can be identified by PCR in the tumour. This is a useful screening test but needs to be viewed in the context of a very common virus that a high proportion of the population carry as a latent infection. More direct evidence can be obtained by Southern blot analysis, in which the number of variable viral terminal repeats can be used as a clonal marker. The presence of deletions within viral genes can also be useful to show that viral integration occurred before neoplastic transformation. Using these methods, about one-third of cases show evidence of a clone of EBV-containing cells. The most definitive evidence to show that EBV is important in the pathogenesis of HD is to show that the virus is active within Reed–Sternberg cells. This is done by detecting viral RNA production using *in situ* hybridization with the EBER probes and by immunocytochemical detection of the latent membrane proteins that are a feature of EBV-transformed B-cells. With these markers, EBV-positive Reed–Sternberg cells are seen in about 25% of cases of NS/MC HD, with some excess in younger patients. This is another area of difference from LPNHD, where no evidence of EBV infection is found. EBV is also rare in anaplastic lymphoma, except possibly in cases associated with AIDS, and the demonstration of EBV may have a role in a few cases as an additional discriminatory marker.

The mechanism of B-cell immortalization by EBV has been extensively studied *in vitro* and the key viral proteins responsible have been identified. The pattern of viral gene expression seen in infected RS cells differs from that seen *in vitro* with absence of the viral transcription factor EBNA2. The viral protein Lmp-1, which may be involved in the inhibition of apoptosis, is usually strongly expressed on RS cells. It is not clear how particular patterns of viral gene expression interact with other genetic abnormalities in producing a malignant cell phenotype.

A major problem in proving the pathologic role of EBV in Hodgkin's disease is that despite intensive efforts to detect the virus it is only present in a subset of cases and by any available criteria these do not seem to be in any way distinctive. It is a distinct possibility that EBV infection is one of several genetic abnormalities that may disrupt the same regulatory pathway, leading to a similar endpoint.

Some of the pathological and clinical features may be due to cytokine production

A number of the characteristic clinical features of the nodular sclerosing and mixed cellularity types of Hodgkin's disease are not due to direct invasion of tissues by tumour. Most common among these effects are the B symptoms of fever, night sweats, weight loss and pruritus. In a large proportion of patients with NS/MC HD there is myeloid and megakaryocytic hyperplasia of the bone marrow. It is not unusual for the marrow to be maximally cellular but this does not appear to correlate with the other classical B-symptoms.

Immune dysregulation is also a common feature of NS/MC HD. This may be clinically manifest as reactivation of Herpes infections (simplex, zoster and CMV) or mucocutaneous fungal infections. In very occasional cases disorders of immunosuppression such as progressive multifocal leukoencephalopathy may occur. *In vitro* immunological tests give little clue as to the pathogenesis of immunodeficiency. In about 30% of patients there is a T-cell lymphopenia, with normal numbers of circulating B-cells. Non-specific B-cell activation and hypergammaglobulinaemia may also occur. Macrophage activation occurs with the formation of granulomas in the liver, spleen and sometimes bone marrow. Although immunosuppression is clearly a feature of Hodgkin's disease, pre-existing immunodeficiency can predispose to Hodgkin's disease. Hodgkin's disease is described in association with HIV, combined variable immunodeficiency and post-transplant immunosuppression.

Much rarer are the non-infiltrative effects of Hodgkin's disease on the liver. Some patients develop cholestasis, hepatocellular atrophy or vanishing bile duct syndrome, leading to hepatic failure without direct infiltration of the liver by tumour (Figure 7.10). These effects can occasionally occur in patients with low bulk or occult disease and may be an early feature of relapse.

This range of clinical effects suggests that a key feature of Hodgkin's disease may be dysregulation of cytokine production. This has been studied by immunocytochemistry and *in situ* hybridization in tissue samples, cell lines and in the serum of Hodgkin's patients. About 75% of RS cells appear to secrete IL-1α, IL-1β or both. TNFα and TGFβ are also commonly found. Increased levels of GM-CSF, IL-3 and IL-6 are also found in some patients. IL-6 secretion may be central to the excess secretion of immunoglobulin but in general there is a poor correlation between clinical symptoms and particular cytokines.

As well as mediating systemic effects cytokine production may govern the interaction between the RS cells and the non-neoplastic cell populations that make up most of the mass of the node. Vascular endothelial cells show enhanced expression of various adhesion molecules such as ELAM-1, which mediates traffic into the node. TGFβ is a potent connective tissue growth factor and may be responsible for the

Figure 7.10 Cholestasis due to HD. This patient had advanced HD with abnormal liver function. There was no evidence of liver infiltration on CT scan but intense cholestasis was seen on liver biopsy (bile is the darkly staining pigment). This is one of a range of presumably cytokine-mediated effects on the liver.

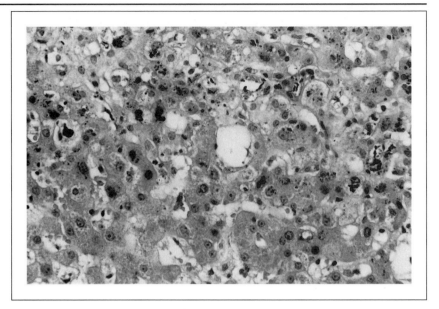

fibrosis in NSHD. Some or all of the production of the cytokines described may be produced by non-RS cells such as macrophages, T-cells or eosinophils.

Although many of the details remain obscure there is good reason to consider that dysregulation of cytokine production is a central feature in the pathogenesis of the clinical and pathological features of Hodgkin's disease.

7.5 Staging and therapy of classical Hodgkin's disease

Clinical examination and imaging studies may underestimate stage of disease

Laparotomy to accurately stage Hodgkin's disease is now rarely undertaken. Most patients will be staged using a combination of routine radiography and CT scanning. Using these methods about 30% of patients with apparently early disease will be reclassified to a higher stage. Staging laparotomy, if carried out, may further increase the stage in some patients. The argument for carrying out a staging laparotomy is that it clearly delineates patients who require chemotherapy from those with localized disease for whom radiotherapy is appropriate. However, disease response to chemotherapy following relapse after radiotherapy alone is so good that laparotomy is now generally considered unnecessary.

Stage of disease is one of the main prognostic factors in Hodgkin's disease (Tables 7.3, 7.4).

As well as the number of anatomical sites involved, disease bulk, especially in the mediastinum, is also important. High-bulk mediastinal disease is defined as greater than 10 cm diameter or more than one-third of the thoracic width on X-ray. Direct invasion of the lung parenchyma by a mediastinal tumour is an additional prognostic factor.

Table 7.3 The Cotswold modification of the Ann Arbor staging criteria for Hodgkin's disease

Clinical stage (CS) criteria
Lymph node involvement
a. Clinical enlargement of a node when alternative pathology may reasonably be ruled out (suspicious nodes should always be biopsied if treatment decisions are based on their involvement)
b. Enlargement on plain radiograph, CT, or lymphography

Spleen involvement
Unequivocal palpable splenomegaly alone, or equivocal palpable splenomegaly with radiological confirmation of either enlargement or multiple focal defects (radiological enlargement alone is inadequate)

Lung involvement
Radiological evidence of parenchymal involvement in the absence of other likely causes, especially infection

Bone involvement
History of pain or elevation of serum alkaline phosphatase, supported by plain X-ray changes or evidence from other imaging studies (isotope, CT or MRI)

Central nervous system
a. A spinal extranodal deposit may be diagnosed on the basis of the clinical history and findings supported by plain X-ray, myelography, CT and/or MRI
b. Intracranial involvement will rarely be diagnosed **clinically** at presentation. It should be considered on the basis of a space occupying lesion in the face of disease in additional extranodal sites

Other sites of involvement
Clinical involvement of other extranodal sites may only be diagnosed if the site is contiguous or proximal to a known nodal site (i.e. an 'E' lesion)

Pathological stage (PS)
Pathological stage depends on histopathological confirmation of specific sites of involvement such as bone, bone marrow, lung, liver and skin

Table 7.4 Staging system for Hodgkin's disease (based on Ann Arbor classification with Cotswold modifications)

Stage I: Involvement of a single lymph node region (LNR) (e.g. cervical, axillary inguinal, mediastinal) or lymphoid structure such as spleen, thymus, Waldeyer's ring or single localized extralymphatic site (ELS)

Stage II: Involvement of two or more LNR or lymphoid structures or one localized ELS plus one or more LNR on the same side of the diaphragm
[Hilar node involvement both sides = Stage II]
[Involvement of both para-aortic and paracaval nodes = Stage II]$_3$
Number of anatomical regions is indicated by a subscript, e.g. II3

Stage III: Involvement of LNR or lymphoid structures of both sides of the diaphragm

Extranodal disease
Involvement of extralymphatic tissue by limited direct extension from adjacent LNR is indicated by the subscript 'E'

Stage IV: Extensive extralymphatic involvement and/or disseminated disease with involvement of liver, bone marrow, bone, plasma, lung or skin

Bulky disease
Criteria: The bulk of palpable lymph nodes is defined by the largest dimension (cm) of the single largest lymph node or nodal mass in each LNR
If ≥ 10 cm = bulky
- Abdominal nodal bulk is defined using CT, MRI, lymphography or ultrasonography
  [Measurement of hepatic or splenic lesions is **not** used for staging purposes]
- Mediastinal masses are defined as bulky when the maximum width ≥ one-third internal transverse diameter of thorax at the T5/6 level (standardized PA chest X-ray taken at maximal inspiration in the upright position at a source–skin distance of 2 m) The subscript X is added to denote the presence of bulky disease

B Symptoms
Criteria:
- Unexplained weight loss of more than 10% of the previous body weight during the 6 months before staging
- Unexplained, persistent or recurrent fever with temperatures above 38°C during the previous month
- Recurrent drenching night sweats during the previous month

The extent of disease may be reflected in elevated serum levels of markers such as LDH and beta-2-microglobulin. Serum CD30 is also being assessed as a prognostic factor; it is possible that this may be of particular value in detecting relapse. The prognostic impact of histological subtypes has been discussed above.

A bone marrow aspirate and trephine biopsy at presentation will reveal involvement in about 1–2% of cases (Figure 7.11).

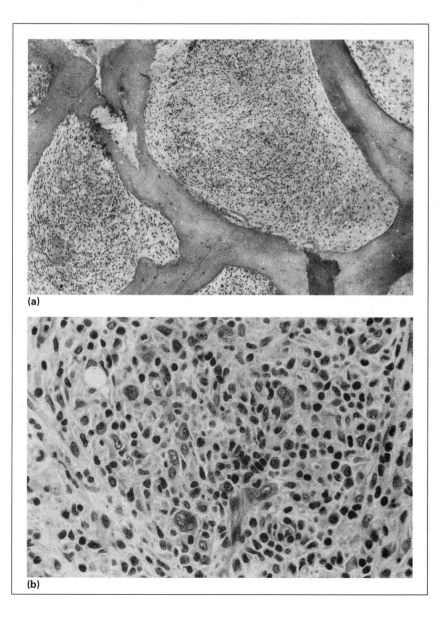

(a)

(b)

Figure 7.11 (a, b) Hodgkin's disease – bone marrow. Bone marrow examination in a patient with advanced Hodgkin's disease showed complete marrow replacement. The infiltrate consists of a background of lymphocytes, plasma cells and macrophages with relatively small numbers of Reed–Sternberg cells.

Despite this low diagnostic yield, it is a useful investigation. If a patient has marrow infiltration at presentation the prognosis is poor. However, if a patient has marrow infiltration by lymphoma but early stage disease on imaging investigation the diagnosis should be reviewed and the possibility of T-cell lymphoma or T-cell-rich B-cell lymphoma should be given further consideration. Infiltration of other extranodal sites also confers a very poor prognosis and with the exception of direct invasion from involved nodes should only be seen in patients with advanced-stage nodal disease. Liver infiltration is a poor prognostic feature but is very rare if the spleen is unaffected. However at the present time the available histological and clinical prognostic factors do not identify at presentation all of the patients who will prove to have refractory disease (Figure 7.12).

Response to treatment on imaging studies and absence of early relapse are among the most important prognostic factors (Table 7.5).

A management problem that may arise is the presence of stable residual masses (Figure 7.13). Given the content of fibrous tissue of many nodes in Hodgkin's disease it is not surprising that they do not entirely disappear with treatment. Size stability can be used to indicate inactive disease. It has recently been suggested that gallium scanning may be useful in this context, but it remains to be validated.

Figure 7.12 Pulmonary infiltration by HD – CT scan. This patient relapsed after treatment and was found on CT to have extensive pulmonary infiltration by Hodgkin's disease.

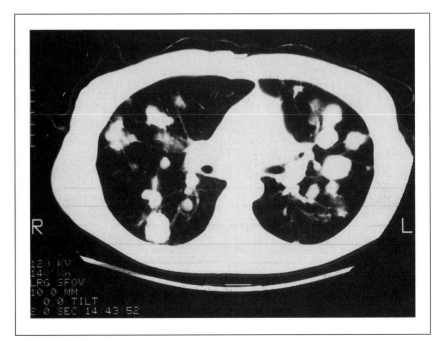

Table 7.5 Poor prognosis factors in Hodgkin's disease

- Higher stage
- NS2/lymphocyte-depleted morphology
- Bulky mediastinal lymphadenopathy (≥ 10 cm or mediastinal lymphoadenopathy more than one-third the diameter of the thorax)
- B symptoms
- Age > 45 years
- Extranodal disease
- Relapse within 1 year post-chemotherapy

Stage and disease bulk determine the choice of radiotherapy and chemotherapy

While radiotherapy has proved an effective treatment modality over many years, the introduction of the MOPP combination chemotherapy regimen in the 1970s significantly enhanced treatment outcomes, particularly in advanced stage disease. The use of these treatment modalities singly or in combination means that most patients with Hodgkin's disease can expect to achieve sustained complete remissions and cure.

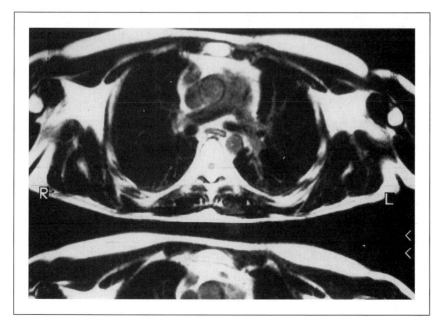

Figure 7.13 Residual mediastinal mass, NSHD – CT scan. This patient had typical NSHD and achieved complete clinical remission. Repeated CT scan showed a stable residual mediastinal mass.

The pattern of contiguous spread that is a central feature of Hodgkin's disease is the key principle governing the choice of therapy and means that patients who have localized disease can be treated by radiotherapy. Patients with stage I and possibly stage IIA non-bulky disease have an excellent response to radiotherapy alone. There is now agreement that chemotherapy is the treatment of choice in stage III and IV disease and in all patients with B symptoms. Many patients with bulky stage IIA disease also receive combination chemotherapy. Radiotherapy has an important adjuvant role in the treatment of bulky mediastinal or other tumour masses, as it reduces the risk of local relapse at sites of previous bulky disease.

A relatively small number of patients have disease refractory to standard treatment or relapse within 1 year of treatment. Some of these patients will respond to second-line chemotherapy and such responses may be consolidated by additional intensive chemotherapy, for example BEAM (BCNU, etoposide, cytosine arabinoside, melphalan), with peripheral blood stem cell support. Bulky disease, systemic symptoms and NS2/lymphocyte-depleted morphology are often features of this group of patients, though about 10% of patients with no adverse features at presentation will have refractory/relapsing disease.

The use of involved-field radiotherapy as a primary treatment for Hodgkin's disease was found to be associated with a high rate of relapse in adjacent lymph node groups. This resulted in the development of extended-field techniques – notably mantle and inverted Y. With the advent of effective chemotherapy to salvage patients who relapse after radiotherapy, involved-field treatments have been revisited for patients with stage IA and IIA disease. While the overall survival for patients treated with localized radiotherapy is the same as those treated with extended-field radiotherapy, the 5-year relapse-free survival for localized radiotherapy is 30–40% compared with 60–70% for extended-field treatment. Despite this risk involved-field radiotherapy remains the treatment of choice for patients not fit to receive extended-field radiotherapy or chemotherapy.

If there is bulky mediastinal disease, chemotherapy is usually preferred in the first instance because the chances of achieving local control with radiotherapy are relatively poor. Also, there may be occult (e.g. para-aortic) disease and the presence of a large mediastinal mass may necessitate irradiating a relatively large volume of lung. Adding a 'para-aortic strip', i.e. increasing the length of irradiated field to cover the para-aortic lymph nodes, will reduce the risk of relapse but does not alter overall survival. This is common practice in the USA and Europe but has found less favour in the UK because it increases acute morbidity and may reduce bone marrow reserve in patients who subsequently require chemotherapy and stem cell harvesting.

Infradiaphragmatic Hodgkin's disease is relatively rare so it is difficult to assess the role of radiotherapy. Because of the increased risk of splenic involvement in patients with para-aortic disease, inverted Y radiotherapy is often confined to those patients with stage IA disease affecting the pelvis/inguinal or femoral nodes.

It is common practice to irradiate sites of previous bulk disease on completion of chemotherapy in Hodgkin's disease. This reduces the risk of recurrence within the irradiated area, but has not been shown to affect the overall survival.

In the attempt to improve remission rates and long-term results, a variety of drug combinations has been evaluated, including the anthracycline-based four-drug regimen ABVD (Adriamycin, bleomycin, vinblastine, dacarbazine) multi-drug hybrid or alternating regimens and weekly schedules. The data that have emerged indicate that better response rates and increased failure-free and overall survival are achieved with the anthracycline-based regimens.

Despite the success of high-dose chemotherapy with autologass stem cell support in the relapse setting, it is not appropriate as first-line treatment because of the difficulty of identifying suitable poor prognosis subgroups with confidence.

Long-term follow-up is needed to monitor complications of therapy and late relapse

A relapsing course is well described in patients with LPNHD but late relapse of other types may also occur, even after 10 years or more of complete remission. The presentation of relapsed NS/MCHD is much more variable than the primary presentations. It has been suggested that relapsed HD is more often associated with Epstein–Barr virus.

Patients treated for Hodgkin's disease have a significant risk of second malignancy, most commonly MDS/AML which may occur after both radiotherapy and chemotherapy; the relationship to alkylating agent therapy has been described extensively. The cumulative risk is around 3% after 10 years. A similar incidence of diffuse large B-cell lymphoma is also noted. What is not clear is whether this is an effect of treatment or transformation of the Hodgkin's disease. DLBC lymphoma is well described in LPNHD but may also occur in NS/MC HD. Some patients have composite lymphomas at presentation – usually NSHD and follicle centre lymphoma. Cutaneous malignancy, sarcomas, breast and thyroid

Table 7.6 Long-term complications of treatment and the related factors

- Pneumococcal sepsis
  - Splenectomy
- Infertility
  - Alkylating agents; procarbazine
- Cardiotoxicity
  - Anthracyclines
  - Radiotherapy
- Lung fibrosis
  - Bleomycin
  - Radiotherapy
- Second malignancy
  - Chemotherapy and radiotherapy

carcinomas also occur in radiotherapy fields. The overall incidence of second malignancy is approximately 13%.

Patients treated for Hodgkin's disease may also show a number of other toxic effects of therapy. Most male patients will be azoospermic and around 80% of female patients will have reduced fertility. Specific long-term toxicity may occur in relation to particular chemotherapeutic agents, for example pulmonary fibrosis in patients treated with bleomycin and cardiomyopathy following anthracyclines. Radiotherapy to the heart may accelerate the progress of ischaemic HD. As a result of these complications patients treated for HD have a significant excess of non-HD-associated mortalities (Table 7.6).

Attention is now being directed towards reducing the late sequelae of chemotherapy, by omitting agents particularly linked with specific complications, though this should not be at the cost of reduced efficacy in control of HD. Trials comparing multi-drug with simpler regimens are currently under way.

7.6 Key references

7.6.1 Diagnosis and classification of Hodgkin's disease

Ashton-Key, M., Thorpe, P. A., Allen, J. P. and Isaacson, P. G. (1995) Follicular Hodgkin's disease. *American Journal of Surgical Pathology,* **19,** 1294–1299.

Pappa, V. I., Norton, A. J., Gupta, R. K. *et al.* (1995) Nodular type of lymphocyte predominant Hodgkin's disease. A clinical study of 50 cases. *Annals of Oncology*, **6**, 559–565.

Schmidt, U., Metz, K. A. and Leder, L. D. (1995) T-cell-rich B-cell lymphoma and lymphocyte-predominant Hodgkin's disease: two closely related entities? *British Journal of Haematology*, **90**, 398–403.

Various authors (1996) Proceeding of the 3rd International Symposium on Hodgkin's disease. *Annals of Oncology*, 7(Suppl. 4).

Von Wasieleski, R., Werner, M., Fischer, R. *et al.* (1997) Lymphocyte-predominant Hodgkin's Disease: an immunohistochemical analysis of 208 reviewed Hodgkin's disease cases from the German Hodgkin's Study Group. *American Journal of Pathology*, **150**, 793–803.

Wickert, R. S., Weisenburger, D. D., Tierens, A. *et al.* (1995) Clonal relationship between lymphocytic predominance Hodgkin's disease and concurrent or subsequent large-cell lymphoma of B lineage. *Blood*, **86**, 2312–2320.

7.6.2 Pathogenesis of Hodgkin's disease

Chan, W. C. and Delabie, J. (1995) Hodgkin's disease. Lineage and clonality *American Journal of Clinical Pathology*, **104**, 368–370.

Falini, B., Bigerna, B., Pasqualucci, L. *et al.* (1996) Distinctive expression pattern of the BCL-6 protein in nodular lymphocyte predominance Hodgkin's disease. *Blood*, **87**, 465–471.

Gereiner, T. C., Gascoyne, R. D., Anderson, M. E. *et al.* (1996) Nodular lymphocyte predominant Hodgkin's disease associated with large cell lymphoma; analysis of Ig gene rearrangements by V–J polymerase chain reaction. *Blood*, **88**, 657–666.

Gruss, H. J., Ulrich, D., Braddy, S. *et al.* (1995) Recombinant CD30 ligand and CD40 ligand share common biological activities on Hodgkin and Reed–Sternberg cells. *European Journal of Immunology*, **25**, 2083–2089.

Hummel, M., Ziemann, K., Lammert, H. *et al.* (1995) Hodgkin's disease with monoclonal and polyclonal populations of Reed–Sternberg cells. *New England Journal of Medicine*, **333**, 901–906.

Kanzler, H., Kuppers, R., Hansmann, M. L. and Rajewsky, K. (1996) Hodgkin and Reed–Sternberg cells in Hodgkin's disease represent the outgrowth of a dominant tumor clone derived from (crippled) germinal center B cells. *Journal of Experimental Medicine*, **184**, 1495–1505.

Kuppers, R., Rajewsky, K., Zhao, M. *et al.* (1995) Hodgkin's disease: clonal Ig gene rearrangements in Hodgkin and Reed–Sternberg cells picked from histological sections. *Annals of the New York Academy of Sciences*, **764**, 523–524.

Orscheschek, K., Merz, H., Hell, J. *et al.* (1995) Large-cell anaplastic lymphoma-specific translocation (t[2;5] [p23;q35]) in Hodgkin's disease: indication of a common pathogenesis? *Lancet*, **345**, 87–90.

Spina, D., Leoncini, L., Close, P. *et al.* (1996) Growth vs. DNA strand breaks in

Hodgkin's disease: impaired proliferative ability of Hodgkin and Reed–Sternberg cells. *International Journal of Cancer*, **66**, 179–183.

Stoler, M. H., Nichols, G. E., Symbula, M. and Weiss, L. M. (1995) Lymphocyte predominance Hodgkin's disease. Evidence for a kappa light chain-restricted monotypic B-cell neoplasm. *American Journal of Pathology*, **146**, 812–818.

Vasef, M. A., Kamel, O. W., Chen, Y. Y. *et al.* (1995) Detection of Epstein–Barr virus in multiple sites involved by Hodgkin's disease. *American Journal of Pathology*, **147**, 1408–1415.

Weiss, L. M., Lopategui, J. R., Sun, L. H. *et al.* (1995) Absence of the t(2;5) in Hodgkin's disease. *Blood*, **85**, 2845–2847.

7.6.3 Staging and treatment of Hodgkin's disease

Armitage, J. O. (1994) Early bone marrow transplantation in Hodgkin's disease. *Annals of Oncology*, **5**(Suppl. 2), 161–163.

Carde, P. (1995) Should poor risk patients with Hodgkin's disease be sorted out for intensive treatments? *Leukemia and Lymphoma*, **15**(Suppl. 1), 31–40.

Crowther, D. and Lister, T. A. (1990) The Cotswold report on the investigation and staging of Hodgkin's disease. *British Journal of Cancer*, **62**, 51–55.

Cullen, M. H., Stuart, N. S. A., Woodroffe, C. *et al.* (1994) ChLVPP/PABlOE and radiotherapy in advanced Hodgkin's disease. *Journal of Clinical Oncology*, **12**, 779–787.

Rosenberg, S. A. (1994) Modern combined modality management of Hodgkin's disease. *Current Opinion in Oncology*, **6**, 470–472.

Sankila, R., Garwiez, S., Olsen, J. H. *et al.* (1996) Risk of subsequent malignant neoplasms among 1641 Hodgkin's disease patients diagnosed in childhood and adolescence: a population-based cohort study in the five Nordic countries. *Journal of Clinical Oncology*, **14**, 1442–1446.

Vivani, S., Bonadonna, G., Santoro, A. *et al.* (1996) Alternating versus hybrid MOPP and ABVD combinations in advanced Hodgkin's disease: ten year results. *Journal of Clinical Oncology*, **14**, 1421–1430.

Peripheral B-cell lymphoproliferative disorders in lymph nodes, spleen, blood and bone marrow

8

Peripheral B-cell lymphoproliferative disorders are tumours that consist of immunocompetent B-cells that have completed the rearrangement of their immunoglobulin genes, as opposed to lymphoblastic disease, which consists of B-cell precursors. This is by far the largest group of lymphoproliferative disorders but as yet there is no satisfactory explanation as to why peripheral B-cells are so much more susceptible to neoplastic transformation than peripheral T-cells. Primary extranodal B-cell lymphoproliferative disorders are distinctive in their clinical presentation, therapy and pathogenesis and are considered separately in Chapter 10. This chapter focuses on B-cell neoplasms that primarily affect lymph nodes, spleen, blood and marrow. Unlike peripheral T-cell lymphomas the principles of classification of peripheral B-cell lymphomas are now largely agreed.

This chapter is, by necessity, the longest in the book and includes the most common types of lymphoproliferative disorder as well as a number of rare entities. The chapter is divided into three main sections according to broad clinical categories. The first section covers tumours in which lymphadenopathy is usually the predominant feature – follicle centre lymphoma, diffuse large B-cell lymphoma and its variants, mantle cell lymphoma and nodal marginal zone lymphoma. The second section deals with the chronic B-cell leukaemias. The third section considers the immunosecretory disorders, including plasma cell myeloma and Waldenström's macroglobulinaemia, where dysregulated secretion of antibody is

Table 8.1 The main categories of peripheral B-cell lymphoproliferative disorders

- Follicle centre lymphoma
- Diffuse large cell lymphoma
- T-cell-rich B cell lymphoma
- Mantle cell lymphoma
- Marginal zone lymphoma
- Chronic lymphocytic leukaemia (lymphocytic lymphoma)
- Prolymphocytic leukaemia
- Hairy cell leukaemia
- Splenic lymphoma with villous lymphocytes
- Waldenström's macroglobulinaemia
- Multiple myeloma

the central feature. Assignment of each type of B-cell lymphoproliferative disorder to one of these categories is, of course, somewhat arbitrary, but may be useful as a broad framework for understanding this group of tumours (Table 8.1).

8.1 Tumours in which lymphadenopathy is the predominant feature

8.1.1 Follicle centre lymphoma

Follicle centre lymphomas are recognized by abnormal follicular microarchitecture

The normal germinal centre is a transient structure where B-cells responding to antigen undergo clonal expansion and mutation of immunoglobulin genes. Cells are selected by antigen-binding affinity to survive and differentiate into memory B-cell and plasma cells.

Follicle centre lymphomas (FCL) consist of neoplastic centrocytes and centroblasts similar morphologically and in most phenotypic features to those seen in a reactive germinal centre but differing in relative proportion and most importantly in the structure of the follicles that the tumour cells form (Figure 8.1).

Centrocytes are usually about 10–12 μm in diameter and have a folded or cleaved nucleus, one or more small nucleoli and minimal cytoplasm. Centroblasts are larger, in the range 15–20 μm, with round nuclei, two or three small basophilic nucleoli located close to the nuclear membrane and distinctive basophilic cytoplasm, which is best seen in a Giemsa-stained section. In some lymphomas these cell types may show much greater variation in size and nuclear configuration. The cells in most follicle centre lymphomas express sIg, although in a significant proportion this may be very weak or even absent. Clonality can sometimes be demonstrated in paraffin sections using immunoglobulin light-chain restriction but this requires excellent tissue preservation. As is the case in normal germinal centre cells, tumour cells may express either IgM or, if class switching has occurred, IgG. Germinal centre cells have a distinctive phenotype with almost every case strongly expressing pan-B-cell markers, including CD19, CD79 and CD20. In paraffin sections almost all tumour cells and their normal equivalents will express CDw75. The expression of CD10 is characteristic although it is a very variable feature of FCL. CD10 is a surface endopeptidase that appears to be involved in the modulation of the activity of peptide cytokines and appears to be inversely expressed with CD23. CD23 is a low-affinity IgE receptor, which is rapidly shed from the cell surface. There is some evidence that this may have an autocrine effect on normal B-cell growth, although its effect on neoplastic cells is not known (Figure 8.2).

The features of follicle centre lymphoma are summarized in Table 8.2.

Neoplastic follicle centre cells either form structurally abnormal follicles or grow diffusely but in practice pure diffuse follicle centre lymphomas are very rare when adequate biopsy material is available. The term 'diffuse centroblastic/centrocytic' was used more frequently in the pre-immunocytochemistry era and it is a matter of conjecture how these cases would now be classified, but they are likely to include mantle cell lymphoma, marginal zone lymphoma and some T-cell lymphoma.

Unlike normal germinal centres, neoplastic follicles do not have a zonal structure and are not confined to the cortex of the node but replace the entire node and spread into the surrounding tissues. In most cases the neoplastic follicle contains a high proportion of centrocytes; the centroblast-rich proliferative zone is lost or may be confined to a rim at the periphery of the follicle. Apoptosis, which is highly characteristic of reactive germinal centres is greatly reduced in neoplastic follicles and there may be no macrophages containing cell debris. The follicular dendritic cell network is very variable in neoplastic follicles: it may appear normal or be greatly reduced and almost absent. The presence and size of the lymphocyte mantle is also a variable feature. In many cases it is completely absent, but in some cases it is partly retained. Interestingly, when a mantle zone is present it can be shown in some cases to be part of the tumour while in others it appears to be a residual normal structure with polyclonal immunoglobulin expression.

Failure of apoptosis is a central feature in the pathogenesis of germinal centre cell lymphoma

In the normal germinal centre a high proportion of cells undergo apoptosis and debris is taken up by the resident macrophage population.

Figure 8.1 Follicle centre lymphoma. In follicle centre cell lymphoma the internal structure of the germinal centre is lost and is replaced in most cases by a relatively monomorphic population of centrocytes **(a)**. These cells have irregular or cleaved nuclei and one or more small nucleoli **(b)**. The follicular growth pattern is clearly seen using a reticulin stain **(c)**. In almost all cases neoplastic follicle centre cells express *bcl-2* **(d)**, which is not found in significant numbers of normal germinal centre cells.

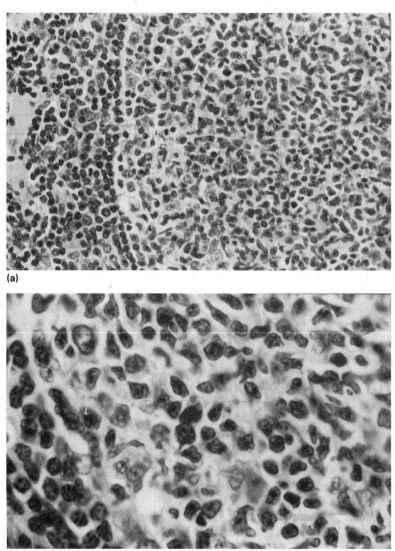

(a)

(b)

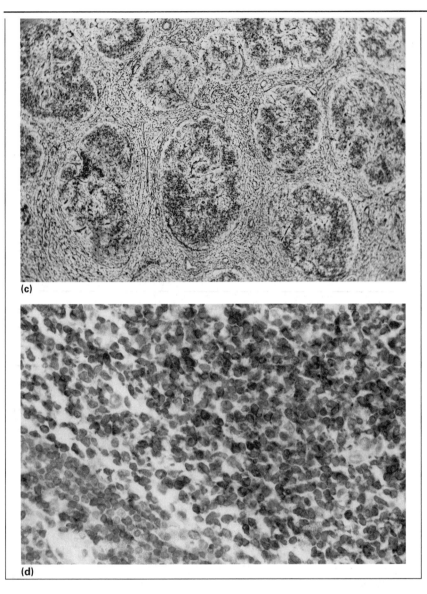

(c)

(d)

Those cells destined to survive as memory or preplasma cells are induced to express Bcl-2. A similar feature is noted *in vitro*, where cultured germinal centre cell cells will only survive for a short time unless Bcl-2 is induced, usually by stimulation of CD40 by its ligand or antibody. Bcl-2 forms homodimers or heterodimers with Bax and the relative proportions of Bax and Bcl-2 determine the probability of apoptosis. In normal lymphoid tissue very few germinal centre cells express Bcl-2, although some express Bax. A very important feature of almost all cases of follicle centre lymphomas is the aberrant expression of Bcl-2. This is now a key

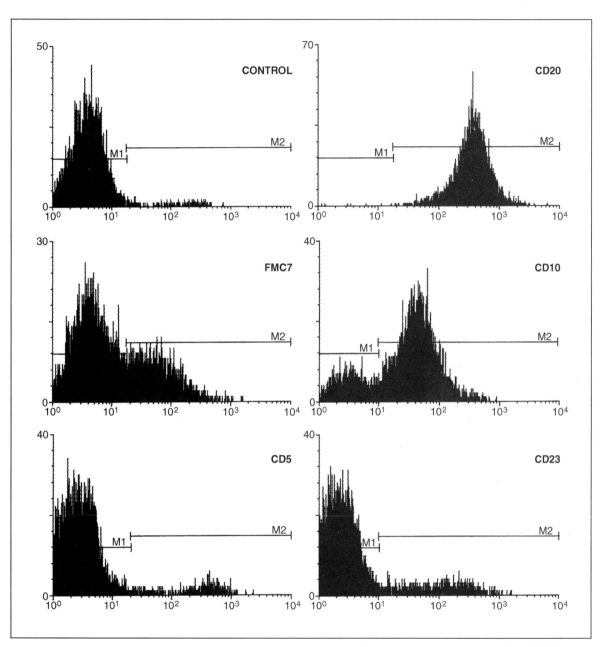

Figure 8.2 Follicle centre lymphoma – immunophenotype. This shows the flow cytometric analysis of a follicle centre lymphoma. There is CD10 expression with absent CD5 and CD23. Otherwise typical cases may show considerable variation in CD10 expression and in some cases CD23 may also be produced by some of the cells. Both CD10 and CD23 are important determinants of B-cell growth and variations in expression of these molecules may in part account for the heterogeneous clinical behaviour of the tumours.

Table 8.2 Follicle centre lymphoma

- **Morphology**: Cells resembling germinal centre centrocytes and centroblasts. Tumours vary in the proportions of these cells and degree of cytological atypia.
- **Immunophenotype**: sIg$^+$ (any heavy chain – usually IgM or IgG), CD19$^+$, CD20$^+$, CD5$^-$, CD10$^{+/-}$, CD23$^{+/-}$ (CD10 and 23 tend to be inversely related), CD38$^{+/-}$, Bcl-2$^+$, CDw75$^+$.
- **Cytogenetics**: t(14;18) with *bcl-2* deregulation in almost all cases.
- **Pattern of disease**: Most cases have stage III or IV nodal disease and marrow disease at presentation. Blood involvement is less common. Wide variation in rate of progression. A proportion of cases transform to diffuse large B-cell lymphoma.

diagnostic feature although some caution is needed in the interpretation of this finding. The T-cells that are a component of both normal and neoplastic germinal centres express Bcl-2 and so it is essential to ensure that the positive cells have typical germinal centre cell morphology and phenotype. The antibody MT-2 (CD45RA) shows a similar pattern of reactivity to anti-Bcl-2 with aberrant expression being a common feature of follicle centre lymphomas. MT-2 is also helpful in delineating a residual mantle zone.

The deregulated expression of Bcl-2 is caused by the translocation of the *bcl-2* gene into the JH region of the *IgH* gene. The translocation involves a breakpoint within the JH region of the *IgH* gene on chromosome 14 and one of two regions close to the *bcl-2* gene on chromosome 18 (Figure 8.3).

Most occur in the major breakpoint cluster (mbr) region, which is in the 3′ untranslated portion of the gene, with a minority in the minor cluster region (mcr) which is 20 kb 3′ of the *bcl-2* gene. Other much less common variants may occur. A high proportion of translocations will be detected by Southern analysis using probes to these regions. PCR is a more practical method of detection and is the only option when fixed tissue is being used, but it should be noted that a much greater number of false negatives are found than with Southern blotting. Demonstration of t(14;18) is seldom of direct importance in the diagnosis of typical follicle centre lymphomas. Its main role is likely to be in disease monitoring but there are some circumstances, such as the diagnosis of unusual morphological variants, when it may have a role.

The translocation also occurs in a proportion of diffuse large cell lymphomas and the value of the t(14;18) as a diagnostic test is further

Figure 8.3 The t(14;18). This involves the translocation of the *bcl-2* gene from chr18 to the *IgH* locus on chr14. About 70% of the breakpoints on chr18 occur within the MBR region and 30% in the MCR region. The effect of this translocation is dysregulation of the expression of Bcl-2 and inhibition of programmed cell death.

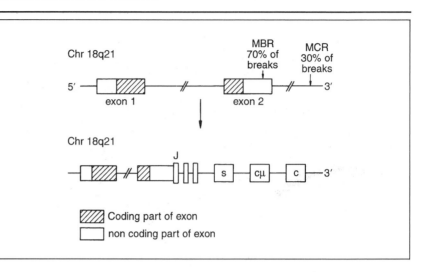

limited by the finding that small clones of lymphocytes bearing this translocation may be found in up to 5% of reactive lymph nodes and peripheral blood samples from individuals who do not have lymphoma. The fate of these cells is unknown and there is no information as to whether this finding carries an increased risk of lymphoma. Somatic mutation is a feature of normal germinal cells and there is evidence that this process may affect the translocated *bcl-2* gene in neoplastic cells. In some cases of transformed follicle centre lymphoma increased levels of *bcl-2* mutation may be found.

A small proportion of cases of FCL appear to lack evidence of a t(14;18) and do not show abnormal Bcl-2 expression. These cases are identical in other respects to Bcl-2-positive cases, which raises the interesting question as to whether an abnormality elsewhere in the apoptotic control pathway may lead to the development of the tumour.

Morphological variants of follicle centre cell lymphoma may cause diagnostic difficulty

The description of classic follicle centre lymphoma above applies to over 95% of cases but a number of rare variants may cause diagnostic difficulties (Figure 8.4).

A degree of sclerosis is often present in FCL but in a few cases this may be extensive. In sclerotic areas the tumour cells are dispersed in small cords or aggregates, but in some cases nodule formation may lead to confusion with nodular sclerosing Hodgkin's disease. Basic cell marker studies and attention to the clinical features should prevent this problem.

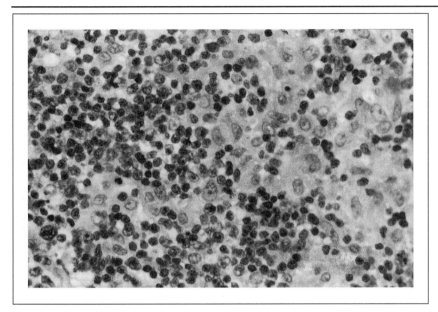

Figure 8.4 Histiocyte-rich follicle centre lymphoma. This is a case of otherwise typical FCL in which the neoplastic follicles contain a high proportion of reactive histiocytes. The differential diagnosis may include Hodgkin's disease and Lennert's-type peripheral T-cell lymphoma.

In some cases of FCL very large numbers of epithelioid macrophages are present and these may form granulomas. This may be difficult to distinguish from lymphocyte-predominant nodular Hodgkin's disease. This is resolved by demonstrating monoclonality in the germinal centre cells, abnormal Bcl-2 expression and a t(14;18).

In the signet-ring-cell variant of FCL (Figure 8.5) the neoplastic centrocytes have a large vacuole that contains an as yet unidentified protein. It is possible that this tumour could be confused with metastatic adenocarcinoma on morphological grounds but this should never occur if appropriate markers are used.

Follicle centre lymphomas are usually disseminated at presentation

Almost all patients with FCL will present with widespread painless lymphadenopathy. On clinical examination the nodes may be large but are usually well circumscribed without obvious invasion and attachment to deep tissues. Further clinical examination and imaging studies will show disseminated stage III or IV disease in almost all patients. It is important to identify the small number of patients with localized disease who may be successfully treated with radiotherapy. A further group of patients who present with abdominal symptoms often have extensive bulky disease within the mesenteric and retroperitoneal nodes without obvious peripheral lymphadenopathy.

Figure 8.5 Signet-ring variant of FCL. In this case of FCL the centrocytes have a large cytoplasmic vacuole and morphologically resemble the signet-ring cells (arrow) seen in some epithelial tumours. The nature of the vacuole contents is unknown.

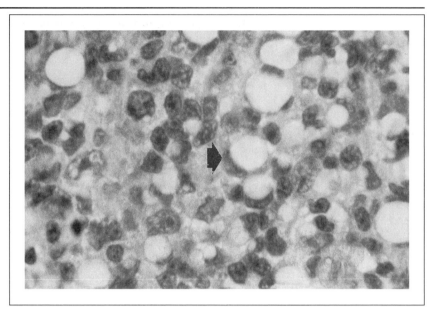

Bone-marrow infiltration is very common in follicle centre lymphoma. In a single marrow aspirate and trephine biopsy over 50% of patients will show infiltration and this proportion is increased by multiple biopsies and the use of PCR techniques to detect monoclonality or t(14;18). Follicle centre lymphoma infiltrates the marrow in a characteristic pattern, which usually consists almost entirely of small centrocytes aggregated in the paratrabecular region. As the disease progresses these areas expand to become confluent. It is important to recognize that although marrow infiltration is very common the extent of involvement varies widely. In many patients only a few small paratrabecular aggregates may be seen. However, in a significant minority the marrow may be completely replaced, which may potentially limit therapy (Figure 8.6).

It should be possible to make a confident diagnosis of FCL on a marrow examination, especially when cells are available for flow cytometry and immunogenetic studies. This may be of value where a CT-guided biopsy of a deep lesion is suggestive of the diagnosis but inconclusive. However, a degree of caution is required as typical FCL in marrow may be present in a patient who has transformed aggressive nodal disease. Close correlation with imaging findings, LDH and beta-2-microglobulin levels are important.

Overt peripheral blood involvement is relatively rare although routine use of flow cytometry and immunogenetic monitoring will detect many more patients with small numbers of circulating cells.

The clinical course of follicle centre lymphoma is variable and difficult to predict at presentation

The criteria that define follicle centre lymphoma are clear and if rigorously applied should lead to a high degree of diagnostic consistency. However, this should not be taken as an indication that this is a homogenous group of tumours. Patients show considerable variation in the disease progression and this is matched by similar variation in a number of cellular features.

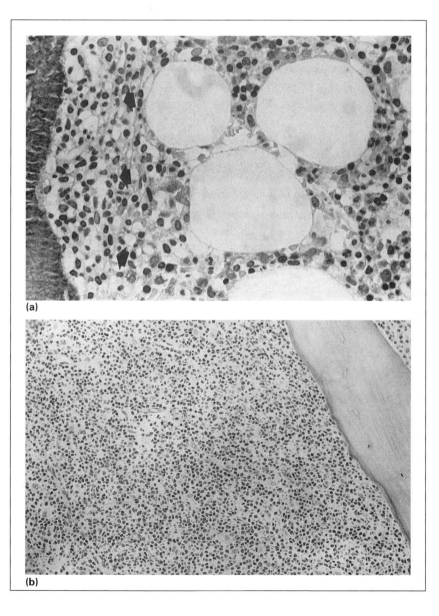

(a)

(b)

Figure 8.6 Bone marrow infiltration by FCL. The extent of marrow infiltration by FCL varies widely from **(a)** a minimal paratrabecular deposit (arrow) to **(b)** marrow replacement. The extent of marrow reserve may affect the delivery of therapy.

The typical patient with FCL has disseminated disease at presentation but will achieve a complete clinical remission with therapy. A protracted clinical course follows, lasting 5–7 years, punctuated by relapses at decreasing intervals. The terminal phase of the disease is usually characterized by progressively increasing disease bulk but some patients may die of intercurrent infections. Alternatively patients may present with high-bulk aggressive disease or develop this shortly after presentation. Despite this variety of natural histories, the majority of cases of follicle centre lymphoma affect elderly patients and a proportion will die of causes unrelated to this malignant process.

In some patients transformation to diffuse large cell lymphoma occurs. This is defined as replacement of all or part of the node by a cohesive infiltrate of centroblasts and immunoblasts. A qualitative change of this type suggests genetic progression. Clinically, this will be apparent as a rapidly expanding node or group of nodes. The incidence of transformation is uncertain. In many trials a high incidence is cited but transformation is defined only as progressive lymphadenopathy without histological confirmation. Transformation of FCL is relatively rare in lymph node biopsies but is much more commonly seen at autopsy. Transformation may also occur prior to clinical presentation with evidence of the underlying FCL being found in bone marrow (Figure 8.7).

Wide variation is also found in a number of the cellular characteristics of follicle centre lymphomas. Many of these variables have been assessed as possible predictors of clinical behaviour. The most widely used are cell size and the relative proportions of centroblasts. The International Working Formulation divides follicle centre lymphomas into low-grade[1] and intermediate-grade on the basis of the proportion of large centrocytes and centroblasts. These criteria are based on the survival characteristics of the patients included in the original multinational study that formed the basis of the classification. In practice this is highly subjective and may be complicated by considerable variation between neoplastic follicles within the same lymph node or between lymph nodes from the same patient. It is possible to devise morphometric methods for measuring cell size and shape but these are very labour-intensive and are not suitable for routine diagnostic use. Although in the context of clinical studies large cell size does seem to correlate with aggressiveness this has not been found to be of value in directing therapy for the individual patient.

Cell proliferation in most follicle centre lymphomas is low and may be considerably less than is seen in a reactive germinal centre. The cell

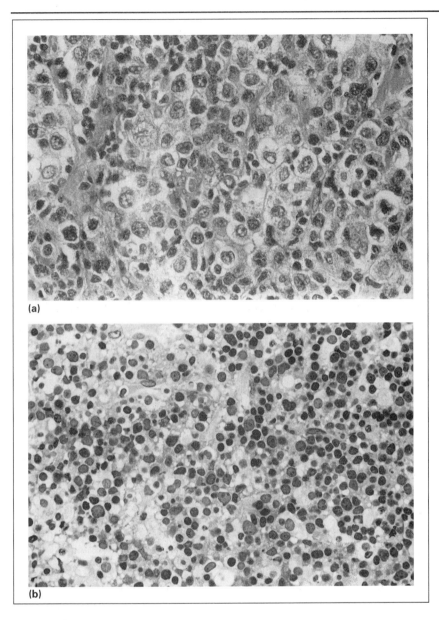

(a)

(b)

Figure 8.7 Transformed follicle centre lymphoma. In most cases of transformation of FCL a node or part of a node is replaced by a diffuse infiltrate of large B-cells **(a)**. In a few cases transformation results in marrow replacement and leukaemia **(b)** with cellular morphology resembling Burkitt's lymphoma. In some of these cases a t(8;14) has been shown, with deregulation of c-Myc.

cycle fraction defined by anti-Ki67 antibodies is routinely used in most laboratories as a convenient measure of cell proliferation. Again, this shows wide variation between different tumours but in some cases there may be up to a fivefold difference between follicles in the same biopsy. The non-random distribution of Ki67 reactivity means that it is difficult to state a single value that accurately describes a particular tumour's cell cycle fraction. As with cell size there appears to be a general correlation with clinical behaviour that is not sufficiently accurate for directing therapy.

Phenotypical variation also occurs in the expression of markers such as CD10, CD23 and Bcl-2, all of which may be important determinants of tumour growth. In normal germinal centres follicular dendritic cells are a key element in the organization of growth and differentiation. Follicular dendritic cells are almost always present in FCL but their number and the size of the dendritic networks formed varies widely.

The reason for this variation in cellular and clinical features is not clear. One explanation may lie in the high incidence of apparently random genetic change that may be seen in these tumours. This can be detected by allelic imbalance and microsatellite instability of repeat sequence loci. It is possible to speculate that these high levels of genetic change may be responsible for the sporadic expression of p53 that occurs in these tumours. A complex interaction between genetic change, cell proliferation and partial or complete inhibition of apoptosis by Bcl-2 may determine the probability of tumour progression. In about 20–30% of transformed cases mutational inactivation of *p53* occurs. When combined with Bcl-2 expression this will greatly facilitate the genetic evolution of the tumour by blocking the removal of cells which acquire new genetic abnormalities, but mutational inactivation or deletion of *p53* is not an essential step in transformation. In a very few cases FCL transforms to a very aggressive tumour that resembles Burkitt's-like large cell lymphoma. These patients show rapid disease progression, often with a leukaemic phase. This pattern of disease progression is sometimes associated with deregulation of c-*myc*, usually due to t(8;14).

At the present time there are no cellular or molecular features that allow accurate prediction of clinical behaviour in the individual patient.

Other lymphomas with a nodular growth pattern need to be considered in the differential diagnosis

A number of other lymphomas have a nodular growth pattern and all of these can be confused with follicle centre lymphoma. The most common differential diagnosis is lymphocyte-predominant nodular Hodgkin's disease (LPNHD). In this condition the nodules are much larger and although they appear to be derived from B-cell follicles the cellular content is much more varied than in follicle centre lymphoma. The B-cell population will be polyclonal. The patient with LPNHD will have localized cervical disease and is very unlikely to have generalized lymphadenopathy. A few cases of classical-type Hodgkin's disease may also have follicular pattern of growth.

The presence of large proliferation centres in CLL/lymphocytic lymphoma may produce a histological pattern that resembles follicle centre lymphoma. The cells in the proliferation centres may also express CD75, CD20 and variable Bcl-2. However, there are several important differences that allow confident distinction of these tumours. Proliferation centre cells are prolymphocytes and immunoblasts with prominent nucleoli. The proliferation centres do not have the reticulin pattern or the follicular dendritic cell network present in follicle centre lymphoma. The surrounding cells in lymphocytic lymphoma are small lymphocytes, which in fixed tissue are weakly CD20, CD43$^+$, CD5$^+$, CD23$^+$ and in fresh tissue express weak sIg and CD5. This phenotype is not seen in follicle centre lymphoma. The diagnosis of CLL will usually be obvious in the peripheral blood or bone marrow.

Other lymphomas produce a nodular pattern by colonizing existing reactive germinal centres. The most important diagnosis to consider is mantle cell lymphoma, which also has cytological similarity to follicle centre lymphoma. Nodal involvement by a marginal cell lymphoma of extranodal origin (MALToma) may also show follicular colonization, again with cytological similarities to follicle centre lymphoma. These cells may also show Bcl-2 expression without a t(14;18). These tumours can be distinguished phenotypically by absence of CD10 and weak or absent CD75 expression, but of greater value is the demonstration of residual fragments of germinal centres or mantle zones. These may be seen on H&E section but are more readily demonstrated using a combination of markers that includes CD75 (germinal centre cells), CD21 (follicular dendritic cells) and IgD (mantle cells). Secondary infiltration of the node by marginal zone lymphoma is most likely to be a diagnostic problem in neck nodes with tumour spreading from salivary gland. At other sites – gastrointestinal and respiratory – the primary tumour is much more likely to be the presenting feature. It is also very unlikely that a marginal zone lymphoma will be widely disseminated or show bone marrow disease.

These differential diagnoses can all be readily resolved by marker studies but also illustrate the value of close correlation of clinical and staging information.

Treatment of follicle centre lymphoma

Typically FCL is slowly progressive and treatment may not be required or indicated initially

While slowly increasing lymphadenopathy is usual, spontaneous remissions or prolonged periods of stability may also be seen and a 'watch and wait' policy can reasonably be adopted in many patients initially. A variety of prognostic factors have been identified – age, the presence of B symptoms, bulk of disease, extent of extra nodal disease, serum beta-2-microglobulin (β_2m) and serum LDH – but treatment strategies have not generally been determined using such information. Systems such as the International Prognostic Index for non-Hodgkin's disease may come to be applied prospectively in developing treatment strategies in the future.

For the 15–20% of patients with clinically localized disease at presentation, radiotherapy is effective treatment with the probability of prolonged disease survival and the possibility of cure. Decisions to treat may often be delayed without significant effect on longer-term outcome. Although the detection of immunoglobulin gene rearrangements or of t(14;18) by PCR in blood or bone marrow indicate that disease is not localized, 'local control' of disease is likely to continue as an acceptable early treatment modality in the absence of definitive curative therapy.

Alkylating agents and corticosteroids have been the mainstay of treatment for many years

Treatment with alkylating agents, corticosteroids or combinations, of patients with non-localized disease usually brings about resolution of symptoms, with reduction in disease bulk of varying degree. There is no good evidence that combinations such as COP (cyclophosphamide, vincristine, prednisolone) or CVP (cyclophosphamide, vinblastine, prednisolone) have any significant advantage over chlorambucil or cyclophosphamide given alone. Treatment is usually given intermittently, partly because continuing treatment after disease regression is not necessary and partly to reduce the long-term mutagenic effects of exposure to alkylating agent therapy. Despite this a relapsing course is usual, with a tendency to shorter remissions, progressive or transformed disease leading ultimately to death. For patients with non-localized disease the median survival is 7–9 years.

The success of anthracycline-containing combinations in the treatment of more aggressive lymphomas encouraged their use in follicle centre lymphoma. Combinations such as CHOP may achieve a greater proportion of complete remissions, as clinically defined, with some prolongation of remission duration, but no clear overall survival benefit has been demonstrated and it has not, as yet, been possible to clearly define patient groups, based on cellular characteristics or prognostic factor information, for whom combination chemotherapy would be more appropriate.

Maintenance therapy to prolong responses has not been shown to confer any advantage, though there has been particular interest in the use of alpha-interferon (IFNα) as a means of delaying disease recurrence or progress. IFN α, which has modest activity in follicle centre lymphoma as a single agent, given as part of induction therapy or as maintenance, has been shown to prolong remissions, though it does not appreciably influence the pattern of eventual relapse or overall survival.

A wide range of cytotoxic agents have demonstrable activity in recurrent follicle centre lymphoma

Alternative combinations to CHOP, e.g. those which include the anthracenedione mitozantrone, have been found to be well tolerated and effective. The purine analogues, deoxycoformycin, fludarabine and 2-chlorodeoxyadenosine (2CDA), all have activity against follicle centre lymphoma. Both fludarabine and 2CDA are well tolerated by patients and have been reported as achieving responses in 50–70% of patients with recurrent disease. An important side effect of such treatment, however, is the sustained suppression of T-cells, which may significantly increase the risk of opportunistic infection (particularly in patients also receiving corticosteroids). The possibility of transfusion-associated GvHD makes the use of irradiated blood products mandatory. Combinations of purine analogues and other active agents that enhance the effect of the purine analogue are being explored, with the possibility of developing more effective relapse schedules that will produce greater numbers of complete responses and hopefully prolong survival.

Monoclonal antibodies may have a valuable role in therapy in the future

The use of anti-idiotype antibodies is an interesting experimental approach for tumours that express surface immunoglobulin, although at present the production of an anti-idiotype antibody is not practical. Unfortunately, in many cases following exposure to antibody and initial response the tumours rapidly grow back but have now lost expression of the epitope on the cell surface and no longer respond. A novel development of this anti-idiotype strategy is to copy and clone the idiotypical determinant using PCR, which is then injected into skeletal muscle, resulting in high-level expression of the antigen and an endogenous anti-idiotype response. B-cell-specific antibodies may also be conjugated with toxins such as ricin, saponin or a radioisotope. Although activity has been demonstrated in phase I trials, repeated treatment is likely to be limited because of the development of antiricin and antimurine antibodies, although humanization of the antibody can circumvent this problem. Humanized anti-CD20 is a promising monoclonal antibody shown to have activity alone or in an yttrium-90-labelled form and also in combination with chemotherapeutic agents. It seems likely that monoclonal antibody therapy will be explored further as part of the development of new strategies for treating follicle centre lymphoma.

More intensive approaches may be feasible and justifiable in younger patients

High-dose therapy with haemopoietic stem cell support is an investigational approach being applied to younger patients with follicle centre lymphoma, justified because of the generally poor results of conventional treatment. In the studies carried out to date follow-up has been too short to demonstrate that any patients are cured and this is not really expected. Widespread clinical application awaits the results of randomized trials of conventional chemotherapy *versus* high-dose therapy with stem cell support, which are being carried out at relapse. The use of peripheral blood stem cells rather than autologous bone marrow in support of high-dose therapy has reduced the initial procedure-related toxicities. However, the high incidence of marrow disease means that in many cases the peripheral stem cell harvest will be contaminated by tumour cells. Heavy contamination can be detected by flow cytometry and low-level contamination by PCR for B-cell monoclonality and presence of the t(14;18). Not all of these cells are clonagenic and capable of regrowing if re-infused but the available evidence would support the use of uncontaminated peripheral stem cells if this is possible. Stem cell harvest can be 'purged' by CD34$^+$ selection; further negative selection with CD19 or other antibody to remove B-cells may prove a useful adjunct. The limited data on allogeneic bone marrow transplantation would suggest that this is at least an option in selected younger patients with highly refractory disease.

8.1.2 Diffuse large B-cell lymphoma

Diffuse large cell lymphomas (DLCL) are a major group of nodal lymphomas being approximately equal in incidence to follicle centre lymphoma. Unlike FCL, about one-third of diffuse large B-cell lymphomas are of extranodal origin and the distinction of nodal and extranodal diffuse large B-cell disease is of great importance from the point of view of clinical presentation, staging, therapy and even in some cases the cause of the tumour.

Diffuse large B-cell lymphomas show considerable morphological variation

In the Kiel classification DLCL are subdivided into immunoblastic and centroblastic types. The centroblastic lymphomas are then further subdivided into monomorphic, polymorphic, multilobated and centrocytoid types. The International Working Formulation divides DLCL into category G (intermediate grade) – diffuse large non-cleaved cell – and category H (high-grade) – immunoblastic. These distinctions are poorly reproducible and should not form the basis for therapeutic decisions. However, the description of these various morphological subtypes is useful as a guide to the morphological heterogeneity that is likely to be seen in this common group of tumours (Figure 8.8).

The typical centroblast is a medium to large lymphoid cell, around 15–20 μm in diameter with a round nucleus, a fine or vesicular chromatin pattern, three or four small peripheral nucleoli and scanty cytoplasm. This is analogous to the normal cells seen in the proliferation zone of the germinal centre. At least 10% of the cells in a tumour must be of this type to make a diagnosis of centroblastic lymphoma according to the Kiel criteria. Tumours in which more than 60% of the cells are of this type are classified by the Kiel classification as monomorphic centroblastic lymphomas. Most centroblastic lymphomas are more varied in cellular content and include immunoblasts, small and large centrocytes and a variety of intermediate forms. These are termed polymorphic centroblastic lymphomas; the Kiel classification includes the further criterion that such tumours should contain more than 10% immunoblasts. Multilobular cells will be found in a number of centroblastic lymphomas. These are a little larger than typical centroblastic cells but have a similar nuclear chromatin pattern and distribution of nucleoli. When more than 10–20% of these cells are present the Kiel classification uses the term multilobated centroblastic lymphoma.

Using the Kiel criteria problems can arise in distinguishing centroblastic from centroblastic/centrocytic (follicle centre lymphoma) in which centroblasts are numerous. The presence of cohesive groups of centroblasts is taken as the critical feature. In the Kiel classification centroblastic lymphomas may have a follicular growth pattern and be regarded as high-grade tumours, but this is very rare.

The fourth category of centroblastic lymphoma is the centrocytoid variant. This consists of smaller, round or irregular-shaped cells described as being intermediate between centroblasts and centrocytes. This category in particular may give rise to confusion with mantle cell lymphoma.

Figure 8.8 Diffuse large B-cell lymphoma. Most cases of diffuse large cell lymphoma contain a pleomorphic mixture of large B-cells with centroblastic or immunoblastic morphology **(a)**. In this case most of the cells have strong expression of CD79a **(b)**. Tumours of immunoblastic type in which almost all the cells have immunoblastic features with prominent large central nucleoli **(c)** are much less common. Clinical and immunogenetic differences between immunoblastic and other types of diffuse large cell lymphoma have not yet been fully documented.

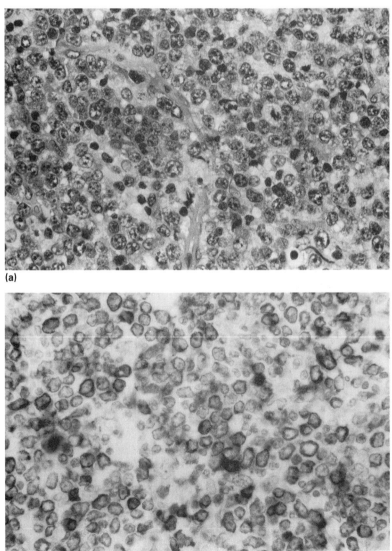

(a)

(b)

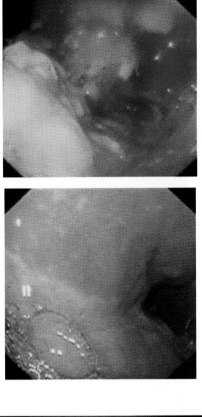

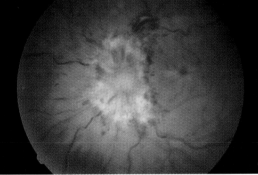

Plate 1 (a),(b) Gastric diffuse large cell lymphoma. At presentation this patient was found to a have a large ulcerated tumour in the pylorus **(a)** which on biopsy was shown to be a diffuse large B-cell lymphoma. After six cycles of CHOP chemotherapy a follow-up endoscopy and **(b)** biopsy showed complete resolution of the tumour.

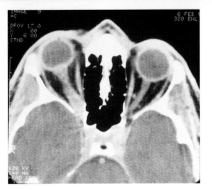

Plate 2 Acute lymphoblastic leukaemia – optic nerve. This adult patient, who was considered to be in remission following treatment for common acute lymphoblastic leukaemia, presented with loss of vision and headache. Examination of the retina **(a)** showed extensive infiltration of the optic disc. On CT scan **(b)** there was thickening of the optic nerve and lymphoblasts were found in the cerebrospinal fluid.

Plate 3 Untreated advanced Hodgkin's disease – cervical nodes. This patient presented with a long-standing progressively enlarging mass in the neck. On biopsy this was found to be nodular sclerosing Hodgkin's disease. Presentation with advanced bulky disease in cervical nodes is now rare.

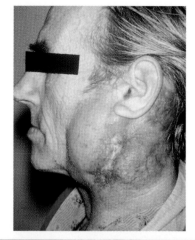

Plate 4 Relapsed Hodgkin's disease – chest wall. This patient, who had been treated by chemotherapy for mediastinal Hodgkin's disease, developed a recurrence, which involved the full thickness of the chest wall.

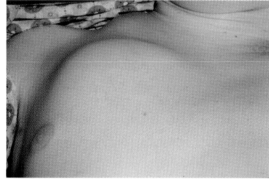

Plate 5 Diffuse large B-cell lymphoma – relapse in breast. This patient, who had been treated for diffuse large B-cell lymphoma, developed an indurated and inflamed mass in the right breast which was found to be due to lymphoma.

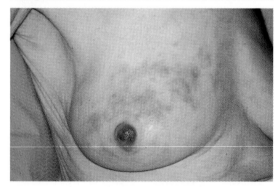

Plate 6 Primary cerebral lymphoma. This patient presented with raised intracranial pressure. A neurosurgical biopsy showed a primary intracerebral lymphoma. At autopsy there was an extensive haemorrhagic mass in the left temporal lobe.

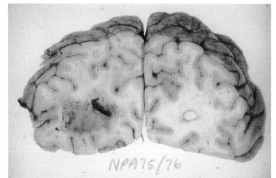

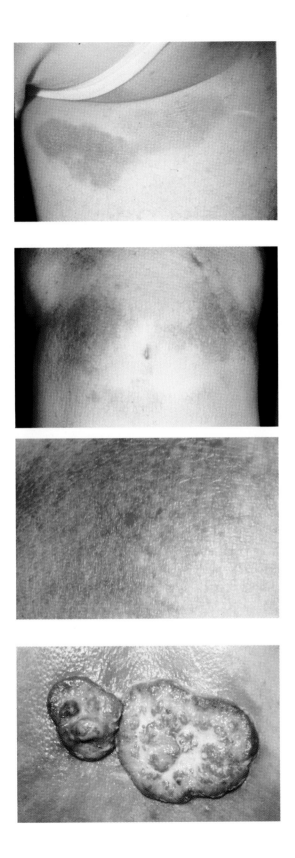

Plate 7 Parapsoriasis *en plaque* – early mycosis fungoides. This patient presented with irregular pruritic scaling plaques on the upper abdomen and was shown on biopsy to have early mycosis fungoides. The differential diagnosis of parapsoriasis *en plaque* includes cases of early mycosis fungoides and chronic superficial dermatitis and in some patients multiple biopsies over a period of time may be required to make a definitive diagnosis of lymphoma.

Plate 8 Mycosis fungoides – anterior abdomen. (a) Patient with extensive involvement of the abdominal skin by mycosis fungoides. Lesions are classified by clinical appearance into patches, plaques and tumour phases. In mycosis fungoides non-exposed skin is often affected. Closer examination of the rash **(b)** shows variable pigmentation, scaling and telangiectasia and degree of infiltration. Small nodules of tumour are present.

Plate 9 Tumour phase mycosis fungoides. This patient with long-standing mycosis fungoides developed multiple rapidly growing ulcerating nodules within plaques. This is a typical feature of late-stage disease and biopsy will often show an increasing proportion of large atypical T-cells and higher rates of proliferation than in plaque phase lesion.

Plate 10   Follicular mucinosis. This is a well circumscribed plaque in which many of the hair follicles are replaced by a plug of mucin. This lesion is caused by infiltration and destruction of hair follicles by mycosis fungoides, which is associated with over-production of mucopolysaccharide. A similar clinical appearance can be caused by chronic dermatitis reactions and fungal infection.

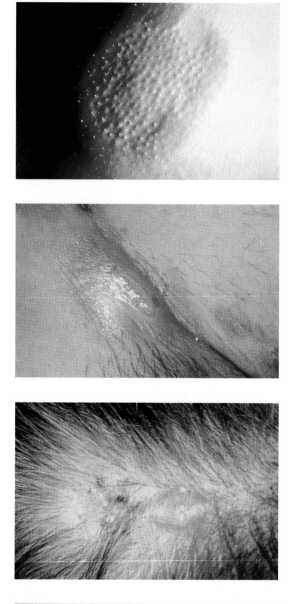

Plate 11   Lymphomatoid papulosis. This patient presented with a rapidly growing nodule in the groin, with central ulceration. A biopsy showed features of lymphomatoid papulosis. If lesions are not excised they undergo spontaneous regression. Relapses may occur over a long period.

Plate 12   Cutaneous lymphoid hyperplasia – scalp. This patient presented with a multinodular indurated lesion on the scalp. Biopsy showed features of cutaneous lymphoid hyperplasia. A direct cause is rarely identified and the lesion may recur. The clinical features are very similar to cutaneous B-cell lymphoma and these conditions can only be distinguished on biopsy.

Plate 13   Orbital infiltration by mantle cell lymphoma. This patient presented with infiltration of the oral mucosa and the extensive intra-abdominal disease. This was shown to be due to mantle cell lymphoma and bone marrow infiltration was presented. After commencing treatment the patient developed an intraorbital mass of lymphoma that extended into the subcutaneous tissue around the orbit.

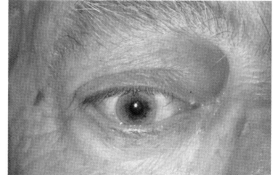

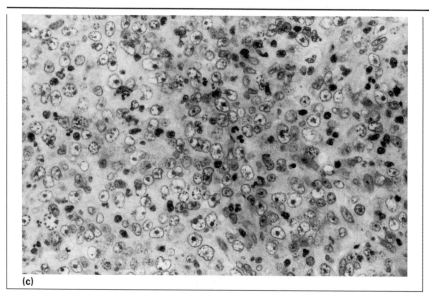

(c)

The morphological variation in centroblastic lymphomas is also reflected in phenotypical heterogeneity. About half of these tumours express moderate or strong IgM, but many are sIg-negative, either by flow cytometry or immunohistochemistry. All cases will be CD19$^+$ and CD20$^+$ but there is wide variation between and within tumours in the expression of germinal-centre-related markers CD10, CD23 and CDw75. Of these CDw75 is the most commonly found and is present on most cells in about 60% of tumours. Some centroblastic lymphomas also express CD43 and CD5, raising the question of the relationship to mantle cell lymphoma: it is not obvious how this relates to the centrocytoid variant. Rarely, CD43 and CDw75 can be coexpressed.

The features of diffuse large B-cell lymphoma are summarized in Table 8.3.

The term 'immunoblastic B-cell lymphoma' is used in the Kiel classification for tumours that consist almost entirely of immunoblasts (> 90%). These are large lymphoid cells with abundant cytoplasm, an oval nucleus and at least one central eosinophilic nucleolus. Tumours with immunoblasts that do not meet these criteria will be in the polymorphic centroblastic category. Many immunoblastic lymphomas will show some evidence of plasma cell differentiation. The immuno-phenotype of immunoblastic lymphomas is similar to centroblastic tumours with the exception of cIg expression. Where there are many preplasma cells some of the pan-B-cell markers may be partially lost. A few cases of DLCL of B-cell type have anaplastic morphology with

Table 8.3 Diffuse large B-cell lymphoma

- **Morphology**: Variable proportion of cells with features of centroblasts or immunoblasts. Large numbers of reactive T-cells may be present.
- **Immunophenotype**: Variable expression of surface and cytoplasmic immunoglobulin and B-lineage markers.
- **Cytogenetics**: t(14;18), t(8;14), 3q27 (*bcl-6*) abnormalities, t(12), *p53* mutation and others.
- **Pattern of disease**: May present with localized or disseminated disease at nodal and extranodal sites.

---

strong expression of CD30 and with cellular features similar to T-cell/null types of ALC lymphomas.

The cell-cycle fraction in DLCL defined by Ki67 may vary from 20–100% and similar differences may also be present in apoptotic rate. Diffuse large cell lymphomas also vary in terms of reactive cells present, with variable numbers of histiocytes and T-cells. In some cases these may be so numerous that the diagnosis is only apparent when the cell populations are separated by marker studies.

Diffuse large B-cell lymphoma may be localized or disseminated at presentation

Patients with diffuse large B-cell lymphomas present with rapidly expanding nodal masses. In most cases there will be a short history of lymphadenopathy, which may be at any site, although the neck is the most common. A proportion of patients may present with localized disease although in most of these cases imaging studies will show evidence of dissemination.

The disease bulk is determined by imaging studies of thorax and abdomen combined with clinical examination. It is interesting that bone marrow involvement and the detection of circulating tumour cells, either by morphology or flow cytometry, is very rare in DLCL at presentation. Despite this, these tumours are usually disseminated at presentation. Patients with high-bulk DLCL are usually symptomatic, with weight loss and classical B symptoms. Equally, patients presenting with early-stage disease may be asymptomatic apart from the presence of lymphadenopathy. β_2m and LDH and non-specific markers such as serum albumin are of value as serological markers of disease bulk and aggressiveness.

An unusual variant of diffuse large B-cell lymphoma shows angio-trophism with the accumulation of tumour cells within capillary beds leading to vascular stasis and ischaemia. This may be due to failure of the expression of adhesion molecules required to exit from blood vessels. The presentation of angiotrophic B-cell lymphomas will reflect the vascular beds involved and can include skin lesions, renal failure or seizures (Figures 8.9, 8.10).

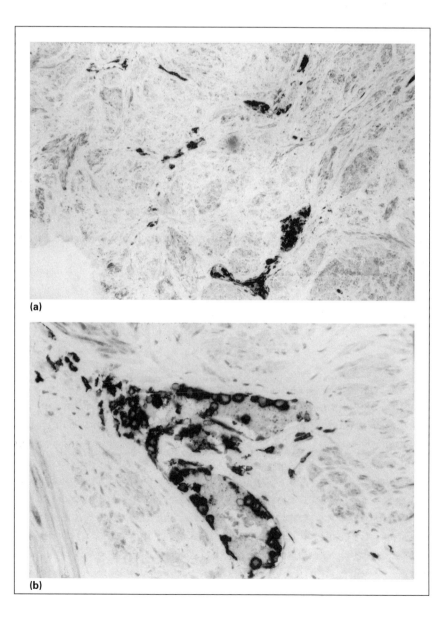

(a)

(b)

Figure 8.9 (a, b) Angiotrophic B-cell lymphoma. This patient presented with systemic symptoms and urinary retention. A resection of the prostate showed many vessels in which the endothelial surface was lined by CD20 large B-cells. CNS symptoms developed later. These tumours are a variant of diffuse large B-cell lymphoma. The angiotrophic behaviour may be due to a decreased ability to exit from vessels.

Figure 8.10 Diffuse large B-cell lymphoma. This patient with diffuse large B-cell lymphoma was found on CT scan to have bulky intra-abdominal disease.

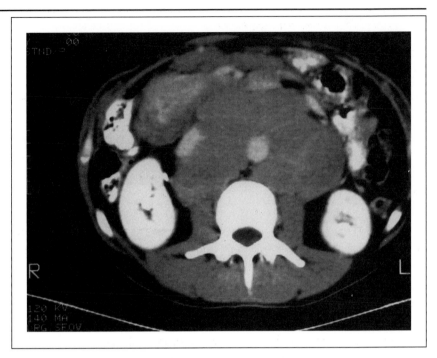

An unknown proportion of diffuse large cell lymphomas arise by transformation of a more indolent tumour

Follicle centre lymphomas are the most likely tumours to transform to DLCL. Transformation typically occurs during the progressive phase in a patient with preceding indolent disease but in some patients evidence of transformation may be present at the time of initial presentation. However, there are several other types of transformed disease with varying clinical consequences. Transformation of CLL is rare but may give rise to a nodal or soft tissue mass; these tumours are usually of immunoblastic type and are reported as frequently showing mutated *p53*.

The relationship of DLCL to mantle cell lymphoma is less clearly defined. An aggressive lymphoblastoid variant of mantle cell lymphoma is well described but it is possible that other less distinctive forms of DLCL lymphoma expressing CD5/CD43 may also be related. DLCL may also arise by transformation of LPNHD. In this case some of the tumour cells will resemble polylobated RS cells with expression of EMA. In many of these cases the disease is localized and should have a good prognosis.

Staging of diffuse large cell lymphoma

Staging of diffuse large cell lymphoma is only useful as part of a general prognostic index

The Ann Arbor staging system (Table 8.4), with its emphasis on anatomical distribution of disease and particularly nodal involvement, correlates much less well with the true extent of disease and progress in diffuse large cell lymphoma than in Hodgkin's disease. A large number of factors have been identified as having prognostic significance and a variety of prognostic models have been proposed.

Multivariate analysis has shown five pretreatment characteristics to be independently significant in the prediction of outcome. These were used as the basis of the International Prognostic Index (IPI). Three of these remained independently significant in patients aged 60 years or younger (Table 8.5). One of the major problems with such approaches is establishing a universally acceptable system that is of practical value in clinical practice. There would be considerable attraction in using simple objective measurements that are easily reproducible and the fact that LDH and beta-2-microglobulins are quite powerful independent prognostic indicators has led to their use in stratification. Currently, the IPI is being adopted in prospective trials of treatment but it may well be superseded in due course. A particular concern is the fact that some younger patients with extensive and bulky, but localized, disease who happen to have a relatively good performance status and/or normal LDH will be assigned to the better prognostic categories.

Poor prognostic features can be identified at presentation

These tend to reflect the bulk of the disease and the host's ability to resist the effects of the tumour and treatment. In one investigation the four IPI risk groups – low, low intermediate, high intermediate and high – were associated with predicted 5-year survivals of 73%, 51%, 43% and 26%. (These categories should not be confused with tumour grade.) Factors associated with a poor 5-year survival are the same as those associated with relapse.

Treatment of large cell lymphoma

Anthracycline-containing combination chemotherapy has been the standard treatment for many years

Although various cytotoxic drugs, notably alkylating agents, have been used in the treatment of lymphoma, the introduction of combination chemotherapy in the early 1970s was a watershed in the development of

Table 8.4 The Ann Arbor staging system

Stage I	I	A single lymph node
	IE	A single extralymphatic site
Stage II	II	Two or more nodal regions on the same side of the diaphragm
	IIE	A single extralymphatic site plus nodal involvement on same side of diaphragm
	IIS	Splenic involvement in addition to lymph nodes on same side of diaphragm
Stage III	III	Lymph nodes on both sides of the diaphragm
	IIIE	A single extralymphatic site with nodes on both sides of the diaphragm
	IIIS	Splenic involvement with nodes on both sides of the diaphragm
Stage IV		Disseminated extralymphatic disease

effective therapy. Complete remission rates in well over half of patients treated became possible, together with the prospect of prolonged disease-free survival and cure. Variations on the CHOP regimen were the most widely adopted, though subsequently many other combinations were investigated.

There was a general acceptance that early exposure to multiple non-cross-resistant chemotherapeutic drugs would increase tumour cell kill and therefore the chance of achieving complete remission encouraged the development of intensive polychemotherapy regimens. Additionally, because disease progression could occur between the cycles of CHOP, strategies employing more frequent treatment were introduced. Some of these were comparable to the induction treatment of acute lymphoblastic leukaemia while others incorporated less myelosuppressive agents given during the period of bone marrow depression as in BACOP (bleomycin, Adriamycin, cyclophosphamide, prednisone), M-BACOD (methotrex-ate–bleomycin, Adriamycin, cyclophosphamide, dexamethasone) and CHOP-Mtx (CHOP–methotrexate). The advent of growth factors to reduce the degree and duration of neutropenia encouraged the further exploration of more intensive chemotherapy, though their use has only a marginal effect on the incidence of side effects and does not significantly improve outcome.

Although much improved response rates were claimed for some of these regimens, it is now clear that the groups of patients being investigated were

Table 8.5 The International Prognostic Index for diffuse large cell lymphoma

Pretreatment criteria ('risk factors')	Score 0		Score 1
Age (years)	≤ 60	versus	> 60
Stage (Ann Arbor)	I or II	versus	III or IV
No. extranodal sites	≤ 1	versus	> 1
Performance status (ECOG scale)	0 or 1	versus	≥ 2
Serum LDH	≤ 1 × normal	versus	> 1 × normal

Risk groups	Risk factors
Low	0 or 1
Low intermediate	2
High intermediate	3
High	4 or 5

Age-adjusted model for younger patients (≤ 60 years)

Pretreatment risk factors	Score 0		Score 1
Stage	I or II	versus	III or IV
Performance status	0 or I	versus	≥ 2
Serum LDH	≤ 1 × normal	versus	≥ 1 × normal

Risk groups	Risk factors
Low	0
Low intermediate	1
High intermediate	2
High	3

very heterogeneous and essentially non-comparable. It is now recognized that these regimens offer no survival advantage over standard CHOP, although their role in certain subgroups has not been fully evaluated. An important point to remember when interpreting historical trials is that where the entry criteria have been intermediate and high-grade NHL according to the Working Formulation, lymphomas as disparate as lymphoblastic disease, Burkitt's lymphoma, mantle cell lymphoma and large cell variants of follicle centre lymphoma may have been included. Additionally, transformed and primary DLCL have usually been treated identically although the chances of cure are less in patients with underlying indolent disease. The age range of patients treated is also very important in view of the significantly poorer prognosis of NHL in the elderly.

Refractory and recurrent disease remains a major therapeutic challenge

The complete range of remission rates reported with a variety of chemotherapy regimes varies from 45–85% with early death rates from 1–15%. The implication of this is that there is a high percentage of patients with primary refractory disease. Of the patients who relapse the majority do so in the first year, fewer in the second year and by the third the curves are approaching a plateau. Regimens to treat these cases have been developed in which chemotherapeutic agents with a different spectrum of action are used initially; the possibility of further intensification of therapy with autologous support is increasingly being adopted, although the true value of this approach is not fully established.

A wide variety of relapse regimens has been investigated. The choice of drugs is influenced by the need for at least partial non-cross-resistance with the first-line anthracycline-containing regimens. Examples are the ifosfamide-containing regimens MIME (methyl-Gag, ifosfamide, methotrexate etoposide) and IM (ifosfamide, mitozantrone), and the *cis*-platinum-containing regimens such as DHAP (dexamethasone, cytosine arabinoside, *cis*-platinum) or attenuated versions of this. Sustained remissions rarely occur and further 'consolidation', usually with intensive myeloablative chemotherapy such as BEAM with autologous support, is given to patients with responsive disease with the aim of amplifying response and achieving more prolonged remissions. The success of intensive high-dose chemotherapy with autologous rescue in the responsive relapses has led to an interest in extending this approach to initial first-line treatment. This approach would be particularly valuable in patients with a poor prognosis identified using the international index. Trials to test this approach are in progress.

Subclassification of DLCL on the basis of genetic abnormalities may lead to more targeted therapy

The preceding discussion has shown that DLCLs are very heterogeneous and that morphological and phenotypical methods of subclassification are both difficult and not very reproducible. Equally, the need for subclassification is apparent in the variable prognosis and response to treatment. The basis of a genetic classification of DLCL is now beginning to emerge and this may be of considerable importance in designing future treatment strategies by the identification of tumours with unusually good or bad prognosis or likely high levels of drug resistance.

Abnormalities of p53 occur in around 20% of cases of DLCL

p53 abnormalities are much more common in DLCL than in other types of lymphoma but is less common than epithelial malignancy. p53 is a nuclear transcription factor that is produced in response to genetic damage and leads to cell-cycle arrest and induction of apoptosis. p53 can be inactivated by mutation or gene deletion or by formation of complexes with other proteins, most notably MDM2. In general, mutated p53 is more stable than its normal counterpart and more readily detected by immunocytochemistry. However, the correlation between detection of p53 and mutation is less clear than in carcinoma. Clearly, a tumour with both alleles deleted will be negative. The consequences of inactivation of p53 are that a tumour will transmit new genetic abnormalities more readily to daughter cells, facilitating tumour progression. Since many drugs and radiation act by causing genetic damage, therapy may be much less effective.

Around 30% of DLCLs express Bcl-2

Around 30% of DLCLs express Bcl-2 but the correlation between expression and the presence of a t(14;18) has not been fully established. The proportion of cases with Bcl-2 expression and a t(14;18) that arise by transformation of a follicle centre lymphoma is unknown. In some cases Bcl-2 expression may be mediated by other genetic mechanisms. The effect of abnormal expression of Bcl-2 is inhibition of apoptosis. This will tend to inhibit the action of normal p53 and act in synergy with mutated or inactivated p53 in preventing cytotoxic-drug-induced programmed cell death. Several studies appear to confirm that Bcl-2 expression is indeed a poor prognostic factor, although a considerable number of questions remain unanswered.

Bcl-6 may be deregulated by translocation or mutation

Bcl-6 is a zinc finger DNA-binding protein that appears to have a critical role in the normal germinal centre. In mice with disrupted Bcl-6 there is failure of germinal centre formation and loss of T-cell-dependent antibody production. This gene may be deregulated by translocation of the 3q27 locus to one of a number of potential chromosomes. Mutation

Figure 8.11 Abnormalities of *bcl-6*. Deregulation of *bcl-6* is a relatively common abnormality in diffuse large B-cell lymphoma. The *bcl-6* gene on 3q27 can form translocations with a wide range of other loci. Although initially reported as a good prognostic factor in diffuse large B-cell lymphoma, the full significance and cellular effects of *bcl-6* rearrangements remain to be determined.

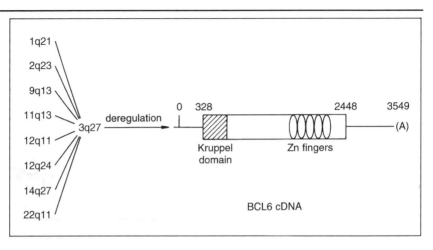

within the regulatory sequence is also described in B-cell lymphoma. These abnormalities and the expression of Bcl-6 protein are common features of diffuse large B-cell lymphoma but the exact incidence and the functional significance remain to be determined (Figure 8.11).

p53, Bcl-2 and Bcl-6 are all part of complex pathways regulating cell division, differentiation and apoptosis and it is likely that many more related genetic abnormalities will be described. Ultimately, classification may be based on defective pathways regulating cell death and proliferation rather than individual genetic abnormalities.

Figure 8.12 T-cell-rich B-cell lymphoma. In this cervical node small T-cells and macrophages predominate **(a)** and in some areas there is a vascular pattern similar to angioimmunoblastic lymphadenopathy **(b)**. The population of neoplastic large B-cells is most clearly seen using anti-CD20 **(c)**.

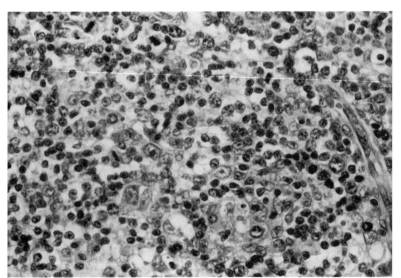

(a)

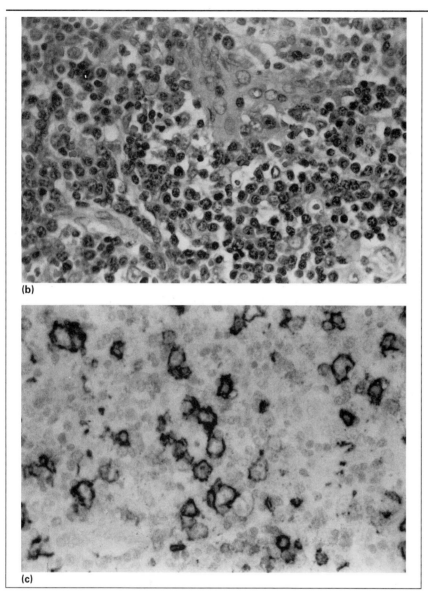

(b)

(c)

8.1.3 T-cell-rich B-cell lymphoma

Almost all diffuse large B-cell lymphomas contain a population of non-neoplastic T-cells. In some cases T-cells may present in large numbers and this has given rise to the concept of T-cell-rich B-cell lymphoma. There are as yet no agreed criteria for this diagnosis. Some authors use the term when the number of T-cells exceeds 55% of the total whereas others place emphasis of the nature of the T-cell infiltrate, with the presence of activated cells, highly endothelial-lined vessels, follicular dendritic cells and macrophages. It is also becoming apparent that T-cell-rich B-cell lymphoma is not a single diagnostic entity but rather a collection of variants of diffuse large cell lymphoma, lymphocyte-predominant nodular Hodgkin's disease, follicle centre lymphoma and possibly other types of B-cell malignancy. For this reason the clinical and prognostic implications of this diagnosis are not clearly defined. Progress in this area awaits better understanding of the interaction between neoplastic B-cells and reactive T-cells (Figure 8.12).

8.1.4 Burkitt's and Burkitt's-like lymphoma

African Burkitt's lymphoma is a distinctive syndrome

African Burkitt's lymphoma is a tumour of young children, which in its most characteristic form presents with involvement of the facial bones. The tumour is morphologically distinctive with a highly monomorphic population of medium to large cells with vacuolated basophilic cytoplasm and multiple small central nucleoli. The tumour has a very high rate of cell proliferation and apoptosis with the cohesive sheets of tumour cells being interspersed by debris containing 'starry-sky' macrophages. Burkitt's lymphomas show a peripheral B-cell phenotype with strong sIgM expression together with CD19, CD20, CD10 and CD38. The strong expression of clonal sIgM and the lack of Tdt are among the features that distinguish Burkitt's lymphoma from tumours of precursor lymphoid cells.

The features of Burkitt's lymphoma are summarized in Table 8.6.

The part played by studies of African Burkitt's lymphoma in understanding lymphomagenesis is hard to underestimate. Almost all

Table 8.6 Burkitt's lymphoma

- **Morphology:** Relatively monomorphic medium to large lymphoid cells with round nuclei and multiple central nucleoli. Basophilic cytoplasm with lipid vacuoles. High rates of cell proliferation and apoptosis.
- **Immunophenotype:** sIgM⁺, CD19⁺, CD20⁺, CD38⁺, CD10⁺, CD23⁻.
- **Cytogenetics:** t(8;14) or t(2;8) or t(8;22) with c-*myc* deregulation. EBV integration in African cases and some HIV-associated tumours.
- **Pattern of disease:** Localized extranodal disease in Africa. Otherwise highly aggressive abdominal disease with overt leukaemia in some cases.

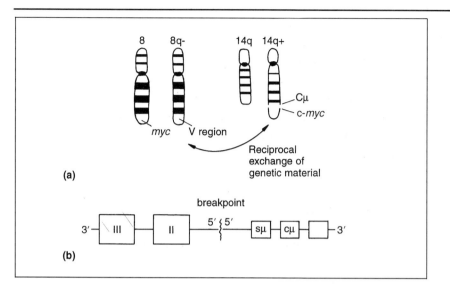

(a)

(b)

Figure 8.13 The t(8;14). This translocation is typical of Burkitt's lymphoma but occurs in other B-cell lymphomas. There is a reciprocal exchange of genetic material between 8q24 and 14q32 **(a)** which produces a fusion gene on chromosome 14 which includes exons II and III of c-*myc* and the immunoglobulin heavy chain locus **(b)**. The translocated c-*myc* gene is deregulated, resulting in increased levels of cell proliferation and apoptosis. A similar effect is produced by translocation of c-*myc* to the light-chain loci (t(2;8) and t(8;22)).

cases have chronic immune stimulation due to malaria and detectable EBV, although often only a restricted range of viral genes are expressed. In almost every case there is deregulation of c-Myc by translocation of the c-*myc* gene into the immunoglobulin heavy-chain locus (t8;14) (Figure 8.13) or less commonly to the light-chain loci (t(2;8) and t(8;21)).

c-Myc is a key transcription factor involved in the induction of cell division. It has also been shown to be a potent inducer of apoptosis. Whether a cell divides or dies depends on the levels of Bcl-2 and other apoptosis-regulating proteins. The very high proliferative and apoptotic rates seen in this tumour correlate well with the known actions of the gene.

A small number of children in Western counties (around 1–2 per million per year) develop a tumour that is morphologically, phenotypically and cytogenetically similar to African Burkitt's lymphoma. Although similar in cellular features only a small proportion of cases have evidence of EBV. These are very aggressive tumours which in most cases present with a rapidly growing abdominal mass that may infiltrate and destroy bowel and other abdominal organs. A small number of patients present with a leukaemic phase of the disease, which needs to be clearly distinguished from precursor-cell lymphoblastic leukaemia/lymphoma. Most of these cases have ALL L3 morphology but a definitive diagnosis can only be made by immunophenotypical studies (Figure 8.14).

Figure 8.14 (a, b) Burkitt's lymphoma in childhood – node biopsy. This child presented with a rapidly growing abdominal mass. Biopsy of the mass showed a diffuse infiltrate of relatively monomorphic cells with round nuclei and multiple small mainly central nucleoli. Cell proliferation and apoptotic rates were high. Phagocytosis of cell debris by macrophages gives rise to the 'starry sky' appearance. The cells showed CD10 and strong surface immunoglobulin expression. There was no evidence of Epstein–Barr virus.

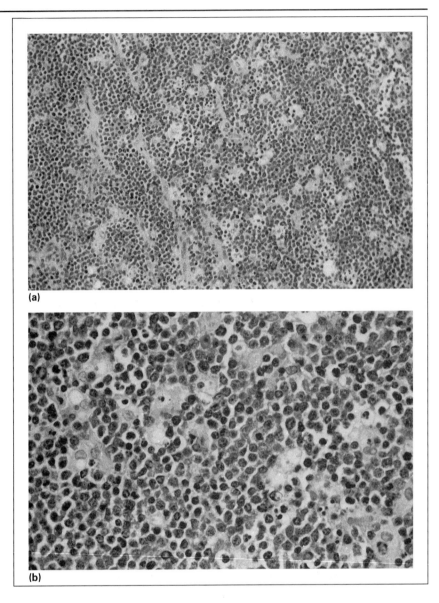

(a)

(b)

Some aggressive diffuse large B-cell lymphomas and acute leukaemias may have Burkitt's-like features

More common than Burkitt's lymphoma are a group of diffuse large B-cell lymphomas and acute B-cell leukaemias, occurring both in children and adults, which have Burkitt's-like features but differ in one or more respects from the classical type of Burkitt's lymphoma described above. In these cases the cells may be more pleomorphic and include cells with centroblastic as well as Burkitt's-like features. Evidence of plasmacytoid differentiation may also be present. A particular problem is that nuclear morphology may be highly sensitive to fixation and that variation within the tumour may reflect penetration of fixative and this contributes to relatively poor diagnostic reproducibility in this group of tumours. The immunophenotype may also show considerable variation and only a minority of cases express CD10. Probably the most reproducible feature of this group is the presence of very high cellular proliferation rates with Ki67 fraction in the range 90–100% often associated with a high rate of apoptosis, as in classical Burkitt's lymphoma. In immunocompetent patients EBV is not found more frequently than in other B-cell lymphomas and the true incidence of c-*myc* deregulation due to t(8;14) and other translocations has not been fully documented. A small proportion of tumours with these features have a t(14;18) translocation and may arise by transformation of a follicle centre lymphoma (Figure 8.15).

It will be clear from this brief discussion that the terms Burkitt's lymphoma and Burkitt-like lymphoma are applied to a diverse group of lymphomas that may share a number of morphological features but differ in pathogenesis, age distribution and in important clinical features such as pattern of spread and response to therapy. For this reason, the value of the term Burkitt-like lymphoma is very doubtful. In designing clinical trials or comparing results it is important that the patients are fully described in terms of other relevant clinical and pathological features.

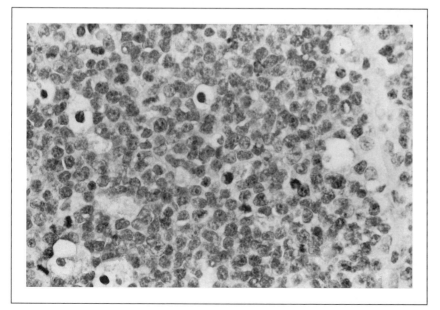

Figure 8.15 Burkitt-like diffuse large B-cell lymphoma. This patient presented with aggressive diffuse large B-cell lymphoma. The tumour had a very high rate of cell proliferation and apoptosis evidenced by the presence of numerous macrophages containing debris.

The treatment of non-endemic Burkitt's and Burkitt's-like diffuse large B-cell lymphomas

The evolution of more intensive chemotherapy from earlier, simpler cyclophosphamide- and methotrexate-containing regimens has resulted in improving rates and duration of remission. Experience gained particularly from the treatment of children indicates that significant improvement in progression-free survival and cure rates can be achieved as a result of intensive chemotherapy even in the presence of the poor prognostic features of bone marrow or CNS involvement. Short-duration, high-dose chemotherapy regimens such as CODOX-M (cyclophosphamide, vincristine, doxorubicin, cytosine arabinoside, high-dose methotrexate) and IVAC (ifosfamide, etoposide, cytosine arabinoside) with concurrent programmes for intrathecal therapy have largely been developed from paediatric experience. The use of such approaches in adult patients is under investigation but the outlook for many of these patients remains poor.

8.1.5 Mantle cell lymphoma

Mantle cell lymphoma has characteristic histological and phenotypical features

The histological and phenotypical features that define mantle cell lymphoma and distinguish it from other nodal lymphomas are now well recognized. The term mantle cell lymphoma is now preferred to diffuse centrocytic or mantle zone lymphoma. Mantle cell lymphoma (MCL) in its typical form consists of a uniform population of cells similar in size and shape to centrocytes with irregular or cleaved nuclei and small nucleoli. The uniformity is one of the key diagnostic features of MCL; blast cells are not dispersed through the tumour as would be seen in follicle centre lymphomas although when residual reactive germinal centres are present the infiltrate may appear more pleomorphic. Morphological variants of mantle cell lymphomas include cases with greater cellular pleomorphism, and a blastic subtype with larger cells with round nuclei and a higher rate of cell proliferation than the common type. In these cases aneuploidy may be more frequent.

The pattern of nodal infiltration was responsible for the earlier name mantle zone lymphoma. In some tumours where there is early nodal infiltration the neoplastic cells surround reactive germinal centres in a broad mantle zone later invading and replacing the follicle, thus forming

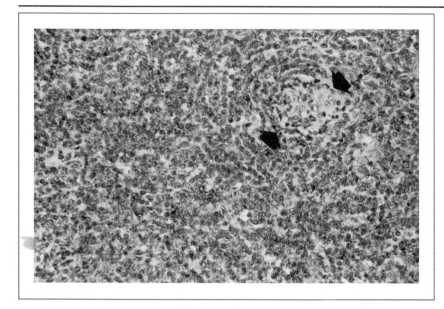

Figure 8.16 Mantle cell lymphoma. In this case of mantle cell lymphoma the tumour has a nodular growth pattern that contains fragments of residual germinal centres (arrows).

a tumour nodule. This pattern then progresses to diffuse nodal replacement (Figures 8.16, 8.17). A feature of the diffusely replaced node is a coarse pattern of reticulin fibres, often with hyalinized vessels and significant numbers of reactive macrophages. The diffuse pattern is by far the most common.

Mantle cell lymphoma has a distinctive immunophenotype. Clonal surface immunoglobulin is expressed at moderate intensity with CD20 CD43 and CD5. CD23 is negative in most of the cells. When examining paraffin section CDw75 (germinal centre cells), Bcl-2 (expressed in mantle cells but not reactive follicles) and CD21 (follicular dendritic cells) will be of particular value in clearly identifying remnants of germinal centres. Cellular proliferation as assessed by Ki67 is very variable in MCL, ranging from minimal numbers to 20–30% positivity.

The features of mantle cell lymphoma are summarized in Table 8.7.

Mantle cell lymphomas have a typical clinical presentation and pattern of spread

Mantle cell lymphoma is a disseminated disease occurring in older patients with a male predominance. Most patients present with lymphadenopathy, which may be rapidly enlarging. There also appears to be a high incidence of involvement of Waldeyer's ring and some patients will present with bilateral tonsillar enlargement.

Figure 8.17 Mantle cell lymphoma. In this case the node is diffusely replaced by mantle cell lymphoma. **(a)** The tumour consists of a monomorphic population of small to intermediate-sized CD5+ B-lymphocytes with irregular or cleaved nuclei. Thick-walled vessels are often a prominent feature of nodes infiltrated by MCL. Although this was an aggressive tumour the cell-cycle fraction, as demonstrated by Ki67 **(b)**, is relatively low.

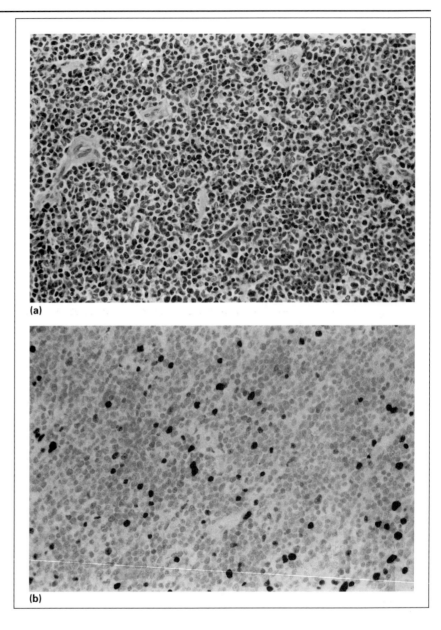

(a)

(b)

Over 70% of patients have marrow involvement at presentation. The pattern of infiltration is similar to that seen in CLL. In the earliest stage of infiltration irregular nodules are present that progress to an interstitial pattern and then to diffuse marrow replacement. The degree of blood involvement is variable and even with a normal lymphocyte count low levels of tumour cells will be often detected by flow cytometry. In the

Table 8.7 Mantle cell lymphoma

- **Morphology**: Monomorphic population of small to intermediate-sized cells with irregular nuclei.
- **Immunophenotype**: sIgM/D⁺, CD19⁺, CD20⁺, CD5⁺, CD23⁻, CD10⁻.
- **Cytogenetics**: t(11;14) with deregulated cyclin D1 in most cases.
- **Pattern of disease**: Nodes, blood and marrow involved in varying proportions. May present with intestinal or Waldeyer's ring tumours.

---

peripheral blood and marrow MCL can clearly be distinguished from CLL cells by being larger and more pleomorphic, with considerable variation in the size and irregularity of the nucleus. There is an increasing number of patients who present with a lymphocytosis and are found to have cells with mantle cell morphology and immunophenotype, but who do not have lymphadenopathy or significant marrow infiltration. The rate of progression of these tumours is not certain.

A significant number of patients with mantle cell lymphoma have multifocal infiltration of the gastrointestinal tract. This may be the presenting and dominant feature of the disease (multiple lymphomatous polyposis, see Chapter 10) or develop as a later complication during the course of therapy.

Overexpression of Bcl-1 (cyclin D1) is a typical feature of mantle cell lymphoma

As mantle cell lymphoma has been become more clearly defined it has become apparent that this group of lymphomas is closely associated with t(11;14) (Figure 8.18). This is detectable in about 50–90% of MCL depending on the technique used. The translocation sometimes occurs in otherwise typical cases of CLL but is very rare by comparison with MCL.

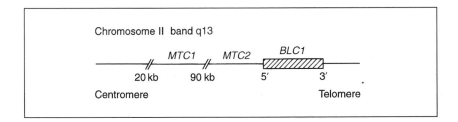

Figure 8.18 The t(11;14). This is the typical translocation of mantle cell lymphoma and results in deregulation of the cyclin D1 gene, which is a key factor in the control of the cell cycle at the G_1/S checkpoint. Breakpoints on ch11 are clustered in a large region 5′ to *bcl-1*. Some are grouped together in two major translocation clusters (MTC). For this reason, PCR will only detect 30% of translocations. It would be expected that this translocation would enhance the propensity of a cell to enter S phase.

It is important to be able to detect the translocation in clinical material. The breakpoint on chromosome 11 is spread over a 100 kb region and as such can not be reliably detected by a standard DNA PCR method. *In situ* hybridization (ISH) methods are now routinely available to detect this abnormality in interphase nuclei and deregulation of the cyclin D1 protein can be readily identified by immunocytochemistry.

The current treatment approaches in MCL are not very effective

MCL has a worse prognosis than follicle centre lymphoma and the other indolent non-Hodgkin's lymphomas. In published series the median progression-free survival is 18 months, with the majority of patients having relapsed by 3 years. However, there does appear to be a subset of patients with mainly bone marrow disease with a rather better prognosis. It is likely that many of these patients have been previously diagnosed as having CLL. Overall there is a median survival of approximately 3 years, with only 30% of patients alive at 6 years. Factors associated with poor prognosis comparable to those in other NHL have been delineated, e.g. greater age, worse performance status, widespread disease, high LDH and low albumin. In addition, high rates of cell proliferation appear to be an independent prognostic factor.

A variety of chemotherapeutic approaches, from single alkylating agent (e.g. chlorambucil) to anthracycline-containing regimens such as CHOP, have been adopted. The evidence to suggest that anthracycline-containing regimens result in higher CR rates and longer survival is minimal and there is a need for prospective studies of carefully delineated patient cohorts in order to test different treatment approaches. On present evidence it would appear that conventional chemotherapy is essentially ineffective and that novel approaches need to be investigated with the aim of obtaining greater numbers of complete responses.

8.1.6 Marginal cell lymphoma

Marginal zone lymphoma rarely occurs as a primary nodal lymphoma; many cases represent nodal spread of primary extranodal tumours

Tumours of marginal zone lymphocytes constitute the majority of extranodal B-cell lymphomas but are very rare as primary nodal lymphomas. Even in cases that do present as lymphadenopathy a proportion will be found subsequently to have a primary extranodal lymphoma, e.g. in the salivary gland.

Involvement of nodes by marginal zone lymphoma is recognized by cellular morphology, phenotype and pattern of infiltration. The cells of marginal zone lymphoma may include a mixture of morphological forms including those with centrocyte-like morphology, cells with monocytoid-like features, plasmacytoid cells and usually small numbers of larger blast cells (Figure 8.19).

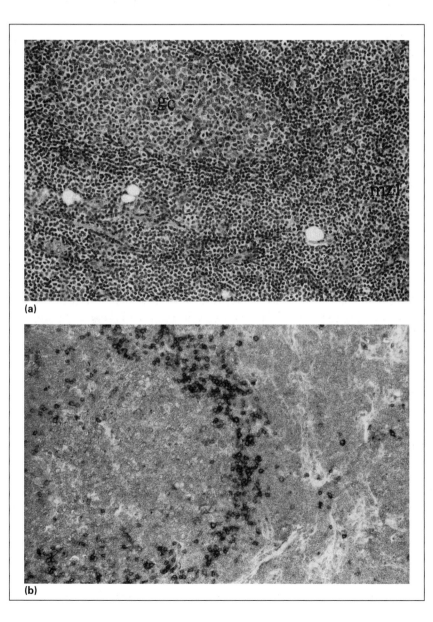

(a)

(b)

Figure 8.19 Marginal cell lymphoma. This patient had a solitary groin node. **(a)** Reactive germinal centres (gc) were surrounded by a broad band of clonal B-cells, most of which had monocytoid features (mzl) with reactively abundant clear cytoplasm. **(b)** The preservation of the follicular mantle surrounding reactive germinal centres is shown using anti-IgD. No evidence of an extranodal B-cell lymphoma was found on staging investigations.

These cells express strong sIgM or IgG, but not IgD, together with the pan-B-cell markers CD19, CD20 and CD79. CD23, CD10, CD5 are negative but cases show variable expression of CDw75. Where plasmacytoid differentiation is present some cells may show cIg. Marginal zone lymphomas may show strong Bcl-2 expression but without t(14;18).

The tumour cells of marginal zone lymphoma invade and expand the interfollicular areas of the node and replace the marginal zone. Reactive germinal centres are usually present and unlike mantle zone lymphoma the follicular mantle is preserved and can be demonstrated using anti-IgD or MT2 (CD45RA). As the disease progresses the follicles become colonized by neoplastic cells, which may then contain a complex mixture of neoplastic and reactive cells. The combination of pattern of nodal infiltration, cellular morphology and immunophenotype should allow nodal marginal zone lymphoma to be distinguished from follicle centre lymphoma and mantle cell lymphoma. However, in a small number of follicle centre lymphomas there may be a proportion of cells with monocytoid features and in these cases distinction from marginal zone lymphoma may be difficult. In such cases the pattern of spread of the disease may be helpful.

The features of marginal zone lymphoma are summarized in Table 8.8.

Primary nodal marginal zone lymphoma is often localized

Dissemination of marginal zone lymphoma can occur and should be excluded by adequate staging but in the majority of cases the tumour is localized. The clinical course is similar to that in extranodal sites and large cell transformation may occur. The treatment of nodal marginal zone lymphoma should include radiotherapy if localized but disseminated disease with symptoms may require either single-agent or

Table 8.8 Marginal zone lymphoma

- **Morphology:** Mixed population of small lymphocytes with irregular nuclei, monocytoid B-cells, plasma cells and occasional blast cells.
- **Immunophenotype:** sIgM(orG)$^+$, sIgD$^-$, CD19$^+$, CD20$^+$, CD5$^-$, CD10$^-$, CD23$^-$.
- **Cytogenetics:** t(3) in an as yet undefined proportion of cases.
- **Pattern of disease:** Most cases arise in extranodal sites with initial spread to local nodes. Marrow and blood involvement is rare.

---

combination chemotherapy. There are insufficient data on the relative efficacy of these treatments, although for most patients the prognosis appears relatively good.

8.2 The chronic B-cell leukaemias

8.2.1 Chronic lymphocytic leukaemia

Chronic lymphocytic leukaemia is the commonest lymphoproliferative disorder with a progressively increasing age-specific incidence from 50 years. Blood, marrow, lymph nodes and sometimes other organs may be involved by CLL and in the past this has given rise to some confusion in terminology. In this discussion CLL and 'lymphocytic lymphoma of B-cell type' are regarded as equivalent and CLL will be used as the preferred term.

The cellular morphology and phenotype of CLL is highly characteristic but the definition of the disease is much less clear

In the typical case of CLL the peripheral blood contains a monomorphic population of small lymphocytes with minimal cytoplasm, a nucleus with dense clumped chromatin and no visible nucleolus. These cells are easily disrupted and this produces smear cells in a blood film. In all cases the diagnosis should be confirmed by immunophenotypic studies. In CLL the cells have weak sIg expression, which in almost all cases is IgD and/or IgM but rare cases which express IgG and even less commonly IgA are described. The B-lineage markers CD19 and CD20 are expressed together with CD5 and CD23; CD11a, CD38 and FMC7 are typically negative (Figure 8.20).

In a proportion of cases, which are in other respects typical, phenotypic variants are found, which most often involve loss of sIg or CD5 expression. The presence of CD38, CD11a or FMC7 is generally associated with atypical morphological features such as irregular nuclei of prominent nucleoli (Figure 8.21). The clinical significance of these variants is not certain.

When sensitive immunophenotypical techniques are used a considerable proportion, perhaps up to 1%, of the adult population can be shown to have small numbers of clonal B-cells with a CLL phenotype on the background of a normal lymphocyte count. Clearly, only a tiny proportion will progress to clinically significant disease. For this reason

Figure 8.20 B-CLL – peripheral blood. This blood film shows heavy infiltration by small lymphocytes which had typical CLL phenotype (low sIg, CD5+, CD19+, CD23+).

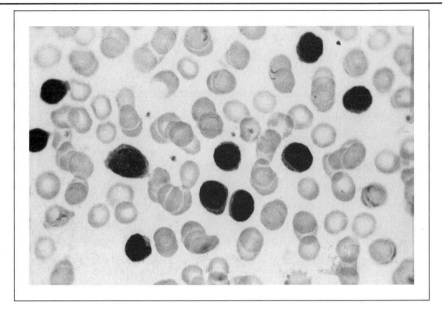

CLL is only diagnosed when there is a persistent lymphocytosis exceeding $5 \times 10^9/l$. It is not clear whether patients who meet these criteria are part of the same population as those with minimal disease. Many patient who have CLL with a moderate lymphocytosis will be detected by a routine blood count and are asymptomatic. It is for these reasons there is no reliable estimate of the incidence of CLL.

The features of B-cell chronic lymphocytic leukaemia are summarized in Table 8.9.

CLL shows a typical pattern of marrow involvement but the extent of disease varies widely

CLL infiltrates the marrow in a series of well defined stages. The earliest stage is the formation of nodules in the medullary space consisting of small lymphocytes. These nodules are not related to bone, which may be helpful in making the distinction from follicle centre lymphoma. As the disease progresses there is an increasing tendency for cells to infiltrate between adipocytes, which results in the diffuse replacement of areas of marrow (Figure 8.22).

At this stage the diffuse sheets of CLL may be interspersed with hyperplastic regenerative marrow. In the final stage there is a packed marrow with progressive replacement of haematopoietic elements. These stages, in particular the first and last, are of prognostic significance. In some cases there is a striking divergence between the extent of marrow infiltration and the peripheral count. This may be most impressive after treatment, when a large reduction in the peripheral lymphocyte count may occur in the continuing presence of a packed marrow.

A number of morphological differences may be seen between the bone marrow and peripheral blood in CLL. Careful examination of trephine biopsy specimens will often show a proportion of cells with plasmacytoid features. When these are numerous the term 'lymphoplasmacytoid leukaemia/lymphoma' has been used in the past, but this can lead to confusion with other tumours which show plasmacytoid features. CLL with plasmacytoid cells has no specific significance and it is not helpful to place them in a separate diagnostic category. Although the type of cells seen in the peripheral blood will be present in the marrow there is often greater polymorphism in the marrow, with cells showing more irregular nuclear contours or prominent nucleoli. Organized proliferation centres containing prolymphocytes and immunoblasts such as are seen in lymph nodes may be present in the bone marrow. There is little correlation between with the numbers of nucleolated prolymphocytes seen in the marrow and those seen in the peripheral blood (Figure 8.23).

Some degree of nodal disease is frequent in CLL and infiltration of other organs may be present

A high proportion of patients with CLL have generalized lymphadenopathy, although the size of the affected nodes varies. It is very rare to have nodal disease with a normal marrow and peripheral blood but in a significant number of cases the initial diagnosis may be made on a lymph node biopsy. The histological features are highly typical but there are pitfalls, which may sometimes lead to confusion with other types of lymphoproliferative disorder. In most cases the nodal architecture is replaced although often the boundaries of the node and some of the sinuses remain. The infiltrate consists of cells similar to those seen in the peripheral blood with scattered proliferation centres (Figure 8.24).

The low levels of sIgM, IgD and CD20 found on CLL cells may mean that these antigens are not detectable in fixed tissue. The phenotype $CD5^+$, $CD43^+$, $CD79^+$, $CD3^-$, $CD23^+$ is the most constant finding in fixed sections. The proliferation centres are strongly CDw75-positive, but this marker is not expressed on cells with small lymphocytic morphology. Most CLL cells express Bcl-2 without a t(14;18).

The nodular appearance of proliferation centres and the expression of CDw75 may suggest the diagnosis of follicle centre lymphoma. CLL

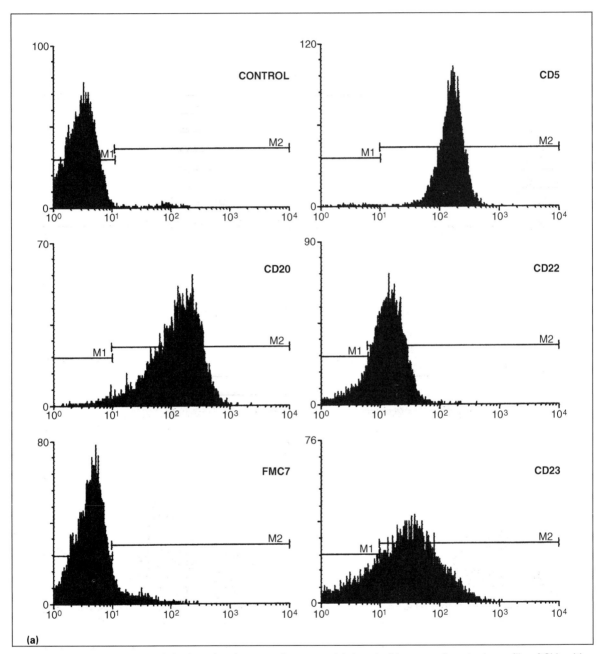

Figure 8.21 Chronic lymphocytic leukaemia – immunophenotype. **(a)** A typical immunophenotypic profile of CLL with coexpression of CD5 and CD23.

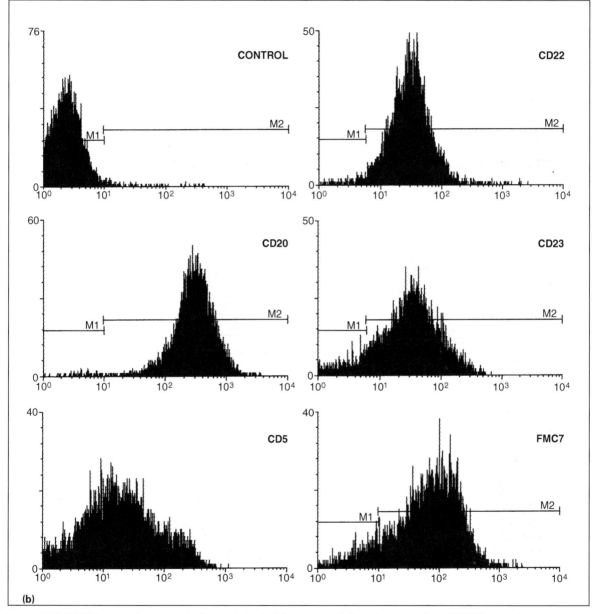

Figure 8.21 (b) This case shows atypical morphological features and there is expression of FMC7, more intense staining with CD20 and a proportion of the cells are CD5⁻.

Table 8.9 B-cell chronic lymphocytic leukaemia

- **Morphology:** Small lymphocytes with variable numbers of larger nucleolated pro-lymphocytes. Organized proliferation centres in nodes and bone marrow.
- **Immunophenotype:** weak sIgM/D$^+$, CD19$^+$, weak CD20$^+$, CD5$^+$, CD38$^-$, CD23$^+$, CD11a$^+$.
- **Cytogenetics:** t(12), 11q–, 13q- and other abnormalities: exact spectrum not well defined.
- **Pattern of disease:** Nodal, blood and marrow infiltration in varying proportions.

---

proliferation centres can be distinguished by cellular morphology, lack of a follicular reticulin pattern, lack of follicular dendritic cells and the nature of the surrounding B-cells. It should be noted that in some cases proliferation centres can be very large and occupy most of the node. Rarely such cases may be confused with large cell lymphoma or transformation of CLL. The size of proliferation centres does not appear by itself to be of prognostic importance and does not correlate with peripheral blood findings.

CLL appears to be a systemic disease and can involve any organ. In liver biopsies CLL cells are seen in small groups within the sinusoids. This is typical but not specific to CLL. Patients with CLL may have skin rashes

Figure 8.22 B-CLL – bone marrow. The extent of marrow infiltration by B-CLL varies widely and may not closely correlate with the peripheral blood count. Some patients may have occasional scattered nodules of CLL **(a)** whereas in other cases there is extensive diffuse infiltration **(b)**. In some cases, proliferation centres containing larger nucleolated cells are found in heavily involved marrows **(c)**.

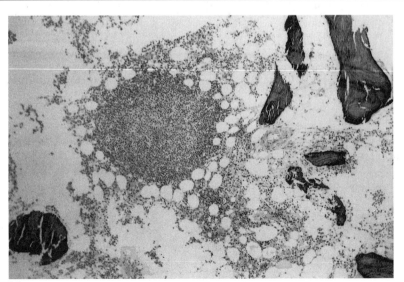

(a)

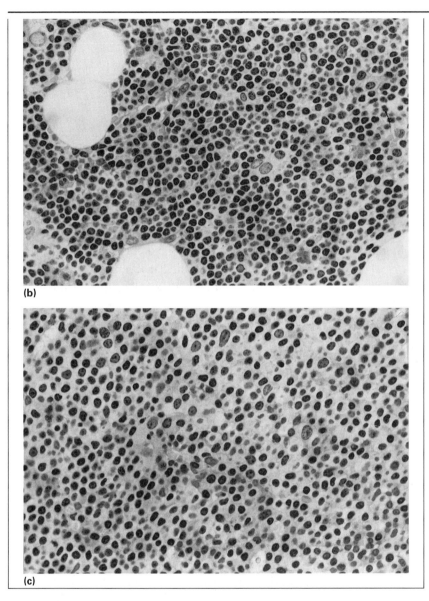

(b)

(c)

but in many cases this is found on biopsy to be a dermatitis reaction rather than infiltration by CLL. Infiltration of non-lymphoid organs by CLL is often found as an incidental finding when biopsies are taken for unrelated disorders such as peptic ulcer disease. A small number of cases of CLL are first diagnosed in surgical resections of epithelial malignancy. It has been suspected that this may be a non-random association but definitive data are lacking. Except where there is organomegaly due to CLL, tissue infiltration appears to be of limited clinical significance.

Figure 8.23 CLL with prolymphocytes – peripheral blood. This patient with CLL had a rising lymphocyte count with relatively large numbers of nucleolated cells in the peripheral blood. The immunophenotype of the cells is typical of CLL, which is helpful in making the distinction from B-PLL.

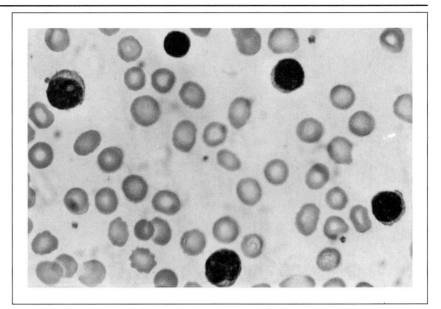

Several molecular abnormalities are typical of CLL

There are a number of genetic abnormalities which have been reported as being consistently associated with CLL although some caution is need in interpreting this data because of varying diagnostic criteria used to separate CLL from other lymphoproliferative disorders. Numerically the most important of these are 13q–, 11q– and trisomy 12. The relevant genes at any of these locations have not been identified. The retinoblastoma gene (*Rb*), which is located at the site of deletion on chromosome 13q, was for a long time considered to be relevant but it is now thought that another linked gene is important. A characteristic feature of these cytogenetic lesions is that they tend to be secondary events and often exist as subclones. As such they are thought to be involved in progression of the disease. Little is known of the primary events in CLL; a translocation t(14;19) was cloned from a case of CLL and a gene *bcl-3* was cloned. Unfortunately, this is only very rarely involved in the pathogenesis of CLL. A variety of translocations involving the IgH locus may occur. The t(11;14) which deregulates cyclin D1 was first reported in CLL but it is now clear that this is very rare and, as described above, this translocation is much more strongly associated with mantle cell lymphoma.

Cellular progression of CLL takes two main forms

The presence of progressive clinical disease with increasing anaemia and lymphadenopathy and decreased sensitivity to treatment is often

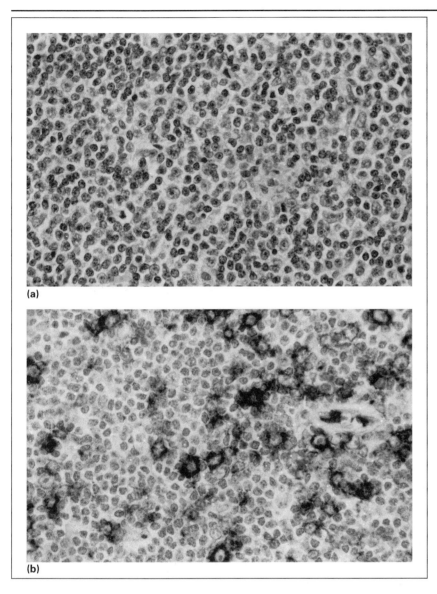

(a)

(b)

Figure 8.24 Chronic lymphocytic leukaemia – lymph node. In lymph nodes replaced by CLL there may be a proliferation centre, which consists of a mixture intermediate sized cells with distinct nucleoli and larger blast cells **(a)**. The proliferation centre blast cells express CD75 **(b)**.

accompanied by rising numbers of cells with prolymphocytic features in the peripheral blood. These cells are larger, with more abundant cytoplasm, and have a prominent single nucleolus. The phenotype is similar to CLL which distinguishes this condition from prolymphocytic leukaemia. When the proportion of prolymphocytes in the peripheral blood exceeds 10% the term CLL-pro is sometimes used and in advanced cases the proportion of prolymphocytes may be in the range 30–50%.

Some patients have rapidly expanding nodes or extranodal masses, which on biopsy show replacement by immunoblastic lymphoma. This is sometimes known by the eponym Richter's syndrome. Although this has been reported in as many as 10% of patients with CLL, the true incidence appears to be much lower. Immunoblastic transformation of CLL has a very poor prognosis.

Immune dysfunction and marrow failure are important clinical features of CLL especially in patients with advanced disease

There is a high incidence of infection in patients with CLL and this may account for about one-third of deaths. The most common problems are respiratory and soft tissue infections with *Haemophilus influenzae, Streptococcus pneumoniae* or *Staphylococcus aureus.* Herpesvirus, *Pneumocystis* and fungal infections are not common in CLL until the terminal phase of the disease or in patients who receive intensive therapy. The increased susceptibility to bacterial infections is due to a combination of marrow failure and immune dysfunction.

Patients with advanced-stage CLL have progressive anaemia, thrombocytopenia and neutropenia. In most cases this is explained by the degree of marrow infiltration. However, in some patients there may be a degree of myelodysplasia. This may be related to treatment with alkylating agents but there also appears to be an association between CLL and MDS that is independent of treatment. The nature of this relationship has not been clarified.

The most important immunological abnormality in patients with CLL is hypogammaglobulinaemia and this is likely to be a major factor in the high incidence of bacterial infections. The mechanism of impaired immunoglobulin production is unknown. There may also be a T-cell lymphocytosis and alteration in the relative proportions of T-cell subsets and NK cells but the significance of these changes is unknown. There is no good evidence that changes in T-cell or NK cell numbers or function are a reflection of an anti-CLL immune response.

There is a high incidence of autoimmune phenomena in CLL

10–35% of cases have a positive Coombs test and about half of these patients have overt haemolysis. ITP is much less common, with an estimated incidence of around 2%. A few patients have antineutrophil antibodies. However, although the low levels of paraprotein which may be detected in CLL are usually IgM, the autoantibodies against red cells and platelets are almost always IgG. CLL cells rarely express sIgG and the source of the antibodies is not apparent. In some patients there is a striking discordance between the apparent tumour bulk and the autoantibody levels, which may persist even after a major degree of cytoreduction has been achieved by therapy.

The antibodies are not produced by the clonal CLL cells themselves and it is postulated that there is a disturbance of idiotypic networks such that lymphocytes producing autoreactive clones are no longer suppressed.

CLL cells and the cells of MCL are B-cells that express CD5 and IgM and may use a limited repertoire of V regions

The tumour cells in CLL and mantle cell lymphoma express CD5 and IgM and a number of studies have indicated that a limited V-region repertoire is used in contrast to most other types of lymphoma. These features suggest homology with the B_1 subset of B-lymphocytes. B_1-cells are present in large numbers in the fetus but decline as the thymic-dependent B_2-cells become dominant. A relative increase in B_1-cells occurs again in later adult life. B_1-cells produce low-affinity polyreactive antibodies, which may be important in early defence against infection; some autoantibodies are also of this type. The balance of evidence appears to suggest that B_1 and B_2 B-cells are separate lineages arising from separate committed precursors. It has been proposed that CLL may be due to the emergence of a clonal B_1-cell population as the thymic-dependent B_2-cells decline in later life. However, there is as yet no definitive evidence in support of this hypothesis. A particular problem is the extent to which CD5 is a lineage marker or whether this can be induced on any type of B-cell given appropriate conditions for activation. There is also a need to account for apparent ethnic differences in the incidence of CLL, for example the rarity of CLL in migrant Japanese, and its apparent familial tendency.

Staging systems in CLL

Defining the stages of the disease delineates prognostic groupings and aids therapeutic decision-making

The stage of the disease at presentation correlates with survival and two most widely adopted staging systems were put forward by Rai and Binet respectively (Tables 8.10, 8.11).

Table 8.10 Staging systems for chronic lymphocytic leukaemia: RAI system

Stage	Clinical characteristics	% of total	Median survival (years)
0	Lymphocytosis only, in blood and bone marrow	30	> 12.5
I	Lymphocytosis with lymphadenopathy	60	8.5
II	Lymphocytosis + splenomegaly ± hepatomegaly	60	6.0
III	Lymphocytosis + anaemia (Hb < 11 g/dl)	10	1.5
IV	Lymphocytosis + thrombocytopenia (platelets < 100×10^9/l)	10	1.5

They incorporate key prognostic information relating to clinical features and define early (Rai 0, Binet A), intermediate (Rai I and II, Binet B) and advanced (Rai III and IV, Binet C) disease. While the life expectancy of patients with early stage disease is not appreciably different from age-matched healthy individuals, the more advanced disease is associated with a median survival of only a few years. The current staging systems are not, however, accurately predictive in the individual. Integration of the Rai and Binet systems to produce a unified system has been put forward by the International Working Group on CLL. The following groupings are generated by such a combined approach: A (0),

Table 8.11 Staging systems for chronic lymphocytic leukaemia: Binet system

Stage	Clinical characteristics	% of total	Median survival (years)
A	No anaemia or thrombocytopenia: less than three lymphoid regions* enlarged	60	> 10.0
B	No anaemia or thrombocytopenia: three or more lymphoid regions enlarged	30	5.0
C	Anaemia (Hb ≤ 10 g/dl) and/or thrombocytopenia (platelets ≤ 100×10^9/l)	10	2.0

* Lymphoid regions considered are cervical, axillary and inguinal lymph nodes (unilateral or bilateral), spleen and liver

Table 8.12 Poor prognostic factors in CLL

- Age
- Male sex
- High stage
- Lymphocyte count > 40–50 $\times$ 10^9
- Diffuse pattern of infiltration
- Response to treatment
- Cytogenetics (t(12), 13q–, 14q+)
- High LDH
- High β_2m

A (I), A (II), B (I), B (II), C (III), C (IV). Other staging systems, such as the total tumour mass index of Jaksic and Vitale, have some merit but are not routinely applied.

Investigative findings that may give useful prognostic information but are not included in these staging systems include absolute lymphocyte count (and lymphocyte morphology), the lymphocyte doubling time, the pattern of bone marrow infiltration, karyotype and cytogenic abnormalities, serum beta-2-microglobulin (β_2m) and lactic dehydrogenase (LDH). Other factors are age and sex with females faring better overall than males (Table 8.12).

Treatment of CLL

In order to assess the results of treatment, particularly in trials, standard definitions of response are required

A complete response (CR) is based on a clinical and haematological assessment of absence of systemic symptoms, lymphadenopathy, hepatosplenomegaly and a normal blood count. Although a percentage of lymphocytes in the bone marrow aspirate (of the order of < 30%) is often quoted as one of the criteria for CR, estimation of the proportion of lymphocytes in a bone marrow aspirate film is an inaccurate procedure. The routine use of trephine biopsies has shown that many patients with an apparently complete response on clinical grounds have a persistent low level of nodular marrow infiltration, though this may not appreciably affect the clinical course. On the other hand, some patients have a very good response in terms of peripheral lymphocyte count and physical

Table 8.13 Standard response criteria

Complete response (CR)
- Absence of lymphadenopathy by physical examination and appropriate imaging
- No hepato- or splenomegaly
- Absence of constitutional symptoms
- Blood count:
    - Neutrophils $\geq 2.0 \times 10^9/l$
    - Platelets $\geq 100 \times 10^9/l$
    - Haemoglobin (without transfusion)
        $\geq 13\,g/dl$ for men
        $\geq 11\,g/dl$ for women
    - Lymphocytes $< 3.5 \times 10^9/l$
- Bone marrow aspirate < 30% lymphocytes; no evidence of lymphocytic infiltration in trephine biopsy

Partial response (PR)
- 50% reduction in lymphadenopathy and/or 50% reduction in the size of the liver and/or spleen
- Blood lymphocytes $< 15 \times 10^9/l$
- Neutrophils $\geq 2.0 \times 10^9/l$ or 50% improvement from baseline
- Platelets $\geq 100 \times 10^9/l$ or 50% improvement over baseline
- Haemoglobin
    $\geq 12\,g/dl$ for men
    $\geq 10\,g/dl$ for women
    or 50% improvement over baseline, not supported by infusion

signs, but have continuing heavy infiltration of bone marrow. Partial responses are difficult to define but a general definition is a 50% improvement in the parameters above (Table 8.13).

In early stage CLL it is unnecessary to institute treatment immediately

CLL is a relatively common lymphoproliferative disease and the diagnosis is often made incidentally (in about 50% of cases) at an early clinical stage of the disease. Many of these patients die from causes unrelated to their leukaemia and treatment has not been shown to be of any benefit or to improve their survival.

Patients with early-stage disease are, therefore, simply monitored until there is evidence of progressive disease, which is characterized by at least one of the following:

- constitutional (B) symptoms;
- development of bulky lymphadenopathy;
- development of (or increase in) hepato/splenomegaly;
- downward trend in Hb level and/or platelet count.

The standard treatment of CLL is single-alkylating-agent chemotherapy with or without corticosteroids

Chlorambucil has long been the treatment of choice in people with advanced or progressive disease and overall response rates (CR + PR) of the order of 60–70% can be expected. In the occasional patient intolerant of chlorambucil (usually because of allergy) cyclophosphamide is an effective alternative. Corticosteroids are active in CLL and are often favoured in patients with evidence of bone-marrow compromise in stage C disease; they also have an important indication in the treatment of autoimmune haemolytic anaemia associated with CLL. Radiotherapy has not been extensively used, even though splenic irradiation is an effective means of reducing spleen size and tumour cell load. More intensive regimens, notably anthracycline-containing combinations such as CHOP, have been reported as achieving more complete remissions and improving survival, though the survival benefit of the addition of an anthracycline is not yet proved and still requires confirmation in a large randomized trial. Combinations such as COP are probably as effective as chlorambucil and a useful alternative in chlorambucil-resistant recurrent disease.

There is accumulating evidence of purine analogue activity and effectiveness

Purine analogues, notably fludarabine and 2-chlorodeoxyadenosine, have been found to be effective agents in the treatment of patients with disease refractory to standard therapy or who subsequently relapse. Fludarabine in particular has been shown to have a high level of activity in these patients, with response rates of the order of 40–60%. There is accumulating data on the use of fludarabine for the treatment of previously untreated patients, with very encouraging results: response rates of up to 80% and a relatively high proportion of apparently complete remission. It is as yet uncertain whether or not this will translate into a significant benefit in terms of overall survival.

Fludarabine is generally well tolerated by patients but there have been concerns about the sustained reduction in T-cells resulting from its use.

In practice, an increased risk of opportunistic infections does not appear to be a major problem, though the incidence of herpetic infection may be increased. Other effects on lymphocyte subsets may explain the occurrence of autoimmune phenomena (haemolytic anaemia, immune thrombocytopenia, red cell aplasia).

The often very considerable reduction in leukaemic cell load resulting from treatment with fludarabine will encourage the exploration of more effective strategies for longer-term disease control in the maintenance setting (incorporating agents such as alpha-interferon) as well as the application of myeloablative radiochemotherapy with autologous stem cell support in younger patients. Allogeneic transplantation may also deserve further consideration.

8.2.2 Prolymphocytic B-cell leukaemia

B-Prolymphocytic leukaemia is a distinctive clinical syndrome

B-PLL is an entity distinct from CLL that affects mainly elderly men and is characterized by bone marrow and splenic infiltration by cells with prolymphocytic morphology. The prolymphocyte count in the peripheral blood is very high and there will be evidence of marrow failure, reflecting the degree of marrow infiltration. In addition the splenic involvement can be massive and in contrast to CLL significant lymphadenopathy is not common although, if examined, nodes will be found to be infiltrated. The prognosis of B-PLL is much poorer than that for CLL.

The cells of B-PLL are immunophenotypically distinct from CLL

Morphologically the cells in B-PLL resemble the prolymphocytes seen in the peripheral blood of patients with progressive CLL or in proliferation centres but they are immunophenotypically distinct. The cells are larger than normal lymphocytes with more cytoplasm. The nucleus lacks the clumped chromatin seen in CLL and there is a prominent large nucleolus (Figure 8.25). The cells in B-PLL express IgM at much higher levels than CLL and do not express CD5. The expression of markers such as FMC7 and CD11c suggests that the cells are at a late stage in B-cell maturation.

The conventional criterion for the diagnosis of B-PLL is a prolymphocyte count greater than 55% and it is often presented as part of a

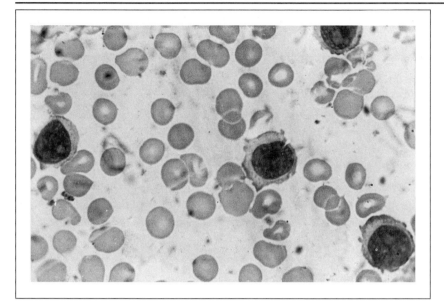

Figure 8.25 B-cell prolymphocytic leukaemia – peripheral blood. This patient presented with a very high lymphocyte count and splenomegaly. In the peripheral blood there was a monomorphic population of large cells with abundant cytoplasm and prominent nucleoli. These cells have strong sIg expression and CD5 was not detected.

spectrum with CLL and CLL-pro. The distinctiveness of the clinical syndrome and the major differences in immunophenotype suggest that this approach is misleading and there is little evidence to suggest that CLL and B-PLL are related or that B-PLL arises by progression of CLL.

The features of B-prolymphocytic leukaemia are summarized in Table 8.14.

The differential diagnosis of B-PLL also includes hairy cell leukaemia and its variant, circulating cells of follicle centre lymphoma, T-PLL and possibly mantle cell lymphoma. The combination of immunophenotype and clinical features should allow B-PLL to be distinguished from these conditions without difficulty in most cases.

Table 8.14 B-prolymphocytic leukaemia

- **Morphology:** Intermediate-sized lymphoid cells with prominent central nucleoli.
- **Immunophenotype:** sIgM⁺, CD19⁺, CD20⁺, CD38⁺, CD10⁻, CD23⁻, CD5⁻, FMC7⁺.
- **Cytogenetics:** No specific abnormality.
- **Pattern of disease:** Spleen, marrow and peripheral blood.

8.2.3 Hairy cell leukaemia

The syndrome of hairy cell leukaemia consists of cytopenia and splenomegaly

This is a rare disease and accounts for only 2–4% of all leukaemias. Most patients with hairy cell leukaemia (HCL) are over 50 years and will present with non-specific symptoms that are related to cytopenia. Although a pancytopenia may be present there is usually a disproportionate reduction in neutrophils and monocytes, which may sometimes by associated with infection. Over 80% of patients will have splenomegaly and 30–40% hepatomegaly at presentation but significant lymphadenopathy is rare and is seen in less than 20% of cases.

The morphology and phenotype of hairy cell leukaemia is highly distinctive

Almost all patients with HCL have peripheral blood infiltration but in some cases the number of cells may be low. The typical hairy cell is larger than a normal lymphocyte with more abundant agranular cytoplasm. The cytoplasmic membrane shows the typical, ruffled hairy pattern, which is best seen by scanning electron microscopy but can be seen by light microscopy. Such cytoplasmic projections are not diagnostic and may be seen in other late B-cell disorders. The nuclei may be oval, bilobular or plasmacytoid with indistinct nucleoli and is usually eccentrically placed within the cell.

In all cases suspected to be hairy cell leukaemia the diagnosis should be confirmed by marker studies

The histochemical demonstration of the tartrate-resistant isoenzyme of acid phosphatase remains in routine use but it gives a variable strength of reaction and has been largely superseded by immunophenotypic analysis. Hairy cells express light-chain restricted sIg together with the B-cell markers CD19, CD20 and CD22. CD5 and CD10 are not expressed. The distinctive features are the expression of the IL-2 receptor CD25, FMC7 and the integrins CD11c/18 and CD103 (HML1, BLY7) (Figure 8.26).

CD103 is an adhesion molecule associated with T-cell-epithelial interactions; the significance of its expression on hairy cells in unknown. Although there is no obvious normal counterpart to hairy cells all the

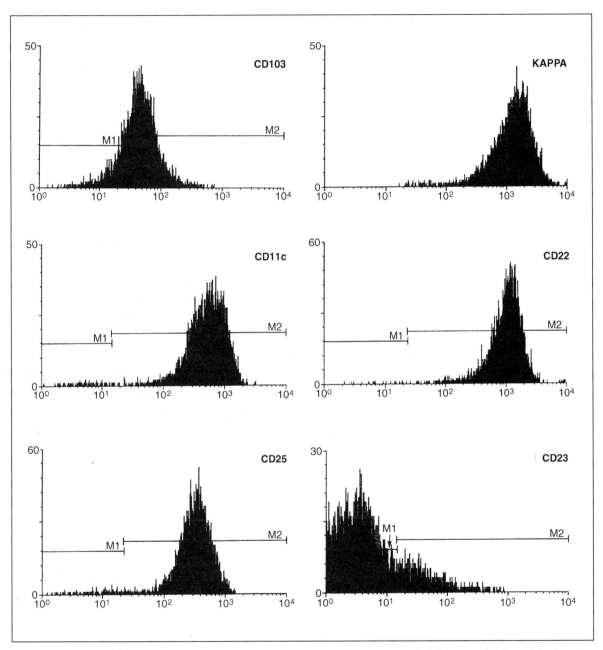

Figure 8.26 Hairy cell leukaemia – immunophenotype. These histograms show typical features of hairy cell leukaemia. All the markers are performed by double labelling with anti-CD19. In addition to expression of sIg, CD19 and CD22, HCL typically shows expression of CD103, CD11c and CD25 and lacks CD5.

Table 8.15 Hairy cell leukaemia

- **Morphology**: Relatively abundant clear cytoplasm, membrane projection, oval or indented nuclei.
- **Immunophenotype**: sIg$^+$ (usually IgM), CD19$^+$, CD20$^+$, CD5$^-$, CD10$^-$, CD23$^{+/-}$, CD38$^+$, CD25$^+$, CD103$^+$, CD11c$^+$, tartrate-resistant acid phosphatase. Variant forms lack acid phosphatase and CD25 and may express sIgG.
- **Cytogenetics**: No specific abnormality known.
- **Pattern of disease**: Spleen, marrow and peripheral blood, with associated cytopenia.

evidence indicates that they are cells in the late preplasma-cell phase of B-cell maturation. In some cases plasmacytoid cells are seen and there may be a low level of IgM paraprotein.

The features of hairy cell leukaemia are summarized in Table 8.15.

In every case there will be marrow infiltration, which will be apparent even when hairy cells are very sparse in the peripheral blood. The morphology and phenotype of aspirated cells are similar to those seen in the peripheral blood but dry taps are very frequent. When the biopsy is examined under low power the marrow appears homogenous with a diffuse infiltrate and the cells appear widely separated. This appearance is due to the relatively large amount of cytoplasm of the hairy cell. The cells appear to have small oval nuclei and the cell membrane is often distinct on an H&E section. A distinctive feature of hairy cell leukaemia is the presence of dilated vascular channels, sometimes with extravasation and pooling of red cells. Normal marrow elements are reduced and in most cases there is a striking reduction in myeloid progenitors. In fixed bone-marrow sections the diagnosis can be confirmed by the expression of DBA44. This antibody reacts with various other B-cells but in the marrow it is relatively specific for HCL. Reticulin staining reveals an excess of fibrous tissue, which explains the difficulty in aspiration of bone marrow.

The spleen in HCL is enlarged due to extensive infiltration of the red pulp by hairy cells

The enlargement of the spleen can be massive in HCL and is almost invariably present at diagnosis. As in the bone marrow, HCL in the spleen is associated with very prominent vascular congestion. So-called splenic pseudosinuses consist of distended spaces filled with red cells but lined with hairy cells rather than endothelium. There tends to be sparing of the lymphoid tissue which is often atrophic and it is uncommon for HCL to cause significant lymphadenopathy or infiltration of other organs although this does occur in a few patients with progressive disease. When present it may be either focal or diffuse involving the interfollicular zone and sinuses. If nodal enlargement is noted a biopsy should be carried out to exclude other causes (Figure 8.27).

Treatment may not be necessary at presentation

About 10% of patients will have stable disease for many years after presentation. Indications for commencing treatment include cytopenia, symptomatic splenomegaly, recurrent infections, extranodal infiltration, leukaemic phase and autoimmune phenomena.

Splenectomy can produce long-term remission in the absence of other treatments

Surgery to remove the enlarged spleen can lead to alleviation of many of the clinical problems associated with hairy cell leukaemia. Cytopenia frequently resolves, although the infiltration of the bone marrow persists. Interestingly it is not the size of the spleen that predicts the response to splenectomy but rather the degree of bone-marrow infiltration, and patients with relatively low levels of marrow infiltration are more likely to benefit. Some patients who respond well may enter a stable phase of the disease that may require no further treatment for many years.

Interferon is a useful agent in HCL

Good responses can be expected with alpha-interferon (IFNα) and at lower doses of the order of $3\,\text{mU} \times 3$/week few side effects are encountered other than minimal 'flu like' symptoms. In 70–80% of cases improvement of blood counts will be seen but complete responses will only be seen in 5% of cases. Significant amounts of residual disease will be expected and relapse should be anticipated in all cases and for these reasons treatment with IFNα should be continued indefinitely as long as the patient is tolerating the treatment.

Purine analogues are becoming increasingly widely used for the treatment of HCL

The introduction of the purine analogues represents a further major advance in the therapy of hairy cell leukaemia. The full effect of these novel agents in improving clinical response is yet to be evaluated as the median survival has yet to be reached. The most active of these agents is deoxycoformycin (DCF), given as a daily infusion for five days every month to maximum response, or 2-chlorodeoxyadenosine (2-CDA), given as a single infusion. The majority (50–80%) of patients achieve complete peripheral blood responses, a much higher percentage than after IFNα. The disease is not completely eradicated and there is frequently

Figure 8.27 Hairy cell leukaemia – marrow and spleen. The bone marrow in hairy cell leukaemia shows diffuse and interstitial infiltration **(a)**. The cells have abundant clear cytoplasm and oval or indented nuclei **(b)**. Intense vascular congestion is often present. The spleen **(c)** shows heavy infiltration of the red pulp.

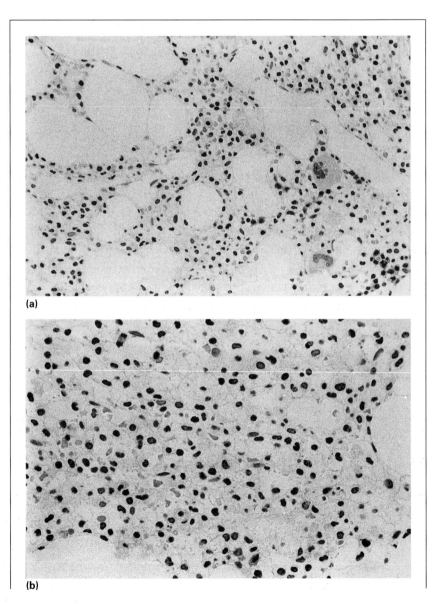

(a)

(b)

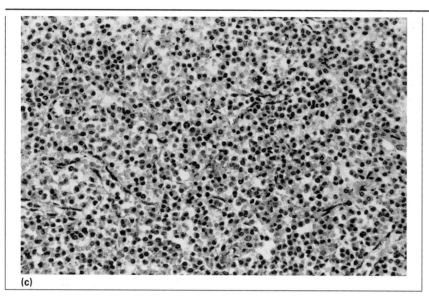

(c)

evidence of residual disease in the bone marrow. The timing of administration of DCF or 2-CDA is not crucial and they can be delivered at presentation, after splenectomy or a period of treatment with IFNα and similar responses can be expected. Side effects are similar to those encountered in the use of fludarabine. Fever is relatively common and opportunistic infections can occur but seem to be relatively infrequent in practice. The routine use of prophylactic acyclovir, co-trimoxazole and fluconazole may, however, be preventing the development of infection in most patients.

Rare variants of hairy cell leukaemia are described

Hairy cell leukaemia is a rare disorder and HCL variants are very rare. Patients have splenomegaly and no significant lymphadenopathy as in typical HCL, but there may be a considerable leukocytosis, which consists mainly of tumour cells. These cells differ from hairy cells in a number of respects. The nuclear morphology and prominent nucleolus may resemble a prolymphocyte and the cells do not express tartrate-resistant acid phosphatase or CD25. There is insufficient data at present on CD103 expression. HCL-variant cells express sIgG and a paraprotein is not seen. The patterns of marrow and spleen infiltration are similar to classical HCL (Figure 8.28).

Figure 8.28 Hairy cell variant – peripheral blood. This patient had a high white count consisting of cells that closely resembled hairy cells but lacked CD25 expression.

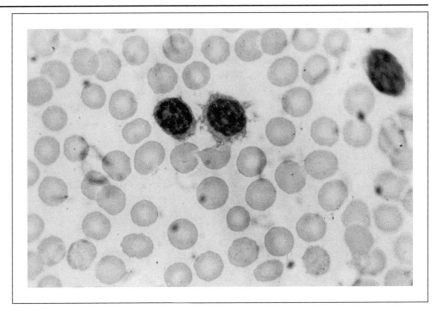

8.2.4 Splenic lymphoma with villous lymphocytes

Patients with splenic lymphoma with villous lymphocytes have significant splenomegaly without lymphadenopathy

The clinical syndrome of splenic lymphoma with villous lymphocytes (SLVL) has a number of features in common with hairy cell leukaemia. SLVL is a rare condition with an incidence that is probably similar to HCL and with a similar age distribution. As with HCL, SLVL patients have splenomegaly without clinically significant lymphadenopathy. Massive enlargement of the spleen with symptoms of abdominal pain and distension may be the presenting problem in some cases along with non-specific general symptoms. There may be changes in the peripheral blood due to hypersplenism but the specific neutropenia and monocytopenia seen in HCL does not seem to be a feature of SLVL. In SLVL the lymphocyte count is typically much higher than in HCL and is reported to be in the range $10–30 \times 10^9/l$.

The features of SLVL are summarized in Table 8.16.

Cellular morphology, immunophenotype and pattern of tissue infiltration differ from HCL

As the name suggests, SLVL was first described on the basis of the cell morphology in the peripheral blood. The typical cell is larger than a

Table 8.16 Splenic lymphoma with villous lymphocytes

- **Morphology**: In the peripheral blood typical cell is a lymphocyte with villous projections at the poles. In marrow and spleen there is more heterogeneous population which includes cells with cleaved nuclei and plasmacytoid cells.
- **Immunophenotype**: sIgM$^+$, sIgD$^{+/-}$, CD19$^+$, CD20$^+$, CD22$^+$, CD38$^+$, CD11c$^+$, FMC7$^+$, CD23$^-$, CD10$^-$, CD25$^-$. Some cases express CD5 and CD103. Tartrate-resistant acid phosphatase$^-$.
- **Cytogenetics**: Trisomy 3 in some cases.
- **Pattern of disease**: Spleen, marrow and peripheral blood. Morphological and phenotypical heterogeneity suggest this may not be a single entity; there is an uncertain relationship to marginal zone lymphoma.

---

mature lymphocyte and has irregular cytoplasmic villi at the poles of the cell. However, there is probably a wider range of morphological appearances than in the other late B-cell syndromes described above. A proportion of nucleolated cells may be present and cells resembling hairy cells may be seen. The cells of SLVL express strong sIgM and in some cases IgD may be present. In many cases an IgM paraprotein may be found, although the cells in the peripheral blood do not express cytoplasmic immunoglobulin. The cells express pan-B-cell markers CD19, CD20 and CD22 and markers of late B-cell differentiation CD38, CD11c and FMC7, and in a few cases CD103. CD23 and CD10 are not expressed. The lack of CD25 and tartrate-resistant acid phosphatase are important distinguishing features from HCL. Most cases of SLVL are CD5$^-$ but a few cases have been reported of otherwise typical cases that appear to express this marker.

In some cases the bone marrow aspirate may show no evidence of infiltration by SLVL but in almost every case tumour is found on a trephine biopsy. The pattern of infiltration is quite different from hairy cell leukaemia, with a nodular infiltrate of cells with centrocyte-like or plasmacytoid features. Examination of the spleen in SLVL shows a variable pattern of involvement. A marginal zone pattern of infiltration with sparing of the germinal centres may be seen. In other cases there may be more diffuse replacement of the splenic lymphoid tissue and in some cases there is nodular and diffuse involvement of the red pulp (Figure 8.29).

It has been suggested that SLVL may represent a spleen and marrow variant of marginal zone lymphoma. However, the variation in immunophenotype seen between cases, including CD5 and IgD expression, suggests that SLVL may not be a single entity but rather a variety of indolent

Figure 8.29 Splenic lymphoma with villous lymphocytes. This patient had typical peripheral blood morphological and immunophenotypical features of SLVL. Splenectomy was carried out to relieve symptoms of massive splenic enlargement. The splenic lymphoid tissue was expanded and replaced by a population of B-cell with irregular or cleaved nuclei and a proportion of larger nucleolated blast cells (a). Anti-CD21 (b) shows fragments of residual follicular dendritic cell networks in germinal centres, which have been replaced by neoplastic cells.

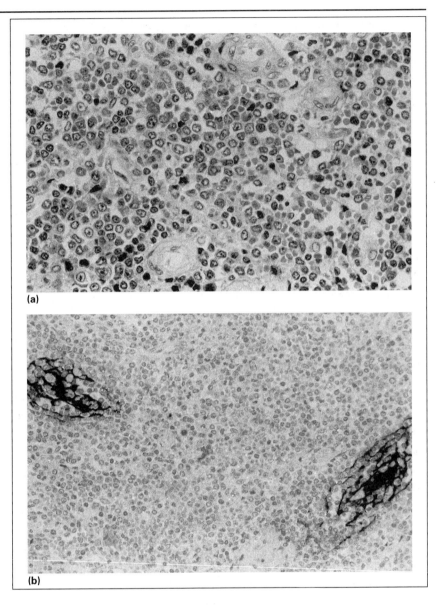

(a)

(b)

B-cell tumours that display a propensity for spleen and marrow infiltration. Equally unclear is the relationship between SLVL and the rare cases of primary splenic marginal zone lymphoma without marrow, blood or nodal disease.

Treatment is directed by clinical symptoms

The clinical course of SLVL is variable but in many patients it will be indolent and treatment should be directed principally towards suppression of symptoms. Many of the symptoms can be relieved by splenectomy but it is important to carry this out when the patients are in good health; they are an elderly group of patients and tolerate operative procedures poorly. Alternative treatments are the judicious use of single-agent oral alkylating agents, which will control disease bulk, or combination chemotherapy, which may increase the response rate but at the expense of more treatment-related side effects.

8.3 The immunosecretory disorders

8.3.1 Waldenström's macroglobulinaemia

In the REAL classification the term lymphoplasmacytoid lymphoma/immunocytoma is used to describe this tumour but terms need to be used with care as they have had different meanings in other classifications.

Waldenström's macroglobulinaemia is a lymphoproliferative syndrome in which most of the clinical features are due to an IgM paraprotein

Waldenström's macroglobulinaemia (WM) may present with a range of problems most of which are attributable either to the production of an IgM paraprotein or to marrow replacement by tumour. IgM forms complexes in the peripheral circulation, which leads to increasing plasma viscosity which may in turn cause a range of non-specific symptoms including fatigue, weight loss and visual disturbances. Increasing plasma viscosity is also associated with disorders of haemostasis, which may occur as a consequence of platelet deficiency or functional abnormality due to marrow infiltration caused by IgM inhibiting platelet agglutination. In some cases the IgM paraprotein behaves as a Type 1 cryoglobulin and precipitation as IgM complexes in the peripheral circulation may cause Raynaud's syndrome. Activation of complement may lead to vasculitis in skin, peripheral nerves or kidney. In around 10% of patients the IgM paraprotein functions as a cold agglutinin, often reacting with the Ia antigen in the peripheral circulation leading to complement activation and chronic haemolysis (Figure 8.30).

The features of Waldenström's macroglobulinaemia are summarized in Table 8.17.

In comparison with myeloma a relatively small proportion of patients develop amyloidosis affecting the heart, lungs, liver and kidney (Figure 8.31). However, in these patients the development of amyloidosis greatly

Figure 8.30 Waldenström's macroglobulinaemia. This patient presented with a IgM paraproteinaemia. The bone marrow was heavily infiltrated by a mixture of light-chain-restricted small B-cells and plasma cells producing IgM **(a)**. The trephine biopsy shows extensive diffuse marrow replacement **(b)**.

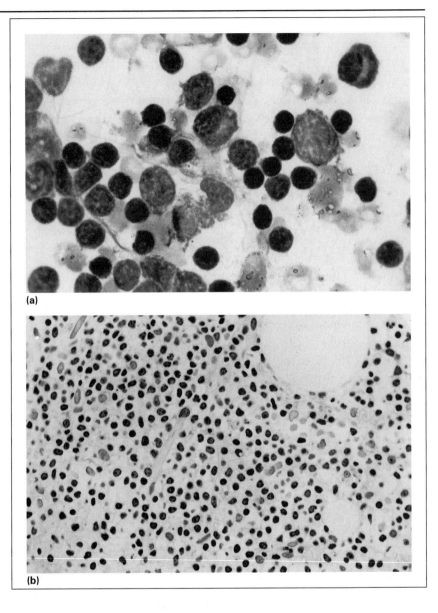

(a)

(b)

increases the risk of death due to cardiorespiratory or renal failure. Nephrotic syndrome and renal impairment may also occur in the absence of amyloid due to the deposition of IgM in the glomerulus.

A small number of patients develop a peripheral sensorimotor neuropathy. In these patients the IgM paraprotein appears to have antimyelin activity. It should be noted that most patients with clonal-IgM-mediated neuropathy have minimal marrow infiltration by lymphoma.

Table 8.17 Waldenström's macroglobulinaemia

- **Morphology**: Small lymphocytes and plasma cells with variable numbers of larger cells with irregular nuclei and occasional blast cells.
- **Immunophenotype**: sIgM$^+$, sIgD$^-$, CD19$^+$, CD20$^+$, CD5$^-$, CD10$^-$, CD23$^{+/-}$ with clonal IgM-secreting plasma cells.
- **Cytogenetics**: No specific abnormality known.
- **Pattern of disease**: Spleen, marrow, nodes and peripheral blood with IgM paraprotein. Hyperviscosity syndrome.

The tumour in Waldenström's macroglobulinaemia consists of mature lymphocytes and plasma cells

Most patients with WM have disseminated disease with varying degrees of peripheral blood, bone marrow, lymph node and sometimes liver and spleen infiltration. In most cases the diagnosis will be made on examination of the peripheral blood and marrow and it is relatively rare to make this diagnosis on a node biopsy. In the bone marrow there is usually an extensive infiltrate, which may form areas of diffuse marrow replacement separated by hyperplastic marrow. The infiltrate consists of mature small lymphocytes that strongly express monoclonal sIgM, pan-B-cell markers and late B-cell differentiation markers such as CD38 and

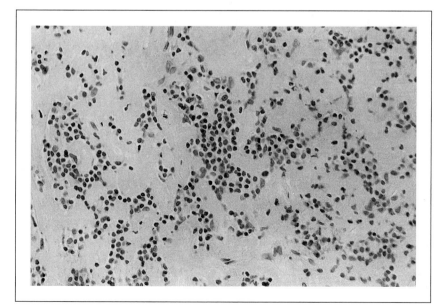

Figure 8.31 Waldenström's – orbital deposit. This patient who had a long history of WM, presented with a space-occupying lesion in the orbit. This consisted of amyloid together with an infiltrate of clonal B-cell and plasma cells.

FMC7; CD5 and CD10 are not expressed. These cells are mixed with varying numbers of plasma cells and plasmacytoid cells, which have monoclonal cIgM with the same light chain as the B-lymphocyte. A few of the cells have a strongly PAS-positive nuclear inclusion known as a Dutcher body. A very common feature is the presence of hyperplasia of bone marrow mast cells, which will be striking in a Giemsa-stained marrow section. A peripheral blood lymphocytosis consisting of B-cells similar to those in the marrow may be present.

In lymph node biopsies the nature of the infiltrate is similar in composition to marrow in most cases but increased numbers of blast cells may be present and it is uncertain if this affects the prognosis. In a few cases large cell transformation with replacement of lymphoid tissue by diffuse monomorphic populations of immunoblasts can occur. Involvement of the spleen can occur and shows an infiltrate centred on the lymphoid tissue if it is examined.

Some other types of lymphoma, including follicle centre lymphoma and marginal zone lymphoma, may contain a mixture of lymphocytes and plasma cells and in CLL a considerable number of cells may have plasmacytoid features. All of these differential diagnosis may be readily resolved by considering the morphological and phenotypical features in the context of the clinical findings. A number of tumours such as CLL and hairy cell leukaemia also produce paraprotein but at levels that do not produce a hyperviscosity syndrome.

Problems rarely arise in making the distinction between Waldenström's macroglobulinaemia and myeloma. In a very few patients clinical features of myeloma may be present with a considerable population of sIgG$^+$ clonal B-lymphocytes in the peripheral blood and marrow. In practice the other clinical features usually determine which cases should be treated as multiple myeloma.

Treatment and prognosis of Waldenström's macroglobulinaemia
This is an indolent disease and treatment is directed towards suppressing the clinical manifestations associated with the IgM paraproteinaemia and the effects of tumour cell infiltration. Plasmapheresis will reduce the effects of hyperviscosity and may be indicated as a short term supportive measure. Low-dose oral alkylating agent therapy, in particular chlorambucil, is widely adopted as a means of reducing the tumour cell load. Long-term usage carries the risk of mutagenesis and this may be reduced by giving pulsed intermittent treatment. There are increasing reports of good responses to therapy with the purine analogues, fludarabine and 2-CDA.

8.3.2 Multiple myeloma

The central feature of myeloma is the accumulation of clonal plasma cells in the bone marrow. However, the progenitor cell that gives rise to these plasma cells may be present in other lymphoid organs.

The incidence of myeloma and monoclonal gammopathy of uncertain significance (MGUS) is difficult to ascertain accurately but it seems to account for 10–15% of all haematological malignancies and 1–2% of all malignant disease. This is equivalent to an incidence of clinically apparent disease of around 3/100 000/year. The incidence of asymptomatic MGUS is much higher. The incidence of myeloma increases with age and only 2% of all cases occur before the age of 40 years.

The diagnosis and assessment of myeloma

Myeloma is a syndrome characterized by lytic bone lesions, paraproteinaemia and marrow failure

The progressive replacement of the bone marrow by neoplastic plasma cells is responsible for the observed clinical features of the disease. The plasma cells show dysregulated immunoglobulin production which, in the majority of cases, results in high concentration of paraprotein in the peripheral blood and suppression of immunoglobulin production by normal B-cells. In about 80% of cases immunoglobulin light chain is produced in excess of heavy chains. The excess light chain is secreted in the urine and is an important cause of nephrotoxicity and in some cases amyloidosis. The infiltrating plasma cells are responsible for disordered bone metabolism, which is the presenting feature in most cases. Finally in the latter stages of the disease there may be progressive marrow replacement and marrow failure.

The diagnosis of myeloma is based on the level of paraprotein levels, the presence of lytic bone lesions and the extent of plasma cell infiltration of the bone marrow

Multiple myeloma is unusual among the haematological malignancies in that the diagnosis is based less on cellular features and more on variables related to disease bulk and its clinical effects. One measure of the extent of disease is the concentration of paraprotein which should exceed 35 g/l for IgG or 20 g/l for IgA (other immunoglobulin types are very rare), with urinary free light chain of more than 1 g/24 h. A serum beta-2-microglobulin concentration of more than 4 mg/l is supplementary

Figure 8.32 Serum beta-2-microglobulin and survival in multiple myeloma. A level of more than 4 mg/l of serum beta-2-microglobulin at presentation is associated with a significantly poorer prognosis in patients with myeloma.

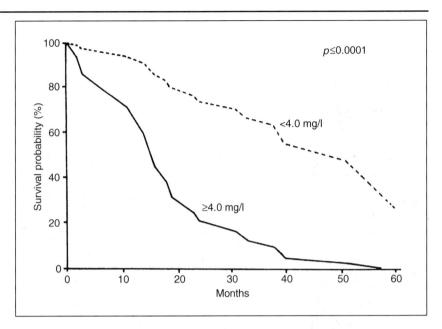

evidence of significant disease bulk (Figure 8.32). In addition, the patient should have one of the typical complications of myeloma – anaemia, hypercalcaemia and bone disease, renal insufficiency or immunosuppression as judged by reduction of the normal immunoglobulin concentration (Figure 8.33).

In most cases of myeloma the number of plasma cells will exceed 10% of the nucleated cells in a bone marrow aspirate and may show a wide range of cytological abnormalities including prominent nucleoli, cytoplasmic vacuolation or nuclear inclusions (Figure 8.34). In every case immunofluorescence studies should be carried out to confirm monoclonality and identify the immunoglobulin type being produced. This should be correlated with the serum paraproteins and urinary light chains.

It is now standard practice to perform a trephine biopsy in every case of suspected myeloma but it is not usually practical to accurately count the proportion of plasma cells in the trephine biopsy. A differential count would be very time-consuming and of doubtful validity because of the non-random distribution of myelomatous plasma cells, and the proportion of cells will be dependent on other marrow elements, i.e. whether it is hyper- or hypoplastic.

Normal plasma cells accumulate around blood vessels in the bone marrow but in the earliest stage of marrow involvement by myeloma this pattern is lost and the neoplastic plasma cells are found as single cells or

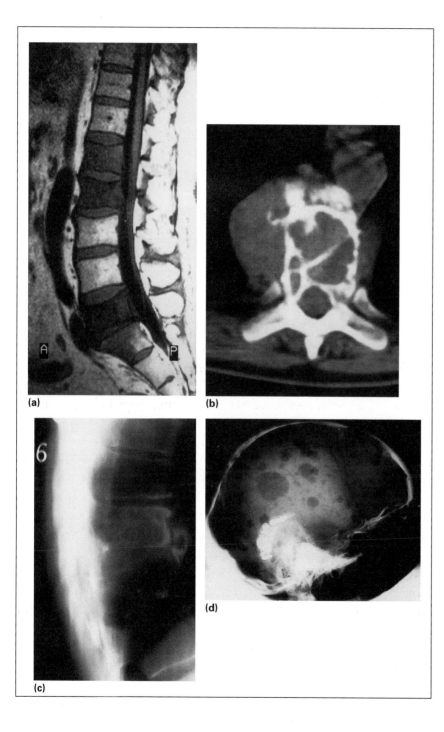

(a)

(b)

(c)

(d)

Figure 8.33 Myeloma – lytic bone lesions. **(a)** MR scan showing replacement of multiple vertebral bodies due to myeloma. **(b)** CT scan showing extensive destruction of a vertebral body with extension of tumour into the paravertebral tissue. **(c)** Lateral X-ray of lumbar spine showing collapse of a vertebral body. **(d)** Lateral X-ray of skull showing multiple lytic lesions.

Figure 8.34 (a, b) Myeloma – bone marrow aspirate. These bone marrow aspirates show infiltration by atypical plasma cells, including binuclear forms.

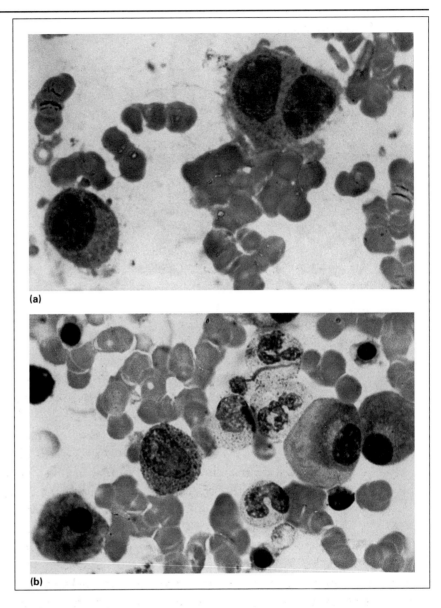

(a)

(b)

small clusters between adipocytes. As the disease progresses, areas of diffuse marrow replacement occur, ending in a packed marrow. These stages broadly correspond to the bulk of marrow disease. Two other patterns of infiltration are seen. In a small number of cases early myeloma shows a paratrabecular distribution similar to follicle centre lymphoma and in some patients with very aggressive disease tumour nodules, often containing very abnormal plasma cells, may be seen. In assessing the pattern of marrow disease in a trephine biopsy it can often be very helpful

Table 8.18 Multiple myeloma

- **Morphology**: Infiltration of the bone marrow by plasma cells, showing a wide range of morphological subtypes. In most cases there will be more than 10% of plasma cells in the marrow aspirate.
- **Immunophenotype**: Clonal cytoplasmsic IgG or IgA or light chain only expression (except in rare cases), sIg⁻, CD20⁻, CD38⁺. Myeloma plasma cells differ from their normal counterparts in having a lower level of CD19 and CD45 and increased expression of CD56 and syndecam-1. IgG or IgA paraprotein and urinary free light chain.
- **Cytogenetic**: Aneuploidy is common, with a wide range of numerical chromosomal abnormalities; 13q-, 11q- and 14q- are said to have prognostic significance.
- **Pattern of disease**: Marrow replacement and lytic bone disease. Immune dysfunction, renal failure and a wide range of other systemic effects. Many patients have a low level of circulating plasma cells.

to use a plasma cell marker such as VS38c or an anti-light-chain antibody, as this will often show much heavier infiltration than is apparent on routine staining (Figure 8.35).

The morphological features of the neoplastic plasma cells seen in trephine biopsies are very variable. In most cases 25% or more of the cells are nucleolated and cells with multiple nuclei or cleaved nuclei may be seen. Cells with abundant foamy or vacuolated cytoplasm may not be readily identified as plasma cells. In some patients with very aggressive disease, especially those in relapse, the marrow may be replaced by large lymphoid cells, resembling immunoblasts, with only a small proportion of cells showing features of plasma-cell differentiation. The cell-cycle fraction can be determined using Ki67 but the proportion of positive plasma cells is very low except in patients with very aggressive disease.

Relatively few B-lymphocytes are present in trephine biopsies infiltrated by myeloma. However, in a few cases one or more large aggregates of small B-cells, admixed with occasional proliferating blast cells may be present. The significance of this finding is not known.

The principal features of multiple myeloma are summarized in Table 8.18.

It is important to distinguish myeloma from the much more common monoclonal gammopathy of unknown significance (MGUS)

As many as 1% of the elderly population have MGUS. In these patients the paraprotein and marrow plasma cell counts do not meet the criteria for multiple myeloma and there is no evidence of bone lesions, anaemia, renal failure or immunosuppression (Table 8.19). In the trephine biopsy a clonal plasma cells population may be present but this is usually very sparse, with an interstitial distribution. A clonal population may sometimes be seen in the aspirate. Some patients with MGUS progress to myeloma and it is not surprising that intermediate or equivocal states exist in which the serological and marrow features of myeloma are present but the patient is asymptomatic with minimal bone lesions. The terms equivocal, indolent or smouldering are used in such cases.

Figure 8.35 Myeloma – trephine biopsy. The pattern of infiltration is a measure of the extent of marrow replacement in myeloma. In early disease **(a)** there is a sparse interstitial infiltrate of atypical plasma, which progresses to marrow replacement **(b)**. In some cases the marrow, especially in relapse, is replaced by highly pleomorphic large nucleolated cells only a few of which are readily identifiable as plasma cells **(c)**.

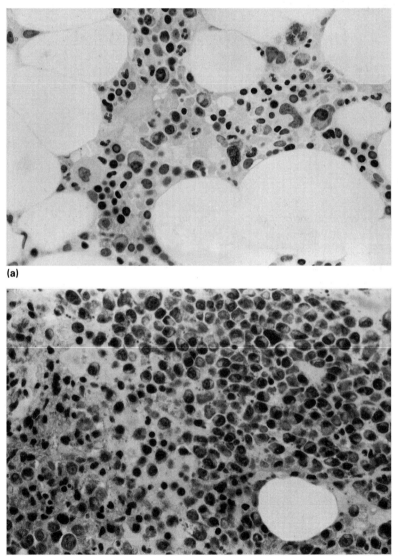

(a)

(b)

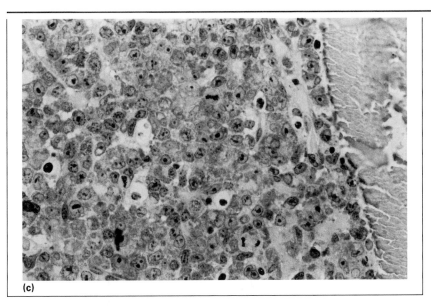

(c)

Table 8.19 Diagnostic criteria for MGUS and myeloma

Monoclonal gammopathy of undetermined significance (MGUS)
- Paraprotein level low and stable (serum IgG $\leq$ 35 g/l, IgA $\leq$ 20 g/l; urinary light chain $\leq$ 500 mg/24 h)
- Marrow plasma cells < 10% (without aggregates/clusters in trephine biopsy)
- No bone lesions
- No anaemia, renal failure or hypercalcaemia
- Additional investigations carried out to exclude multiple myeloma should confirm a normal serum beta-2-microglobulin and absence of light-chain isotype suppression; detailed imaging with CT or MRI should also exclude bone lesions

Multiple myeloma
- Paraprotein (serum IgG > 35 g/l, IgA > 2 g/l, urinary light chains $\geq$ 1.0 g/24 h)
- Bone marrow plasma cells $\geq$ 10% (or clusters in trephine or plasmacytoma in tissue biopsy)
- Additional findings (at least one and not attributable to another disease state):
  - Immunosuppression (normal IgM < 5 g/dl; IgA < 10 g/dl; IgG < 60 g/dl)
  - Lytic lesions (or osteoporosis with plasma cells > 30% in marrow)
  - Anaemia
  - Renal insufficiency
  - Hypercalcaemia
  - Serum β_2m > 4 mg/l

In patients with established myeloma a number of variables may be used to assess tumour load in an attempt to predict outcome

A variety of staging systems have been suggested but the most widely used is the Durie–Salmon staging system, which is based on assessment of bone lesions and paraprotein levels. Although useful in the context of clinical trials this staging system is not highly accurate in predicting the prognosis in the individual patient.

In addition to serum paraprotein levels the beta-2-microglobulin β_2m concentration has been found to be the most powerful prognostic indicator in a number of trials. β_2m is the light chain of class 1 major histocompatibility proteins and as such is present on all nucleated cells. Free serum and urinary β_2m is probably derived from cell membrane turnover. At presentation the β_2m concentration appears to correlate with tumour bulk although the mechanism underlying this relationship is not well understood. The power of β_2m measurement has been shown to be further increased when combined with measurement of the proliferative fraction in the plasma cells, either by pulse labelling or by the use of Ki67. This prognostic value of β_2m/proliferative fraction is independent of other known prognostic factors. A number of other prognostic markers, such as cytogenetic abnormalities and expression of P-glycoprotein, have been proposed but have not gained wide acceptance.

Recently defined and potentially useful prognostic factors that are independent of β_2m have been described. These include the serum level of IL6, the level of the soluble IL6 receptor and the level of soluble gP130. As yet the clinical value of these is not fully established.

A major prognostic variable is the response to initial therapy, especially anthracycline regimes such as VAD (vincristine, Adriamycin, dexamethasone) and VAMP (vincristine, Adriamycin, methylprednisolone). The increasing interest in the use of intensive therapy has greatly increased the need to identify subgroups of patients who will benefit most.

The pathogenesis of multiple myeloma
The central problem in myeloma is that the plasma cells that accumulate and replace the bone marrow are terminally differentiated with a very low rate of cell division. The nature of the progenitor cell that gives rise to these plasma cells remains controversial. In many patients it is possible to detect cells belonging to the myeloma clone in the peripheral blood by PCR but the majority of these cells appear to be plasma cells or preplasma

cells. B-cells are greatly reduced in number in the peripheral blood of myeloma patients and are not phenotypically distinct.

Much can be implied about the origin of the myeloma clone by studying IgH gene rearrangements in MGUS and myeloma

Somatic hypermutation occurs in the germinal centre and, if the cell of origin of myeloma occurred prior to passage through this structure, multiple somatic mutations would be expected in the myelomatous clone. If, however the transformed cell is post-germinal-centre then although somatic hypermutation will be present there will be no intraclonal variation. What is seen in myeloma is clonal IgH rearrangements with identical somatic mutations and no intraclonal diversity, which implies that the bulk of the clone has arisen from a transformed cell that has passed through a germinal centre. Like many other types of tumour it is possible that myeloma may develop through a multistep process and one or more of these antecedent steps may involve the transformation of pre-germinal-centre cells. If so, it would be expected that at least a small proportion of the myeloma clone would contain the same V region fused to mu heavy chain. The finding of such rearrangements has been claimed in some cases of IgG myeloma lending some support to this idea, though contradictory results have also been reported.

If MGUS, a premyelomatous condition, is examined in a similar fashion, multiple somatic mutations are found and it is easier to detect preswitch cells. These data are consistent with a model where the initial immortalized cell in MGUS is a pre-germinal-centre cell or possibly a marginal zone memory B-cell. Such clones may be multiple and the transition to myeloma is accompanied by further genetic change, leading to the growth advantage and clonal predominance of a single clone at the level of differentiation of a post-germinal-centre cell in which class switching has already occurred.

Myeloma plasma cells differ from their normal counterparts in a number of respects

Myeloma plasma cells can be distinguished from normal cells by their immunophenotype. The features of myeloma plasma cells include lower expression of important signal transduction molecules such as CD19 or CD45 and increased expression of the adhesion molecules

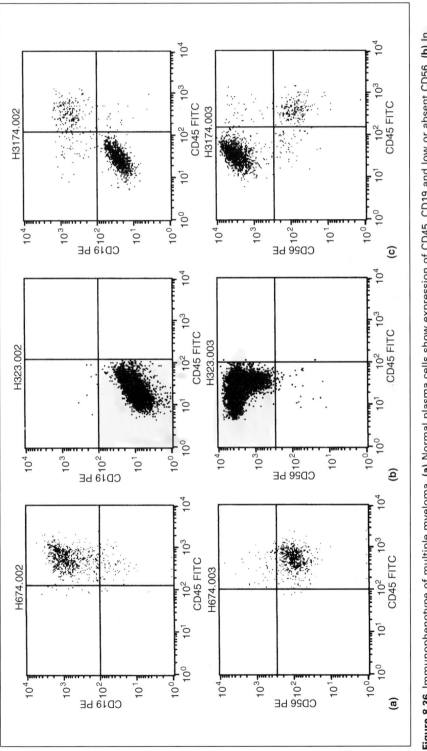

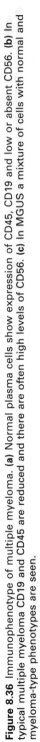

Figure 8.36 Immunophenotype of multiple myeloma. **(a)** Normal plasma cells show expression of CD45, CD19 and low or absent CD56. **(b)** In typical multiple myeloma CD19 and CD45 are reduced and there are often high levels of CD56. **(c)** In MGUS a mixture of cells with normal and myeloma-type phenotypes are seen.

CD56 and syndecam 1 (CD138). The exact immunophenotypic identification of plasma cells is difficult and three-colour flow cytometric methods are essential using a combination of CD38 and syndecam 1 (CD138) together with a third antibody to identify subsets. These immunophenotypic differences represent major changes in cell adhesion and cell signalling pathways and may be the key to understanding the invasive properties of myeloma plasma cells in bone marrow. In patients with MGUS it is usual to find a mixture of plasma cells with both normal and abnormal immunophenotypical features (Figure 8.36).

IL-6 is a critical cytokine in the pathogenesis of myeloma

The cytokine IL-6 is now regarded as being central to regulation of myeloma growth (Figure 8.37).

Although IL-6 was described as a cytokine that could induce immunoglobulin secretion by B-cells, it does not appear to fulfil this role in myeloma and instead IL-6 appears to promote the growth of the myeloma clone. The evidence from *in vitro* studies suggests that in most cases the source of IL-6 is the bone marrow stroma or macrophages. In culture, IL-6-mediated promotion of growth is seen mainly in cells derived from patients with active disease; cells from

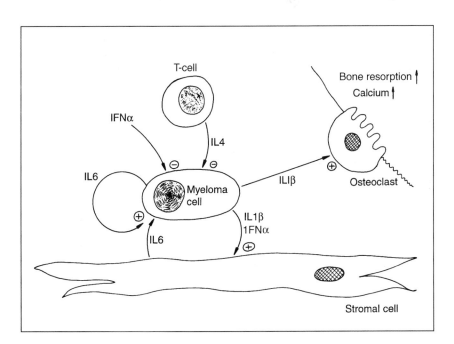

Figure 8.37 Cytokine interactions in myeloma. A key element in the pathogenesis of myeloma is the cytokine interactions that take place between the neoplastic plasma cells and the bone-marrow stromal cells, T-cells and osteoclasts. Abnormal cytokine production may determine the growth of the myeloma cells and be responsible for bone destruction.

plateau phase are less responsive. This effect is enhanced by several other cytokines such as G-CSF and IL-3 and exposure to gamma-interferon can abolish the response.

On the basis of these *in vitro* culture experiments there has been speculation as to whether the stromal cells in myeloma are abnormal or whether they are in turn responding to cytokines produced by the myeloma cells. One example of such a cytokine, produced by at least some myeloma cells and able to upregulate IL-6 production by bone marrow stroma, is IL-1β.

Although this paracrine stimulation of myeloma cells by IL-6 from stromal cells is regarded as the predominant mechanism, some myeloma-derived cell lines show autocrine production and stimulation by IL-6. Recently, it has been shown that in myeloma, but not in most cases of MGUS, there is a population of bone marrow stromal cells infected with the HHV-8 virus, which is also associated with Kaposi's sarcoma and body-cavity-based B-cell lymphoma. This virus has been shown to produce a homologue of IL-6 and it has been suggested that HHV-8-infected stroma may be a critical factor in the progression of MGUS to myeloma.

A range of molecular abnormalities is described in myeloma but most are present in only a small number of cases

Unlike many types of lymphoproliferative disorder there are no genetic abnormalities that are characteristic of myeloma. However, a range of abnormalities have been described, usually in a minority of cases. Numerical abnormalities are relatively common, although highly variable, chromosomes 3, 7, 9 and 11 being the most commonly detected.

Conventional cytogenetic analysis has identified translocation involving 14q23 (the immunoglobulin heavy-chain locus) in a small proportion of cases of myeloma. However, when this has been combined with more detailed molecular cytogenetic studies the proportion of cases appears higher, at least in myeloma cell lines. Unlike most translocations involving this locus in other B-cell lymphoproliferative disorders the IgH switch region is involved and it has been suggested that these abnormalities occur at the time of immunoglobulin class switching in the germinal centre. The partner locus in these translocations is highly variable. Among the most common is the *bcl-1* locus at 11q13, which leads to dysregulation of cyclin D1; this may be present in up to 25% of cases. Another commonly involved gene is *FGFR3* (4p16), which is a receptor for fibroblast growth factor. Plasma cells expressing this gene may receive aberrant growth signals from stromal cells producing FGF.

Mutational activation of N-*ras* and K-*ras* has been reported in up to one-third of patients with myeloma. These mutations disrupt the regulation of cell-signalling pathways and may lead to an enhanced response to IL-6 and protection from steroid induced apoptosis. Mutation of *p53* has also been described in some cases, but this appears to be a feature of advanced disease.

Based on the data summarized above a pathogenic model of MGUS and multiple myeloma is now emerging. The initial event in the development of MGUS is likely to be at the level of the germinal centre, where an immortalized clone of pre-germinal-centre B-lymphocytes or memory B-cells continues to pass through a germinal centre and produce increased numbers of paraprotein-producing bone-marrow plasma cells, which are heterogeneous in their pattern of somatic hypermutation. Further genetic change leads to clonal expansion at the plasma-cell or preplasma-cell stage and recirculation of these cells leads to widespread marrow infiltration. The neoplastic plasma cells are stimulated by stroma-derived IL-6, possibly of viral origin. Cytokines produced by the plasma cells affect the bone marrow stroma and lead to abnormal bone turnover and lytic bone lesions. The relationship of the various molecular abnormalities to these stages of development is not yet clear.

Diagnostic problems in myeloma

Solitary plasmacytoma of bone is closely related to and may progress to myeloma

A small group of patients present with a solitary bone lesion which on biopsy is found to be a plasmacytoma. In the majority of cases the lesion is in the vertebral body and causes a vertebral collapse fracture, often with spinal cord compression. The diagnosis of solitary plasmacytoma depends on the demonstration that the lesion consists of a population of clonal plasma cells and that there is no evidence of disseminated disease by bone marrow aspirate, trephine and skeletal survey or MRI (Figure 8.38).

Some, but not all, patients with solitary plasmacytoma have a paraprotein, though with lower levels than is usual in multiple myeloma; associated immunoparesis is uncommon. However, patients with solitary plasmacytoma of bone have a high rate of progression to multiple myeloma, indicating that these are variants of the same disease process. Good disease control and sometimes cure can be achieved with local radiotherapy. Before embarking on such treatment it is important to

Figure 8.38 Solitary plasmacytoma. This patient presented with a lytic bone lesion due to infiltration by neoplastic plasma cells. Bone marrow investigation showed no evidence of generalized marrow disease. Many of these cases will eventually progress to overt myeloma.

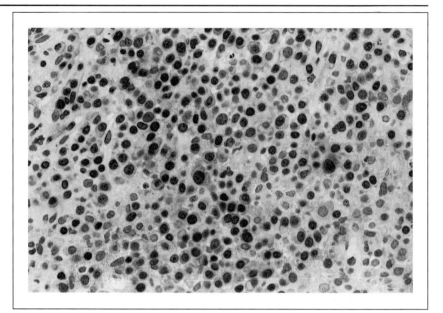

exclude other lesions by MRI. If all of the lesion can be incorporated into a radiation field the median survival is around 10 years, a much better prognosis than for multiple myeloma.

An area of confusion is the relationship of solitary plasmacytoma of bone to plasmacytoma at other sites. The upper respiratory tract is the most common extraskeletal site, but plasmacytomas are seen in skin, lymph node, thymus and at almost any other site. In resolving this confusion it is important to remember that most types of B-cell lymphoma can show some evidence of plasma cell differentiation and in a few cases plasma cells may predominate, e.g. in marginal zone lymphoma (MALToma). Secondly, unlike plasmacytoma in bone, plasmacytomas at other sites do not progress to myeloma. This should not be confused with nodal or soft tissue spread of myeloma which occasionally occurs in the context of advanced disease.

Some aggressive B-cell lymphomas may be confined to bone marrow and may show plasmacytoid differentiation

A small number of patients present with bone-marrow failure with or without lytic bone lesions. Bone marrow examination shows replacement of normal marrow by a diffuse large cell lymphoma consisting of rapidly proliferating cells, centroblastic-, immunoblastic- or plasmablastic-type morphology. Only a minority of the cells express cIg and a paraprotein is

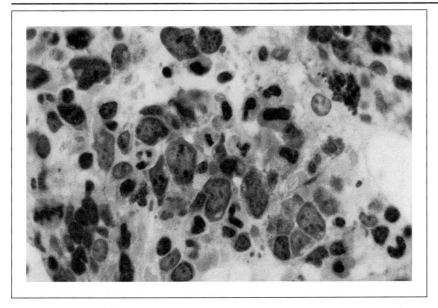

Figure 8.39 Diffuse large B-cell lymphoma localized to marrow. This patient presented with cytopenia but no evidence of nodal disease or other tumour masses. The marrow was replaced with large B-cells that expressed sIg and showed no evidence of plasma-cell differentiation. A complete remission was achieved with CHOP chemotherapy.

often absent. The tumour cells express CD20 and do not have the typical the immunophenotype of myeloma plasma cells. Limited studies suggest that these tumour may respond well to CHOP (Figure 8.39).

Plasma cell leukaemia is a rare complication of myeloma but may occur without preceding disease

In a small number of patients with myeloma an overtly leukaemic phase develops with rising plasma cell counts in the peripheral blood and bone marrow failure. This represents progressive disease and should not pose a diagnostic problem. However, plasma cell leukaemia may occur as a cause of acute bone marrow failure without a well documented history of preceding multiple myeloma. What may give rise to considerable diagnostic problems is the presentation of plasma cell leukaemia with bone marrow failure without preceding myeloma. The cells in the peripheral blood may be of lymphocyte size without clear evidence of plasma cell morphology and in some cases monotypical sIg expression may be present which will tend to obscure the detection of cIg. In these instances the key to diagnosis is the identification of other phenotypical features of plasma cell differentiation such as CD38 and Syndecam-1 positivity with loss of pan-B-cell markers (Figure 8.40).

The distinction of myeloma from Waldenström's macroglobulinaemia has been described above.

Figure 8.40 Plasma cell leukaemia. This patient presented with cytopenia and a very high white cell count with no history of myeloma. The cells were larger than small lymphocytes, with a rim of basophilic cytoplasm. The cells had a plasma cell immunophenotype with very high CD38 expression. No bone lesions were present.

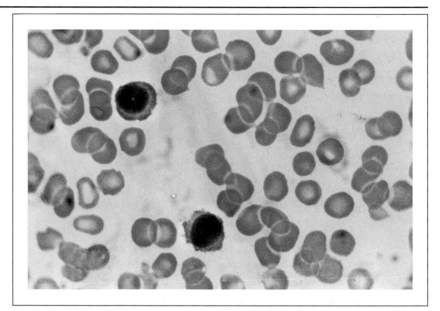

Systemic effects of multiple myeloma

Many of the clinical features of multiple myeloma are brought about by the interaction of the plasma cells with the osteoclasts of the bone matrix

Lesions of the skeleton represent the most frequent presenting symptom of myeloma. Typically, these are punched out lytic lesions, which are frequently multiple and distributed throughout the skeleton and correspond to focal plasma cell expansions. In addition to this there is usually generalized osteoporosis, which is a contributory factor underlying pathological fractures. Collapse fractures of the vertebral column are frequently contributed to by erosive bone lesions and diffuse osteoporosis.

The underlying abnormality is excessive bone resorption that is not matched by a comparable amount of bone formation – an imbalance between osteoclastic and osteoblastic activity. The abnormal osteoclastic activity results from increased recruitment of osteoclasts and their stimulation, largely brought about by cytokine – originally termed 'osteoclast activating factor' – secreted by the plasma cells. It is now known that the major active factor in this is IL-1. There are several important features of this activity. Osteoblasts are not activated and there is no sclerosis in the bone lesions (as occurs when epithelial malignancies metastasize to bone). Consequently, radioisotopic active bone scans, which rely on the uptake of activity in new bone formed by osteoblasts, do not detect the bone lesions in myeloma. There is excess calcium resorption from the bone and, if this is not matched by renal clearance, hypercalcaemia will result. This may be further aggravated by nephrogenic diabetes insipidus and the dehydration that typically accompanies infection with further impairment of calcium excretion. The 'classical' clinical features are muscular weakness, nausea, vomiting, polyuria, polydipsia, thirst and dehydration. Encephalopathic features can range from drowsiness, disorientation and irrational behaviour to stupor. If hypercalcaemia persists it will result in renal dysfunction and lead to dehydration, increasing hypercalcaemia and causing irreversible renal damage.

Very small numbers of cases of myeloma are found that have an osteosclerotic rather than a lytic pattern of bone disease. Some of these cases are associated with peripheral neuropathy and other systemic effects not normally seen in classical myeloma.

Amyloidosis can occur as a complication of myeloma or can be related to an occult B-cell proliferation

Amyloidosis is a consequence of the deposition of protein fibrils in a variety of tissues. It may result in organ dysfunction, of which renal failure and cardiac failure are the most important. Amyloid is defined by its birefingent properties when stained using Congo red and by the presence of non-branching 10–15 nm fibres on electron microscopy. Amyloid may result from the metabolism of a wide range of proteins of which free light chains produced by myeloma are an important example. In amyloid production the primary event is the proteolytic cleavage of the molecule into fragments, which can then form insoluble beta-pleated sheets. This process is probably mediated by macrophages acting on the circulating protein, although it may also occur within tumour deposits. The protein type in myeloma-associated amyloid is called AL (L for light chain) and is in contrast to the AA form found in secondary amyloid, where protein A is deposited. The formation of fibrils requires two other components, which are common to all forms. These are glycosaminoglycans and serum amyloid P component (SAP). SAP is a normal serum protein, produced in the liver, that appears to be an important component of normal basement membrane. It is thought that SAP may have the effect of greatly increasing the resistance of amyloid to further degradation.

The tendency of a given case of multiple myeloma to produce amyloid is a function of the type of light chain produced and it has been shown that lambda light chains are much more likely to give rise to amyloid. In routine biopsy material it is often difficult to demonstrate light chain within amyloid deposits by immunocytochemistry, probably because most antibodies react mainly with parts of the molecule degraded during the formation of amyloid. This does not cause significant diagnostic difficulties when the patient has overt myeloma. However, some patients develop amyloid when only a very small plasma cell clone is present, detectable only by immunogenetic methods. A few patients with Waldenström's macroglobulinaemia may also develop light chain amyloidosis.

The typical pattern of disease in light chain amyloidosis is involvement of nerves, heart and other mesenchymal tissues, although biopsies of rectum, bone marrow or kidney may be valuable in diagnosis. In most cases amyloid is initially deposited around blood vessels and nerves and in some cases a large tumour mass consisting mainly of amyloid protein may develop.

The primary diagnosis of amyloidosis is made on a biopsy specimen, but recently scintigraphy using iodine-labelled SAP has been developed. This technique allows the extent of the disease to be assessed. Working from this method, it has been suggested that amyloid may regress if the primary source of the protein is removed. In myeloma this involves cytoreduction and if possible induction of complete remission. Where light-chain-associated amyloid is present without myeloma there may also be a role for chemotherapy, although this has not yet been substantiated by clinical trials.

Renal failure may be due to the toxic effects of light chain or hypercalcaemia

Nephrotic syndrome and renal failure in myeloma may result from amyloid deposition in the renal glomeruli or arterioles but this is relatively rare, occurring in about 5–10% of cases, and is only one of several possible mechanisms of renal damage in myeloma, which can be seen in some 50% of patients. A further and more common mechanism of renal damage is the effect of free light chain on the renal tubules. Infection or dehydration may lead to the precipitation of free light chain in the tubular lumen. This obstructs the nephrons affected and causes necrosis of tubular epithelial cells. Extrusion of the light chain leads to a macrophage reaction and scarring and may lead to a rapid deterioration in renal function. Free light chain may also become deposited in the glomerular basement membrane and mesangium, where it leads to proliferation of mesangial cells and increased matrix. These deposits do not have the staining features of amyloid. Light-chain deposition of this type leads to chronic renal failure and proteinuria.

Hypercalcaemia may also cause or contribute to the renal insufficiency seen in myeloma. The primary effect of the increased serum calcium is tubular dysfunction, leading to nephrogenic diabetes insipidus with consequent dehydration. Long-term uncontrolled hypercalcaemia may proceed to nephrocalcinosis and be a precipitating factor in the production of renal calculi. In addition to the effects of free light chain and hypercalcaemia, renal damage may also result from the effects of urinary tract infection and sometimes from hyperuricaemia.

Each of these factors may interact to produce accelerated injury: for example a renal calculus may cause obstruction and infection, which in turn could cause the formation of light-chain casts. Renal damage may also be aggravated by the use of some drugs (e.g. non-steroidal anti-inflammatory agents) and exacerbated by contrast imaging and the hyperuricaemia that may follow cytoreductive chemotherapy (Table 8.20).

Cryoglobulins may result in vasculitis

Cryoglobulins are immunoglobulins which precipitate at low temperature. The precipitate may contain only a monoclonal immunoglobulin or may contain complexes of polyclonal and monoclonal immunoglobulins. The pure monoclonal form may be found both in multiple myeloma and MGUS. The commonest effect of cryoglobulins is to cause leukocytoclastic (allergic) vasculitis in the skin. Much more rarely,

Table 8.20 The causes of renal failure in myeloma

- Hypercalcaemia
- Dehydration
- Cast formation
- Light-chain nephropathy
- Renal calculi
- Infection
- Amyloid
- Uric acid nephropathy

cryoglobulins are deposited in the glomeruli and cause a form of proliferative glomerulonephritis.

There are a number of mechanisms through which myeloma can result in symptoms and signs in the nervous system

Myeloma can have a number of specific and non-specific effects on the nervous system. A variety of mechanisms can lead to confusion, including hypercalcaemia, hyperviscosity, renal failure and intercurrent infection, either general or meningeal. Ophthalmoscopy should be carried out to exclude hyperviscosity or other causes of a raised intracranial pressure. Meningeal involvement with myeloma is very rare but intracranial plasmacytomas are more common and can cause focal neurological signs (Table 8.21).

The peripheral nervous system can be affected in a number of specific ways. The most common of these is due to spinal cord compression brought about by either a collapsed vertebra or an erosive plasmacytoma encroaching on the spinal cord. These lesions occur most commonly in the thoracic vertebrae and result in a sensory deficit level corresponding to the site of cord compression and a paraparesis below the level of the lesion, with bladder disturbance. The investigation of

Table 8.21 Myeloma and the nervous system

Central
- Confusion
  - Hypercalcaemia
  - Hyperviscosity
  - Infection
- Space-occupying lesion
  - Plasmacytoma

Peripheral
- Spinal cord compression
  - Plasmacytoma/fracture
- Sensorimotor neuropathy
  - Amyloid
  - Specificity of paraprotein
  - Treatment-related
- Carpal tunnel syndrome
  - Amyloid

these lesions is designed to define the level of obstruction. It can be done by either myelography or MRI scanner. The treatment of these lesions is often a matter of great urgency, requiring surgical decompression. Peripheral sensorimotor neuropathy in multiple myeloma may arise through a number of mechanisms, including the deposition of amyloid, infiltration by the paraprotein or as a result of the specificity of the paraprotein.

Treatment of multiple myeloma

Oral alkylating agents have been the mainstay of treatment but more intensive treatment is now being advocated

In most patients with one or more lytic lesions there will be evidence of disease progression within 1 year. In patients with a low malignant cell load, without bone lesions on X-ray or excess urinary light-chain excretion and with relatively low levels of paraprotein in the serum, the disease often remains stable for several years. There is no evidence to suggest that these patients benefit from the early introduction of treatment. For the remainder, who have symptomatic disease, the options include the use of oral alkylating agents, combination chemotherapy and high-dose stem-cell-supported therapy.

A major development in treatment of myeloma was the introduction of the oral alkylating agent melphalan in the early 1960s, following which the overall median survival increased from less than 1 year to 2 years. Despite attempts to improve on this by adopting a variety of regimens including other active agents, notably corticosteroids, cyclophosphamide and vincristine, there was no good evidence of a superior induction regimen during the following 20 years in a series of clinical trials. Despite this, much information accrued about key aspects of the disease and important principles of management were defined. Of particular importance was the recognition of the importance of hydration. It became apparent that, although the mechanisms underlying renal dysfunction were complex, the relatively simple approach of instituting a regimen of high fluid intake could reverse renal failure in many patients, even in the face of persisting proximal tubular dysfunction and light chain excretion. Similarly, vigorous hydration was shown to be effective in the treatment of hypercalcaemia, with a reduced risk of secondary renal damage. The recognition that infection, a reflection of the often severe immunosuppression, was frequently a causal factor in the morbidity and mortality in the disease, led to earlier and more effective treatment of infective episodes.

The development of combination chemotherapy during the 1980s represented another stage in the evolution of treatment for multiple myeloma. Agents incorporated into these regimens include the anthra-cyclines and nitrosoureas. As in other haematological malignancies, useful information as to likely effectiveness emerged from relatively small studies in patients with relapsed and recurrent disease – in particular on alternative modes of administration (continuous infusion *versus* bolus) and dose levels (escalation of doses of the most active agents such as melphalan and corticosteroids). These approaches resulted in regimes that achieved greater cytoreduction and a higher incidence of more 'complete responses'. The higher doses of melphalan, in particular, usually resulted in considerable reduction in tumour load. There also appeared to be a therapeutic gain in terms of symptom relief. However, there was no good evidence at that stage of a survival benefit.

Another active agent – alpha-interferon (IFNα) – emerged at that time. Early studies suggested a dose–response relationship but also indicated that a higher dose regimen would not be widely applicable because of unacceptable side effects. IFNα alone or in combination is effective and its role as part of induction therapy is being investigated. It was, however, the demonstration of activity in maintaining disease stability and thereby survival which raised the possibility of a valuable application in overall management of myeloma. Again its role in that respect is still being clarified in therapeutic trials (Figure 8.41).

An important concept to emerge as a result of the study of tumour regression following treatment was that of plateau phase, during which the tumour bulk remains constant. In contrast to the active presentation and relapse phases, most forms of chemotherapy are likely to be ineffective and unnecessary during plateau. Plateau may be considered to have been reached when patients are asymptomatic or have minimal symptoms, do not require blood transfusions and have stable serum paraprotein, urinary light-chain output and serum β_2m levels (as assessed, usually, at 3-monthly intervals) (Table 8.22).

While 'standard' treatment with the lower-dose melphalan-contain-ing regimens (or equivalent) is likely to result in the plateau state in about half the patients so treated, the degree of cytoreduction is generally appreciably less than following more intensive treatment regimens. With the escalation of dose levels, 'complete remission' (CR) – defined as the disappearance of paraprotein from serum and

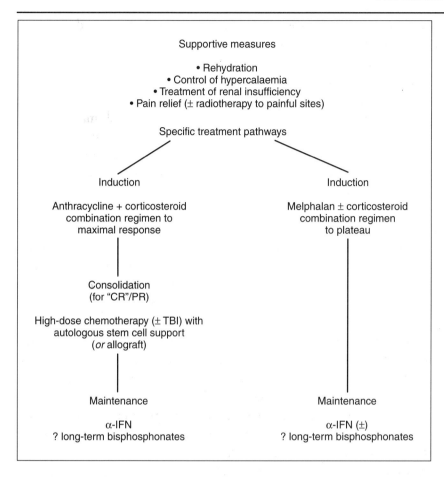

Figure 8.41 Management of patients with multiple myeloma.

urine and reduction in the bone marrow myeloma cell population to below 1% – could be achieved in as many as 50% of patients. The advent of peripheral blood stem-cell-supported intensive therapy, which reduces the morbidity and mortality of the intensive chemotherapy, represents a further development, which is being further refined – as, for example, in the positive selection of CD34+ cells – with the aim of removing clonal myeloma cells. Early therapeutic trials suggest that intensive cytoreductive regimens, which include high-dose melphalan (with or without TBI), are more effective in terms of response rate, duration of response and survival than 'standard' conventional treatment, but further data are required. The perceived benefits in the quality of life also require substantiation. Allogeneic BMT, although not likely to be widely applicable because of toxicity and availability of donors, may offer the possibility of curative therapy.

Table 8.22 Definitions of disease response in myeloma

- Plateau
  - Minimal and stable symptoms
  - Stable paraprotein
  - Stable urinary light chain
  - Stable β_2m
  - Stable haematologically
- Complete response
  - Paraprotein absent from serum and urine
  - Marrow plasma cells less than 1%

Management of bone lesions and disorders of calcium metabolism is an important component of the treatment

The standard treatment of elevated serum calcium is fluid replacement and this can be combined with a forced diuresis using diuretics. This will be sufficient to control hypercalcaemia in the majority of cases but the addition of corticosteroids can improve this number. If hypercalcaemia does not respond to these simple measures then there are a number of therapeutic options. These are only temporary measures until a response to chemotherapy occurs. Bisphosphonates have tended to replace therapy with either mithramycin or calcitonin. These agents bind to calcium in the bone matrix and inhibit osteoclast resorption of the bone. They have also been used to prevent the long-term bone damage seen in myeloma. Further developments may come from the ability to modify the cytokine network involving IL-6.

Radiotherapy has an important role in the management of symptomatic bone lesions

Myeloma is a relatively radiosensitive condition. Isolated painful bone lesions may be treated with palliative radiotherapy. The majority (approximately 90%) of patients will have pain relief with a single fraction or short course of radiotherapy to the affected area. Postoperative radiotherapy is also advisable for patients who have had pathological fractures, spinal cord compression or imminent pathological fractures treated surgically. Sequential hemibody irradiation, irradiating the upper half or lower half of the body with a single fraction of radiotherapy followed by a further single treatment to the other half of the body some weeks later, can be used. It is an effective treatment but does compromise bone marrow reserve. Total body irradiation is being used in some centres as part of high-dose therapy prior to stem cell rescue. There is no evidence as yet that high-dose treatment regimes containing total body irradiation are more effective than those based on cytotoxic chemotherapy alone.

8.4 Key references

8.4.1 Follicle centre lymphoma

Barrans, S., Randerson, J., Evans, P. *et al.* (1995) Heterogeneity in cell proliferation and expression of *p53* and *bcl-2* during the indolent phase of germinal centre cell lymphoma: an explanation for clinical variability. *British Journal of Haematology,* **90,** 830–836.

Gordon, J. (1995) CD40 and its ligand: central players in B lymphocyte survival, growth, and differentiation [review]. *Blood Reviews,* **9,** 53–56.

Horning, S. J. (1994) Treatment approaches to the low-grade lymphomas. *Blood,* **83,** 881–884.

Ji, W., Qu, G. Z., Ye, P. *et al.* (1995) Frequent detection of bcl-2/JH translocations in human blood and organ samples by a quantitative polymerase chain reaction assay. *Cancer Research,* **55,** 2876–2882.

Johnson, P. W., Price, C. G., Smith, T. *et al.* (1994) Detection of cells bearing the t(14;18) translocation following myeloablative treatment and autologous bone marrow transplantation for follicular lymphoma. *Journal of Clinical Oncology,* **12,** 798–805.

Levasseur, M., Middleton, P. G., Angus, B. *et al.* (1995) c-*MYC* gene abnormalities in high grade and centroblastic-centrocytic non-Hodgkin's lymphoma. *Leukemia and Lymphoma,* **18,** 131–136.

Matolcsy, A., Casali, P., Warnke, R. and Knowles, D. M. (1996) Morphologic transformation of follicular lymphoma is associated with somatic mutation of the translocated *bcl-2* gene. *Blood,* **88,** 3937–3944.

Petrasch, S. (1995) Follicular dendritic cells in malignant lymphomas. *Current Topics in Microbiology and Immunology,* **201,** 189–203.

Rohatiner, A. and Lister, T. A. (1994) Management of follicular lymphoma. *Current Opinion in Oncology,* **6,** 473–479.

8.4.2 Diffuse large B-cell lymphoma

Bolwell, B. J. (1994) Autologous bone marrow transplantation for Hodgkin's disease and non-Hodgkin's lymphoma. *Seminars in Oncology,* **21,** 86–95.

De Wolf-Peeters, C. and Pittaluga, S. (1995) T-cell rich B-cell lymphoma: a morphological variant of a variety of non-Hodgkin's lymphomas or a clinicopathological entity? *Histopathology,* **26,** 383–385.

Dent, A. L., Shaffer, A. L., Yu, X. *et al.* (1997) Control of inflammation, cytokine expression and germinal centre formation by *bcl-6*. *Science*, **276**, 589–592.

Johansson, B., Mertens, F. and Mitelman, F. (1995) Cytogenetic evolution patterns in non-Hodgkin's lymphoma. *Blood*, **86**, 3905–3914.

Kocialkowski, S., Pezzella, F., Morrison, H. *et al.* (1995) Mutations in the *p53* gene are not limited to classic 'hot spots' and are not predictive of p53 protein expression in high grade non-Hodgkin's lymphoma. *British Journal of Haematology*, **89**, 55–60.

Maestro, R., Gloghini, A., Doglioni, C. *et al.* (1995) *MDM2* overexpression does not account for stabilization of wild-type p53 protein in non-Hodgkin's lymphomas. *Blood*, **85**, 3239–3246.

Mendoza, E., Territo, M., Schiller, G. *et al.* (1995) Allogeneic bone marrow transplantation for Hodgkin's and non-Hodgkin's lymphoma. *Bone Marrow Transplantation*, **15**, 299–303.

Ye, B. H., Lo Coco, F., Chang, C. C. *et al.* (1995) Alterations of the *BCL-6* gene in diffuse large-cell lymphoma. *Current Topics in Microbiology and Immunology*, **194**, 101–108.

8.4.3 Mantle cell lymphoma

Alkan, S., Schnitzer, B., Thompson, J. L. *et al.* (1995) Cyclin D1 protein expression in mantle cell lymphoma. *Annals of Oncology*, **6**, 567–570.

Argatoff, L. H., Connors, J. M., Klasa, R. J. *et al.* (1997) Mantle cell lymphoma: a clinicopathological study of 80 cases. *Blood*, **89**, 2067–2078.

De Wolf-Peeters, C. and Pittaluga, S. (1994) Mantle-cell lymphoma. *Annals of Oncology*, **5**(Suppl. 1), 35–37.

Harris, A. W., Bodrug, S. E., Warner, B. J. *et al.* (1995) Cyclin D1 as the putative *bcl-1* oncogene. *Current Topics in Microbiology and Immunology*, **194**, 347–353.

Norton, A. J., Matthews, J., Pappa, V. *et al.* (1995) Mantle cell lymphoma: natural history defined in a serially biopsied population over a 20-year period. *Annals of Oncology*, **6**, 249–256.

Ott, G., Kalla, J., Ott, M. M. *et al.* (1997) Blastoid variants of mantle cell lymphoma: frequent bcl-1 rearrangements at the major translocation cluster region and tetraploid chromosome clones. *Blood*, **89**, 1421–1429.

Vandenberghe, E. (1994) Mantle cell lymphoma. *Blood Reviews*, **8**, 79–87.

Williams, M. E., Nichols, G. E., Swerdlow, S. H. and Stoler, M. H. (1995) In situ hybridization detection of cyclin D1 mRNA in centrocytic/mantle cell lymphoma. *Annals of Oncology*, **6**, 297–299.

Zucca, E., Roggero, E., Pinotti, G. *et al.* (1995) Patterns of survival in mantle cell lymphoma. *Annals of Oncology*, **6**, 257–262.

Zukerberg, L. R., Yang, W. I., Arnold, A. and Harris, N. L. (1995) Cyclin D1 expression in non-Hodgkin's lymphomas. Detection by immunohistochemistry. *American Journal of Clinical Pathology*, **103**, 756–760.

8.4.4 Chronic lymphocytic leukaemia

Catovsky, D. (1995) Chronic lymphoproliferative disorders. *Current Opinion in Oncology*, 7, 3–11.

Cuneo, A., Balboni, M., Piva, N. *et al.* (1995) Atypical chronic lymphocytic leukaemia with t(11;14) (q13;q32): karyotype evolution and prolymphocytic transformation. *British Journal of Haematology*, 90, 409–416.

Matutes, E., Oscier, D., Garcia-Marco, J. *et al.* (1996) Trisomy 12 defines a group of CLL with atypical morphology: correlation between cytogenetic, clinical and laboratory features in 544 patients. *British Journal of Haematology*, 92, 382–388.

O'Brien, S., del Giglio, A. and Keating, M. (1995) Advances in the biology and treatment of B-cell chronic lymphocytic leukemia. *Blood*, 85, 307–318.

Oscier, D. G. (1994) Cytogenetic and molecular abnormalities in chronic lymphocytic leukaemia. *Blood Reviews*, 8, 88–97.

Pott-Hoeck, C. and Hiddemann, W. (1995) Purine analogs in the treatment of low-grade lymphomas and chronic lymphocytic leukemias. *Annals of Oncology*, 6, 421–433.

Wolowiec, D., Benchaib, M., Pernas, P. *et al.* (1995) Expression of cell cycle regulatory proteins in chronic lymphocytic leukemias. Comparison with non-Hodgkin's lymphomas and non-neoplastic lymphoid tissue. *Leukemia*, 9, 1382–1388.

8.4.5 Other B-cell lymphoproliferative disorders

Dimopoulos, M. A. and Alexanian, R. (1994) Waldenström's macroglobulinemia. *Blood*, 83, 1452–1459.

Gollard, R., Lee, T. C., Piro, L. D. and Saven, A. (1995) The optimal management of hairy cell leukaemia. *Drugs*, 49, 921–931.

Mandelli, F., Arcese, W. and Avvisati, G. (1994) The interferons in haematological malignancies. *Baillières Clinical Haematology*, 7, 91–113.

Sun, T., Susin, M., Brody, J. *et al.* (1994) Splenic lymphoma with circulating villous lymphocytes: report of seven cases and review of the literature. *American Journal of Hematology*, 45, 39–50.

8.4.6 Multiple myeloma

Alexanian, R. and Dimopoulos, M. (1994) The treatment of multiple myeloma. *New England Journal of Medicine*, 330, 484–489.

Bakkus, M. H., Van Riet, I., van Camp, B. and Thielemans, K. (1994) Evidence that the clonogenic cell in multiple myeloma originates from a pre-switched but somatically mutated B cell. *British Journal of Haematology*, 87, 68–74.

Barlogie, B. (1997) *Multiple Myeloma: Hematology/Oncology Clinics of North America*, W. B. Saunders, Philadelphia, PA.

Bataille, R. (1996) The management of myeloma with bisphosphonates. *New England Journal of Medicine*, 334, 529–530.

Berenson, J. R., Vescio, R. A., Hong, C. H. *et al.* (1995) Multiple myeloma clones are derived from a cell late in B lymphoid development. *Current Topics in Microbiology and Immunology,* **194**, 25–33.

Bergsagel, P. L., Smith, A. M., Szczepek, A. *et al.* (1995) In multiple myeloma, clonotypic B lymphocytes are detectable among CD19+ peripheral blood cells expressing CD38, CD56, and monotypic Ig light chain. *Blood,* **85**, 436–447.

Bergsagel, P. l., Chesi, M., Nardini, E. *et al.* (1996) Promiscuous translocations into the immunoglobulin heavy chain switch regions in multiple myeloma. *Proceedings of the National Academy of Sciences of the USA,* **93**, 13931–13936.

Biggs, D. D., Kraj, P., Goldman, J. *et al.* (1995) Immunoglobulin gene sequence analysis to further assess B-cell origin of multiple myeloma. *Clinical and Diagnostic Laboratory Immunology,* **2**, 44–52.

Bjorkstrand, B., Ljungman, P., Bird, J. M. *et al.* (1995) Autologous stem cell transplantation in multiple myeloma: results of the European Group for Bone Marrow Transplantation. *Stem Cells,* **13**(Suppl. 2), 140–146.

Child, J. A. (1994) Evolving strategies in the treatment of myelomatosis. *British Journal of Haematology,* **88**, 672–678.

Cigudosa, J. C., Calasanz, M. J., Odero, M. D. *et al.* (1994) Cytogenetic data in 41 patients with multiple myeloma. Karyotype and other clinical parameters. *Cancer Genetics and Cytogenetics,* **78**, 210–213.

Hawkins, P. N. (1995) Amyloidosis. *Blood Reviews,* **9**, 135–142.

Herrinton, L. J. (1996) The epidemiology of monoclonal gammopathy of unknown significance: a review. *Current Topics in Microbiology and Immunology,* **210**, 389–395.

Joshua, D. E., Gibson, J. and Brown, R. D. (1994) Mechanisms of the escape phase of myeloma. *Blood Reviews,* **8**, 13–20.

Kishimoto, T., Akira, S., Narazaki, M. and Taga, T. (1995) Interleukin-6 family of cytokines and gp130. *Blood,* **86**, 1243–1254.

Klein, B. (1995) Cytokine, cytokine receptors, transduction signals, and oncogenes in human multiple myeloma. *Seminars in Hematology,* **32**, 4–19.

Klein, B., Zhang, X. G., Lu, Z. Y. and Bataille, R. (1995) Interleukin-6 in human multiple myeloma. *Blood,* **85**, 863–872.

Lai, J. L., Zandecki, M., Mary, J. Y. *et al.* (1995) Improved cytogenetics in multiple myeloma: a study of 151 patients including 117 patients at diagnosis. *Blood,* **85**, 2490–2497.

McSweeney, P. A., Wells, D. A., Shultz, K. E. *et al.* (1996) Tumour specific aneuploidy not detected in CD19+ B-lymphoid cells from myeloma patients in a multidimensional flow cytometric analysis. *Blood,* **88**, 622–632.

Moulopoulos, L. A., Dimopoulos, M. A., Smith, T. L. *et al.* (1995) Prognostic significance of magnetic resonance imaging in patients with asymptomatic multiple myeloma. *Journal of Clinical Oncology,* **13**, 251–256.

Rettig, M. B., Ma, H. J., Vescia, R. A. *et al.* (1997) Kaposi's sarcoma associated Herpesvirus infection of bone marrow dendritic cells from myeloma patients. *Science*, **276**, 1851–1854.

Sahota, S. S., Leo, R., Hamblin, T. J. and Stevenson, F. K. (1996) Ig VH gene mutational patterns indicate different tumor cell status in human myeloma and monoclonal gammopathy of undetermined significance. *Blood*, **87**, 746–755.

Sailer, M., Vykoupil, K. F., Peest, D. *et al.* (1995) Prognostic relevance of a histologic classification system applied in bone marrow biopsies from patients with multiple myeloma: a histopathological evaluation of biopsies from 153 untreated patients. *European Journal of Haematology*, **54**, 137–146.

Schey S. (1996) Osteosclerotic myeloma and 'POEMS' syndrome. *Blood Reviews*, **10**, 75–80.

Varterasian, M. L. (1995) Biologic and clinical advances in multiple myeloma. *Oncology*, **9**, 417–424.

Witzig, T. E., Kimlinger, T. K. and Greipp, P. R. (1995) Detection of peripheral blood myeloma cells by three-color flow cytometry. *Current Topics in Microbiology and Immunology*, **194**, 3–8.

9 Peripheral T-cell lymphoproliferative disorders in lymph nodes, spleen, blood and bone marrow

9.1 Introduction

T-cell lymphoproliferative disorders are classified into tumours of precursor T-lymphocytes discussed in chapter 6 (lymphoblastic leukaemia) and those of peripheral or immunocompetent T-lymphocytes. There is less consensus about the subclassification of peripheral T-cell tumours than exists for equivalent groups of B-cell tumours. There are several well defined extranodal T-cell lymphomas, such as intestinal (enteropathy-associated) T-cell lymphoma and the cutaneous T-cell lymphomas, and a much more heterogeneous group of tumours that affect mainly peripheral blood, bone marrow and lymph nodes but may also involve extranodal sites. All these tumours are rare, accounting for around 10–15% of lymphoid malignancies.

Peripheral T-cell malignancy can be broadly divided into those that mainly affect the blood and marrow and those that form solid tumours. T-cell large granular lymphocyte proliferations (LGL), T prolymphocytic leukaemia (T-PLL) and adult T-cell leukaemia lymphoma (ATLL) typically present as leukaemia although solid tumour deposits may occur, mainly in nodes, skin, liver and spleen. The remaining types of tumour usually present as nodal masses but in up to half of cases there may be extranodal spread at some stage of the disease.

9.2 T-cell lymphoproliferative disorders that are mainly leukaemic

9.2.1 T-cell granular lymphocyte proliferations

Increased numbers of peripheral blood large granular lymphocytes are found in acute viral infections

Large granular lymphocytes (LGL) are a normal component of the peripheral blood and marrow and are phenotypically a mixture of T-cells (both CD4 and CD8) and natural killer (NK) cells. NK cells are recognized phenotypically by absence of surface CD3 and T-cell receptors (TCR) and by the presence of a group of adhesion and Fc receptors known collectively as NKa antigens (CD11b, CD16, CD56, CD57). LGL of both T-cell and NK cells types are larger than normal lymphocytes with abundant basophilic cytoplasm containing azurophilic granules of variable size. The granules contain a mixture of perforins and other enzymes capable of permeabilizing cell membranes, activating the programmed cell death pathway of target cells. The cells may also express the Fas ligand (CD96) on their cell surface and are capable of triggering apoptosis in the wide range of cells which express Fas (CD95). Cytotoxic T-cells recognize their target through the antigen-specific T-cell receptor, whereas NK cells may recognize and kill cells lacking expression of MHC molecules – a feature of some virus-infected cells. The principal function of LGL appears to be the removal of virally infected cells and acute viral infections are the main cause of transient expansion of LGL populations in the peripheral blood. Diagnostic problems arise when there is a persistent LGL expansion in the peripheral blood without obvious viral or other infective causes.

Most persistent LGL proliferations are asymptomatic and benign

Persistent expansions of LGL appear to be common in the elderly although the exact prevalence could only be established by population screening, which has not yet been carried out. The typical patient will have been found on a routine examination of the peripheral blood to have a slightly raised lymphocyte count. This is rarely greater than 10×10^9/l, with increased numbers of LGL on the blood film; mild anaemia may also be present. On periodic review the number of peripheral blood LGL may remain elevated but in most cases there will be no apparent adverse clinical features.

Neutropenia, rheumatoid disease and B-cell malignancy are the main associations with persistent LGL proliferations

LGL proliferations have been recorded in a wide range of diseases, most of which are likely to be coincidental but there are a number of consistent clinical associations. A subset of patients with LGL proliferations have chronic neutropenia, sometimes with mild anaemia (Figure 9.1). Although a pathogenic mechanism has not been demonstrated it has been postulated that the neutropenia may be a consequence of aberrant cytokine production by the LGL. In a few patients with marked neutropenia symptomatic infections sometimes occur, which occasionally may be life-threatening.

LGL proliferations are also strongly associated with rheumatoid disease and in particular with Felty's syndrome (neutropenia and splenomegaly associated with rheumatoid disease). The pathogenic significance of this finding remains unclear and there is no apparent relationship between the LGL count and disease progression. A proportion of patients with asymptomatic LGL expansions are rheumatoid-factor-positive without having joint disease. There is also a significant association between peripheral blood LGL expansions and B-cell malignancy, and it should not be assumed that lymphadenopathy is due to the LGL proliferation. Part of this association may be due to the relatively high frequency of both LGL proliferations and B-CLL in elderly patients. It has also been suggested that LGL expansions may occur in association with occult epithelial malignancy.

Figure 9.1 Large granular lymphocytosis. This is a blood film from a patient with neutropenia and a slightly raised lymphocyte count. The lymphocytes have abundant cytoplasm and prominent granules. The cells express CD3, TCR-2, CD8 and the NKa markers CD16, CD56 and CD57.

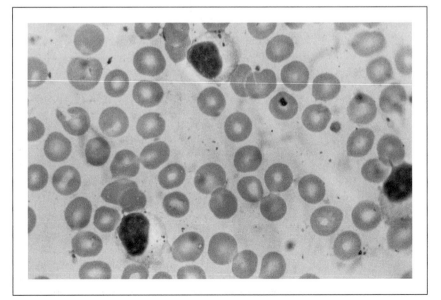

Persistent LGL expansions are phenotypically diverse but are almost always T-cells rather than NK cells

Normal LGLs include a range of cell types from T-cell and NK cell lineages but almost all persistent LGL expansion consists of T-cells. A high proportion of cases express CD3 in conjunction with the alpha/beta TCR receptor or more rarely the gamma/delta receptor. Over 60% of cases express CD8 and 30% CD4. A few of the CD4-positive cases have weak CD8 expression and some lack both CD4 and CD8. Cells that lack both CD4 and CD8 usually express CD3 in association with TCR-gamma/delta. A highly characteristic feature of this group of disorders is the expression of natural-killer-associated (NKa) markers (CD16, CD11b, CD56, CD57) in various combinations. The expression of NKa markers, in particular CD16 (Fc receptor) is frequent in cases associated with neutropenia and rheumatoid disease (Figure 9.2).

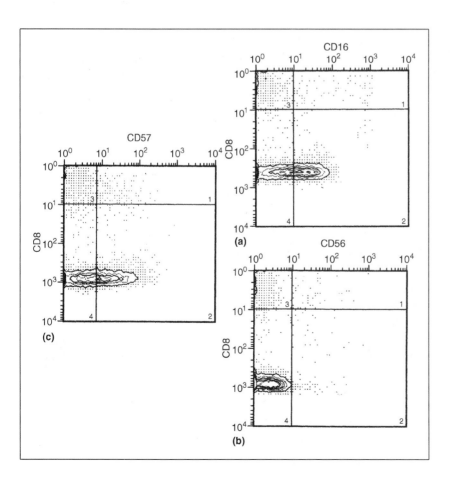

Figure 9.2 Large granular lymphocytosis – immunophenotype. A flow cytometric analysis of a case of a persistent LGL proliferation. Coexpression of CD8 and CD16 is seen in **(a)**, absence of CD56 in the same population in **(b)** and the presence of CD57 in **(c)**. This is one of several patterns seen in LGL proliferations.

Table 9.1 Large granular lymphocytosis

- **Morphology**: Large lymphocytes with relatively abundant cytoplasm containing granules.
- **Immunophenotype**: Most cases are CD8$^+$ T-cells with CD3/TCR2 expression. The presence of NKa markers CD11b, CD16, CD56, CD57 is variable. Monoclonal populations are commonly CD16$^+$, CD56$^-$.
- **Cytogenetics**: None described.
- **Pattern of disease**: Asymptomatic lymphocytosis, which may be associated with neutropenia.

A few patients have persistent expansions of T-cells expressing NKa markers but without obvious morphological evidence of cytoplasmic granulation. In these cases granules below the level of resolution of light microscopy can usually be demonstrated cytochemically using the granule-associated enzyme benzylcarbonyl-L-lysine thiobenzyl esterase or by the use of antiperforin antibodies.

The features of large granular lymphocytosis are summarized in Table 9.1.

Only a proportion of persistent LGL expansions are monoclonal

The immunophenotype CD3$^+$ TCR-alpha/beta$^+$, CD8$^+$, CD16$^+$, CD56$^-$ is strongly predictive of a monoclonal expansion of LGLs as shown by T-cell receptor gene rearrangements. Monoclonality is also found in cases where the cells have abnormal phenotypes such as CD4/8 coexpression. In the rare cases of LGL proliferations with NK cell features that lack CD3 and have germline TCR genes it is possible to demonstrate monoclonality in some cases using X-linked polymorphisms. The terms T-CLL and LGL leukaemia have been used to describe this group of disorders. It is doubtful whether this is a useful nomenclature. Progressive malignant disease is rare and there is little difference in the risk of its occurrence between those with monoclonal and polyclonal proliferation and between those with a T-cell or NK-cell phenotype. Even in patients with significant neutropenia there is usually only a minimal increase in bone marrow T-cells. The use of the terms monoclonal or polyclonal granular lymphocyte proliferation with further specification of the phenotype, would seem more appropriate (Figure 9.3).

Most patients with clonal granular lymphocyte proliferations have stable benign disease that requires no treatment. In the few patients with

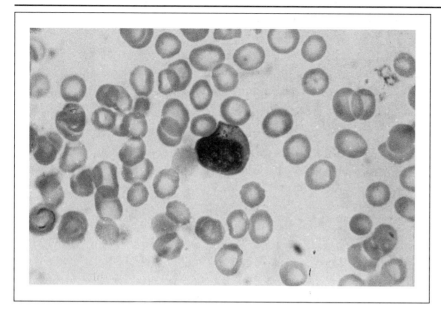

Figure 9.3 Aggressive large granular lymphocyte proliferation – peripheral blood. This patient had a peripheral lymphocytosis consisting of large atypical lymphocytes with prominent granulation. These cells had a CD8+ T-cell phenotype. Multiple tissue deposits were present.

symptomatic infections due to neutropenia treatment with antibiotics and G-CSF is usually sufficient. The very small number of patients with progressive disease are treated with single-agent or combination chemotherapy although there is little consensus as to choice of treatment and little evidence of a beneficial effect. In these rare patients the prognosis is poor (Figure 9.3).

9.2.2 T-prolymphocytic leukaemia

T-prolymphocytic leukaemia is a distinctive clinical syndrome with a poor prognosis

T-prolymphocytic leukaemia (T-PLL) is a rare disorder, with an incidence in Western populations of around $1/1\,000\,000$/year or less. Even the largest centres will see only an occasional case. The usual presenting features are a combination of rapidly progressive lymphadenopathy, splenomegaly and either diffuse or papular skin eruptions. These clinical features together with a lymphocyte count that may be as high as 100×10^9/l should strongly suggest the diagnosis of T-PLL. There is no clear consensus on treatment, though some patients may transiently respond to combination chemotherapy such as CHOP. Purine analogues have also been tried but with little success. Few patients achieve a complete remission and the median survival is only 7 months.

The morphological features of T-PLL are not specific and the diagnosis can only be made by immunophenotypical investigations

The classical forms of both B- and T-prolymphocytic leukaemias are morphologically similar. The cells are medium-sized with round nuclei and variable agranular cytoplasm. The characteristic feature is the presence of a central prominent nucleolus. A proportion of cases of T-PLL consist of smaller cells, which have condensed nuclear chromatin and less prominent nucleoli, although the clinical features and prognosis are similar (Figure 9.4).

Most cases of T-PLL have a normal peripheral T-cell phenotype with expression of CD3/TCR-alpha/beta, CD2, CD5 and strong CD7. Lack of CD1a and Tdt can be used to distinguish the cells from T-lymphoblasts in the occasional case where this may be a problem. In almost every case the neoplastic T-cells express CD4; coexpression of CD4 and CD8 or CD8 alone is much less common. This immunophenotype, together with the morphological and clinical features described above, will be sufficient for a definitive diagnosis in almost every case. T-PLL cells may vary in the expression of T-cell activation markers such as CD71, HLA-DR, CD38 and CD25, but NK-associated determinants – CD16, CD11b, CD56, CD57⁻ – are not present.

inv 14 (q11: q32) is the most characteristic cytogenetic abnormality seen in T-PLL

About 75% of cases of T-PLL will show an inv 14 and over half have trisomy 8. These do not appear to identify prognostically significant subsets. In most cases it is possible to demonstrate a clonal T-cell rearrangement by PCR or Southern blotting although this is not essential for the diagnosis in the presence of the other features described above.

9.2.3 Adult T-cell leukaemia/lymphoma

Adult T-cell leukaemia/lymphoma is strongly associated with HTVL1 infection and has a characteristic geographical distribution

The clinical and morphological features of adult T-cell leukaemia/lymphomas (ATLL) are distinctive and this led to the recognition of its occurrence with a relatively high incidence in the islands of south-west

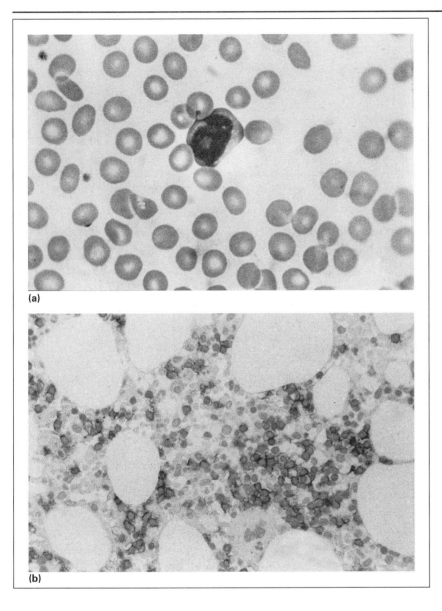

(a)

(b)

Figure 9.4 T-prolymphocytic leukaemia. This patient presented with splenomegaly and a very high lymphocyte count. **(a)** The lymphocytes are relatively large, with a single prominent nucleolus and rim of cytoplasm. The bone marrow biopsy **(b)**, stained with anti-CD3, shows an extensive infiltrate of T-cells similar to those seen in the peripheral blood.

Japan. Clusters of the disease were later described in the Caribbean and in South America. The development of the capability to maintain neoplastic T-cells from ATLL in culture led to the isolation of the retrovirus HTLV1 in the late 1970s. In addition to ATLL the virus was later shown to play a role in the pathogenesis of tropical spastic paraparesis (HTLV1-associated myelopathy). HTLV1 is transmitted by blood transfusion, sexual intercourse or breast-feeding. The incidence of latent infection is high in the endemic areas of Japan and the Caribbean, but even in the UK the incidence rate in blood donors may be as high as 4%. Over a 20–30-year period those infected have 2–5% risk of developing ATLL.

After infecting a T-cell the RNA genome of HTLV1 is reverse transcribed to double-stranded DNA, which integrates into host chromosomes (Figure 9.5).

A number of viral proteins can exert a major effect over the function of the host lymphocyte. TAX is involved in the regulation of viral gene expression and can affect the activity of a wide range of growth factors and their receptors, including IL-1, IL-2, GM-CSF, TGFβ, PDGF, IL-2Rα. One effect of this may be the establishment of autocrine stimulatory loops in which the virus infected cell produces and responds to IL-2. This may lead to failure to return to G_0 after removal of antigenic and other stimuli. TAX may also be able to stabilize p53, which may predispose to the accumulation of random mutations. The viral protein REX regulates the genes responsible for viral replication but may also affect the function of the IL-2 pathway. A number of other proteins are generated by alternative splicing of the viral px region. These include: p21 (REXIII), a cytoplasmic protein of unknown function; p12, which may affect the IL-2 pathway; and the nuclear proteins p13 and p30. The overall effect of virus is to produce clonal expansion of infected T-cells, which have some resistance to apoptosis as a result of genetic damage. When overt leukaemia develops the cells may no longer require the expression of viral genes to sustain a malignant phenotype.

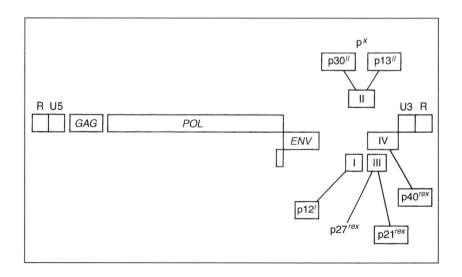

Figure 9.5 HTLV1 genome. This is a schematic representation of the genomic organization of HTLV1 showing the major genes common to all retroviruses – *GAG, POL* and *ENV* – and the HTLV1 genes that are involved in the pathogenesis of ATLL.

ATLL is morphologically and phenotypically distinctive from other types of T-cell lymphoproliferative disease. The presence of positive HTLV1 serology is required for the diagnosis

Most cases of ATLL are diagnosed by examination of peripheral blood or bone marrow. The lymphocyte count is usually increased, but may range from normal to $500 \times 10^9/l$. The circulating cells vary in size but are characterized by highly convoluted or clover-leaf-type nuclei with small nucleoli and basophilic agranular cytoplasm. Almost all cases have a $CD4^+$ peripheral T-cell phenotype with CD3/TCR-alpha/beta and CD45RO expression (Figure 9.6).

CD7 is often absent. The expression of T-cell activation markers such as Class II MHC, CD71 and CD38 is variable but expression of the IL-2 receptor CD25 is a constant feature. This molecule is shed from the cell surface and can be measured in serum. Tdt is always negative. The cell cycle fraction defined by Ki67 is a useful marker to identify patients who are likely to have a rapidly progressive clinical course. In a high proportion of cases aneuploidy can be detected by DNA cytometry although there are no consistent cytogenetic abnormalities. Changes in the degree of aneuploidy present can be used as a further marker of disease progression. In all cases integrated virus can be demonstrated using Southern blotting and patients have high levels of anti-HTLV1

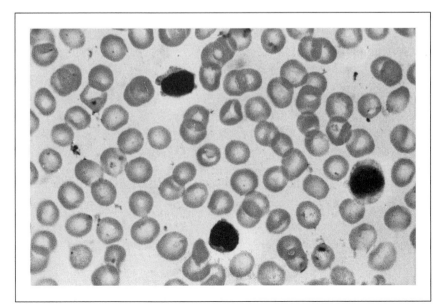

Figure 9.6 Adult T-cell leukaemia and lymphoma – peripheral blood. This patient, who had serological evidence of HTLV1 infection, presented with lymphocytosis. Large numbers of atypical $CD4^+$ T-cells were present in the peripheral blood but with no evidence of hypercalcaemia or solid tumour deposits.

Table 9.2 Adult T-cell leukaemia and lymphoma

- **Morphology**: Circulating cells have highly convoluted nuclei with small nucleoli and basophilic cytoplasm.
- **Immunophenotype**: Peripheral T-cell phenotype with expression of CD3/TCR-alpha/beta and lymphocyte activation markers including CD25 and MHC class II. Ki67-positive fraction correlates with disease progression. Serological evidence of HTLV1 infection and integrated virus can be demonstrated by Southern blotting.
- **Cytogenetic**: High incidence of aneuploidy but no specific abnormality.
- **Pattern of disease**: Most cases present with high lymphocyte count, evidence of tissue infiltration and hypercalcaemia. Clinical variants are classified as smouldering, chronic or lymphoma-type.

antibodies. One or other of these features should be regarded as an essential diagnostic feature of the disease

The features of ATLL are summarized in Table 9.2.

Patients with ATLL may have disseminated multisystem disease

Patients with ATLL frequently have infiltration of lymph nodes (60%), liver (25%) and spleen (20%). Osteolytic bone lesions and associated hypercalcaemia are seen in one-third of patients at presentation and is more common in patients with progressive disease. Extensive skin infiltration may also occur and is seen in about 40% of cases. Pulmonary complications are frequent and occur in the majority of patients. These include pulmonary infiltration by tumour, fibrosis and infection. In some cases there may be involvement of the pleural surfaces.

It is possible to classify ATLL into four prognostic groups

1. **Acute**: This is the classic syndrome of ATLL described above, which has a poor prognosis and often does not respond to chemotherapy. The white cell count is high, there is extensive tissue infiltration, the LDH will be elevated and hypercalcaemia may be present.
2. **Smouldering type**: These cases have a near normal lymphocyte count but with 8% or more cells of typical morphology and immunophenotype in the peripheral blood. The cell-cycle fraction defined by Ki67 is low. The extent of the disease is limited, as evidenced by no hypercalcaemia, LDH only slightly elevated and no lymphadenopathy. Skin or pulmonary lesions may be present.

3. **Chronic type**: There is a lymphocytosis in this group with more than $3.5 \times 10^9/l$ of neoplastic T-lymphocytes. There is no hypercalcaemia, bone, CNS, gastrointestinal or pleural disease but lymphadenopathy may be found. The LDH can be twice the normal value.

4. **Lymphoma type**: In this type there is a presentation with tumour masses in nodes or at other sites without involvement of the peripheral blood.

Treatment of ATLL is directed by the type of lesion

Patients with acute and lymphoma-type presentations are treated with combination chemotherapy with the aim of achieving a cure; however 50% of these patients will be dead within 6 months. The smouldering and chronic types of ATLL are often treated with alkylating agents and have longer survival than the acute and lymphoma types. It is uncertain whether treatment benefits these cases and morbidity and mortality associated with intensive chemotherapy may actually shorten their survival.

9.3 T-cell lymphoproliferative disorders that mainly present as solid tumours

Peripheral T-cell lymphoproliferative disorders that present mainly as solid tumours are very heterogeneous and there is no firm consensus on subclassification. A small number of cases have distinctive morphological features, such as anaplastic large cell lymphoma, or form part of a recognized clinical syndrome, such as angioimmunoblastic lymphadenopathy, but the remainder are difficult to subclassify by conventional morphological and phenotypical criteria and are best considered as peripheral T-cell lymphomas of unspecified or common type.

9.3.1 Nodal peripheral T-cell lymphomas – unspecified type

Peripheral T-cell lymphomas are morphologically heterogeneous and can only be reliably separated from their B-cell counterparts by immunophenotypical analysis

On lymph node biopsy peripheral T-cell lymphomas show complete replacement of the nodal architecture although in a few cases there may be partial sparing of the B-cell areas. One of the features of this group of tumours that make morphological classification difficult is that they contain variable numbers of small, medium and large lymphoid cells (Figure 9.7).

It is usual for the neoplastic T-cells to show a high degree of nuclear pleomorphism, with wide variation in the size and shape of the nucleus, chromatin pattern and number of nucleoli. T-immunoblasts may be distinguished by their abundant clear cytoplasm. In some cases multinucleated cells resembling Reed–Sternberg cells may be present. A

Figure 9.7 Nodal peripheral T-cell lymphoma. Most cases of nodal peripheral consist of a pleomorphic population of intermediate and large tumour cells, which may be difficult to distinguish morphologically from diffuse large B-cell lymphoma (a). In this case most of the cells express CD3 (b). A small proportion of peripheral T-cell lymphomas consist of a relatively monomorphic population of small to intermediate-sized lymphocytes (c).

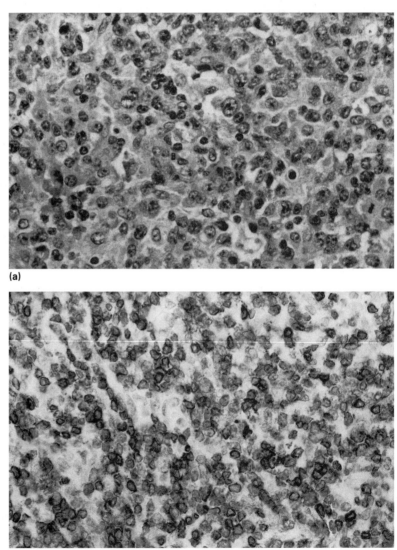

(a)

(b)

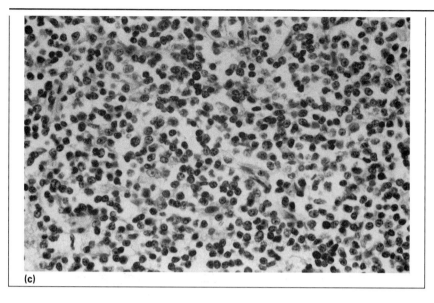

(c)

highly distinctive feature of peripheral T-cell lymphomas is that they often contain large numbers of reactive cells, most commonly macrophages and eosinophils. In some peripheral T-cell lymphomas there may be infiltration and destruction of blood vessels, with resulting necrosis and tissue destruction. This appears to be most characteristic of tumour deposits at extranodal sites (Figure 9.8). The differential diagnosis of angiodestructive tumours includes lymphomatoid granulomatosis and NK lineage tumours in the upper respiratory tract (Chapter 10).

The features of peripheral T-cell lymphoma are summarized in Table 9.3.

The phenotype may be highly abnormal with loss of expression of many of the antigens that characterize normal peripheral T-cells

Most cases are $CD2^+$, $CD3^+$, $CD4^+$, $CD5^+$ but coexpression of CD4 and CD8 may occur or the cells may express neither of these antigens. The expression of T-cell activation markers is also highly variable. Except in anaplastic lymphomas, it is unusual to find significant numbers of cells expressing CD30. Almost all T-cell lymphomas express the lymphocyte adhesion molecule CD43 but this is not lineage-specific and is present in a proportion of B-cell tumours, including B-CLL, mantle cell lymphoma and some diffuse large cell lymphomas.

Figure 9.8 Peripheral T-cell lymphoma with angiodestructive features – breast. **(a)** This patient presented with a large necrotic breast lump. **(b)** There was extensive infiltration and destruction of vessels by CD3+ atypical T-cells.

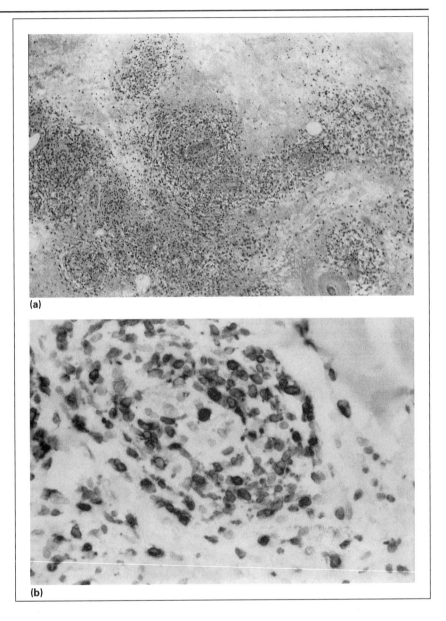

(a)

(b)

CD43 is also strongly expressed in normal macrophages. Normal peripheral blood and nodal T-cells express either CD45RA or RO depending on whether they have previously encountered antigen, but the majority of peripheral T-cell lymphomas express only CD45RO, indicating that these are derived from post-antigen-stimulated T-cells. In fixed tissue sections this antibody is often used as evidence of T-cell lineage but again this is not lineage specific.

Table 9.3 Peripheral T-cell lymphoma

- **Morphology:** Highly variable – most cases have a mixture of intermediate and large lymphoid cells with highly pleomorphic nuclei. Angioimmunoblastic and Lennert's type distinguished by background reactive cell population.
- **Immunophenotype:** May have normal peripheral T-cell phenotype but many cases have loss of one or more pan-T-cell antigens. The majority of cases are CD4$^+$, CD45RO$^+$.
- **Cytogenetics:** No specific abnormalities.
- **Pattern of disease:** Disseminated nodal and extranodal disease.

Peripheral T-cell lymphomas present with advanced nodal and extranodal disease

Most patients with peripheral T-cell lymphomas have extensive nodal disease at presentation. In addition extranodal infiltration appears to be more common than in B-cell lymphomas and this gives rise to a variety of unusual clinical presentations which may lead to diagnostic difficulty (Figures 9.9–9.11). Patients may also have a diverse range of systemic symptoms, including fever and cytopenia, possibly related to cytokine production by the tumour cells. In patients entered in clinical trials of combination chemotherapy the complete remission rate for large T-cell lymphomas appears to be similar to that for B-cell lymphomas, but a number of studies have suggested less stable remissions and shorter periods of disease free survival.

9.3.2 Common variants of peripheral T-cell lymphoma

Angioimmunoblastic T-cell lymphoma

Angioimmunoblastic T-cell lymphoma (AIL) is a syndrome with distinctive clinical features

AIL is a disorder that mainly occurs in elderly patients. In most cases the clinical presentation is dominated by systemic manifestations and lymphadenopathy, which, although usually present, may be relatively minor. The majority of patients have fever, weight loss and non-specific skin rashes. A high plasma viscosity with hypergammaglobulinaemia is usual with electrophoresis showing a polyclonal pattern, although in some patients small paraprotein bands may occur. A positive Coombs test

Figure 9.9 Peripheral T-cell lymphoma – liver and bone. **(a)** MRI scan showing extensive liver infiltration by peripheral T-cell lymphoma. This patient later developed massive bone involvement with extensive destruction of pelvic bones **(b)**. This illustrates the unpredictable pattern of spread of many peripheral T-cell lymphomas.

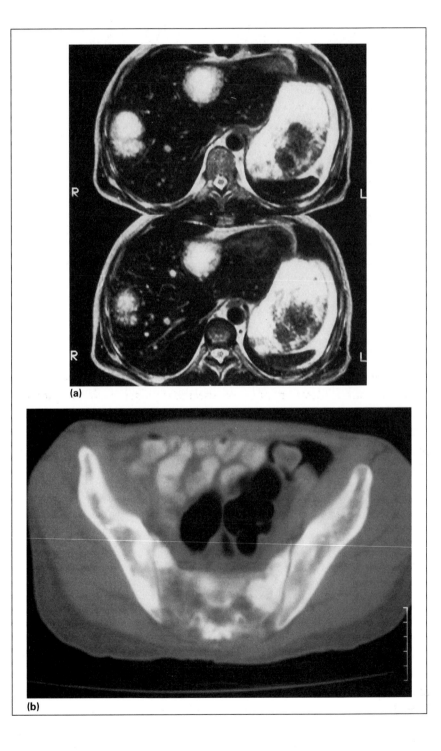

(a)

(b)

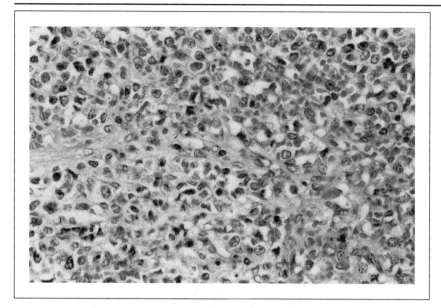

Figure 9.10 Peripheral T-cell lymphoma – spleen. This patient presented with splenomegaly. The spleen was almost completely replaced by a highly pleomorphic population of large T-cells. At laparotomy extensive nodal and gastrointestinal disease was present.

is a common finding and a few patients have overt haemolytic anaemia. Gastrointestinal symptoms including both dyspepsia and diarrhoea may be present at the onset of the disease. These are not usually related to direct tumour infiltration but non-specific changes such as epithelial hyperplasia may be seen in colonic or gastric biopsies and oesophageal ulceration may be present. It is probable that aberrant cytokine production by the tumour cells is central to the pathogenesis of these clinical features.

AIL is a CD4 T-cell proliferation with characteristic histological features

AIL causes loss of nodal architecture and spreads into adjacent perinodal tissues. The most striking feature, which is often apparent on low-power examination of the node, is the presence of an extensive network of blood vessels (Figure 9.12).

These vessels are typically lined by high endothelial cells with extensive polysaccharide deposition in the vessel walls that can be demonstrated by PAS staining. The lymphoid infiltrate is polymorphic, with a wide variety of cell types including mature small lymphocytes, larger cells with more irregular nuclei and T-immunoblasts. The immunoblasts seen in this condition often have abundant clear cytoplasm and have a peripheral T-cell phenotype with expression of CD4+. The number of immunoblasts

Figure 9.11 (a, b) Peripheral T-cell lymphoma – skin. This patient presented with a large cutaneous nodule which on biopsy showed extensive dermal infiltration by peripheral T-cell lymphoma. The patient rapidly developed generalized disease.

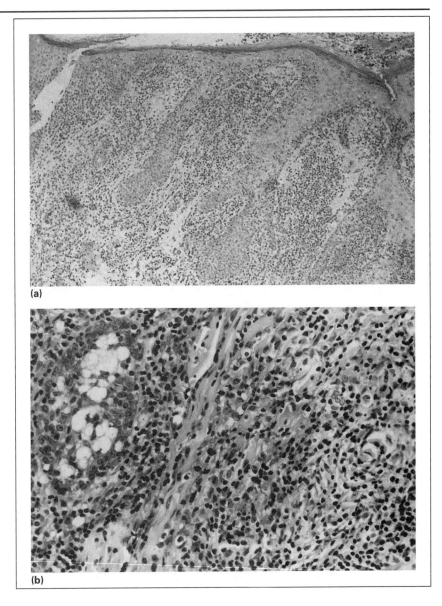

varies considerably between patients and this has been used in some classifications as a basis of distinction between reactive states and true lymphomas. Although this is a general index of disease progression there appears to be little clinical value in making this type of distinction. Cases in which large numbers of immunoblasts are present are more likely to have an abnormal phenotype.

The role of Epstein–Barr virus in the pathogenesis of this condition is uncertain but using a combination of *in situ* hybridization and

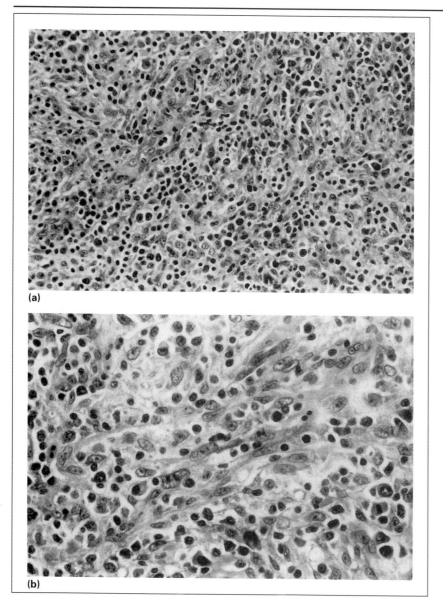

(a)

(b)

Figure 9.12 (a, b)
Angioimmunoblastic T-cell lymphoma – lymph node. This node showed replacement of architecture by a population of lymphocytes, plasma cells, macrophages and lymphoid blast cells with a background of proliferating vessels.

immunohistology it has been possible to demonstrate virus gene expression within the T-cells in AIL. However, in the majority of cases only sporadic cells are involved and the pathogenic significance of this finding is not yet clear.

In addition to the malignant T-cell population large numbers of macrophages, plasma cells and sometimes eosinophils are present. It is unusual to find B-cell follicles with germinal centres in AIL but marker studies almost always show aggregates of mature B-lymphocytes. The use of CD21 or CD35 markers will show an extensive proliferation of follicular dendritic cells, which may be related to the abnormal vessels. This is now regarded as an important diagnostic feature of AIL. In a majority of cases clonal TCR gene rearrangement will be present.

Reactive T-cell proliferations may be difficult to distinguish from AIL

Hypersensitivity reactions may cause lymphadenopathy with histological features that raise the possibility of AIL. Drug reactions, most notably to phenytoin, are the most common cause. A useful histological feature in making the distinction between hypersensitivity reactions and AIL is the presence of reactive germinal centres. As described above these are rare in AIL and their presence, although not an infallible guide, should suggest a reactive cause of lymphadenopathy. The demonstration of T-cell monoclonality by PCR is not by itself diagnostic of malignancy.

AIL is difficult to treat and the prognosis is poor

There is no consensus as to the most appropriate treatment for AIL. The lack of information available from clinical studies is compounded by the extended debate that took place as to whether AIL was a reactive or neoplastic disorder. In the absence of treatment the clinical course is characterized by multiple remissions and relapses, death eventually ensuing as a result of infection or other complications. It is usual to include corticosteroids, which in many cases will control symptoms, as a component of initial treatment before progressing to combination chemotherapy. The clinical outcome may be paradoxical: patients with progressive symptoms may have a quick demise, yet with little evidence of bulky disease, whereas others with bulky disease may remit on treatment; but despite this the overall prognosis is poor.

Lennert's lymphoma

Lennert's lymphoma is a histiocyte-rich form of peripheral T-cell lymphoma

Patients with Lennert's lymphoma usually present with advanced-stage disease, often with involvement of spleen, liver, Waldeyer's ring and marrow. Fever and weight loss are common. In contrast to AIL, tumour bulk rather than systemic symptoms usually predominates. Lennert's lymphoma is distinguished from other types of peripheral T-cell lymphomas by the presence in affected nodes of very large numbers of epithelioid-type macrophages, which may include multinucleate giant cells. The diagnosis depends on the recognition of the neoplastic population of CD4$^+$ T-cells within this background of histiocytes (Figure 9.13).

In most cases these are intermediate-sized cells with irregular or convoluted nuclei and minimal cytoplasm. Cell proliferation as demonstrated by Ki67 is usually low but in some cases increased numbers of proliferating immunoblasts are seen. The nature of the interaction between T-cells and histiocytes in this condition is not understood.

Lennert's lymphoma is classified in the Kiel classification as a low-grade lymphoma; this classification is based on the size of the tumour cells and not on clinical behaviour. However, in most patients this is a clinically aggressive disorder and although there may be an initial response to chemotherapy (e.g. CHOP) the prognosis is poor.

The differential diagnosis of Lennert's lymphoma includes Hodgkin's disease and B-cell lymphoma

The histological differential diagnosis of Lennert's lymphoma includes both mixed cellularity and diffuse lymphocyte-predominant Hodgkin's disease. Increased numbers of blast cells and the presence of eosinophils and plasma cells may make the distinction difficult on H&E-stained sections. However, the use of marker studies should readily resolve this problem in almost every case. A small number of B-cell lymphomas have a large histiocyte component and include variants of follicle centre and diffuse large B-cell lymphomas.

Anaplastic large cell lymphoma (ALCL) – T-cell-type

The term anaplastic lymphoma is used to describe tumours in which the cells show a high degree of cytological atypia and do not resemble identifiable normal lymphoid cells. The majority of these tumours can be shown to be of T-cell lineage although the term can also be used to describe a subtype of diffuse large B-cell lymphoma. A further defining feature is the presence of CD30 expression.

One of the most characteristic features of T-lineage anaplastic large cell lymphoma is the pattern of nodal infiltration

In the early phase of nodal invasion tumour cells proliferate within nodal sinuses, later forming more confluent masses. The cells are large and often appear cohesive, and have abundant cytoplasm, large nuclei with open chromatin and multiple nucleoli. In most cases a proportion of cells with multilobular nuclei are present; these may resemble Reed–Sternberg cells and characteristically some of the cells have a horseshoe-shaped group of multiple nuclei. The pattern of invasion and cellular morphology in many cases strongly resembles metastatic carcinoma or melanoma and it is likely that many anaplastic lymphomas were diagnosed as metastatic tumours before reliable marker techniques were available. The cellular

Figure 9.13 Lennert's lymphoma – lymph node and marrow. This patient presented with generalized lymphadenopathy. The node was replaced by small to intermediate-sized atypical T-cells associated with numerous epithelioid histiocytes (**a, b**). A bone marrow biopsy showed a solitary marrow deposit of T-cell lymphoma (Lel) (**c**).

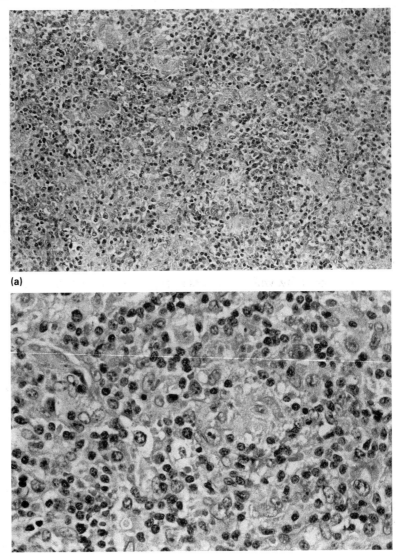

(a)

(b)

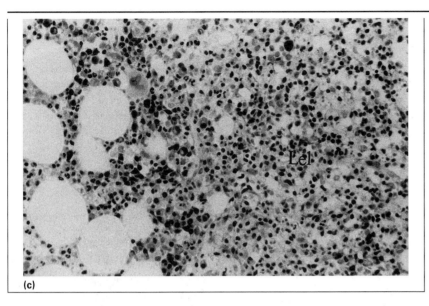

(c)

morphology has also led to some of these cases being diagnosed as histiocytic lymphoma.

The expression of CD30 by the majority of tumour cells is the most characteristic immunophenotypical feature of ALC lymphoma

Almost all ALC lymphomas express CD30. The use of the CD30 antibody Ki-1 in early studies of this group of tumours gave rise to the synonymous term Ki-1 lymphoma. CD30 is a member of the TNF-receptor superfamily, which includes a range of molecules, such as CD40 and Fas, that are key regulators of lymphocyte proliferation and cell death. In normal lymphoid tissue CD30 is expressed as an activation-related marker in a small number of T- and B-cells usually found around the edges of B-cell follicles. The exact function of the molecule is not yet well understood. In addition to CD30 it is usual for ALC to express a range of other lymphocyte activation markers including CD71, CD25 and class II MHC.

The features of anaplastic large cell lymphoma are summarized in Table 9.4.

When unfixed tissue is available expression of CD2 and CD5 is the most consistent feature of T-cell lineage. When only fixed tissue is available CD43 and CD45RO are usually positive although neither is unequivocal evidence of T-cell differentiation (Figure 9.14).

CD3/TCR is much less commonly seen. In many cases the presence of protein constituents of cytotoxic granules has led to the suggestion that

Table 9.4 Anaplastic large cell lymphoma

- **Morphology**: Highly pleomorphic large lymphoid cells with abundant cytoplasm. A proportion of multilobular or multinucleated cells are often present. Infiltration of sinuses seen in early nodal disease.
- **Immunophenotype**: CD30, MHCII and other activation markers, CD43 and highly variable expression of pan-T-cell markers.
- **Cytogenetics**: t(2;5) is present in 50% of cases. A fusion protein with tyrosine kinase activity is produced.
- **Pattern of disease**: Disseminated nodal and extranodal disease. Needs to be distinguished from primary cutaneous anaplastic lymphoma.

anaplastic lymphomas may be derived from cytotoxic T-cells. In paraffin sections at least one-third of cases do not have detectable CD45 expression, which may lead to problems in the distinction between ALC lymphomas and non-haemopoietic tumours or Hodgkin's disease. The expression of epithelial membrane antigen (EMA) is a feature of some ALC lymphomas and may be helpful in differential diagnosis although the incidence has been found to be relatively low. It has recently been suggested that detection of H-blood group by the antibody BNH9 may also be helpful in the diagnosis of ALC lymphoma. In the majority of cases a clonal TCR-beta rearrangement can be detected irrespective of whether there is unequivocal phenotypical evidence of T-cell differentiation. For this reason T-cell and null cell tumours are best regarded as a single group.

A number of variant forms of ALC lymphoma have been described

Variant forms of ALC lymphoma can cause considerable diagnostic difficulty. In such cases the tumour cells are associated with variable numbers of reactive cells, including granulocytes, histiocytes and plasma cells; in a few cases histiocytes may predominate and may be confused with malignant histiocytosis. The tumour cells can be relatively small but have similar immunohistological features to the classical type. A rare sarcomatoid variant has also been described in which some of the cells have spindle-shaped morphology.

t(2;5) is the most consistent cytogenetic finding in anaplastic large cell lymphoma

The t(2;5) involves a tyrosine kinase gene (*ALK*) on chromosome 2 and the gene for nucleophosmin (*NPM*), which is a nucleolar protein, on chromosome 5. The product of this translocation is an abnormal tyrosine

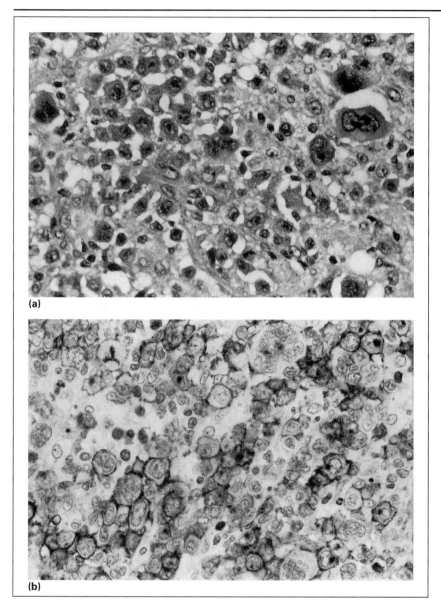

(a)

(b)

Figure 9.14 (a, b) Anaplastic large cell lymphoma – node. This lymph node biopsy shows replacement by a highly pleomorphic population of large lymphoid cells, many of which have multilobular nuclei. The cells show strong expression of CD30 together with CD45 and CD43. A proportion of the cells were CD3$^+$.

kinase fusion protein (ALK is not normally expressed in lymphoid cells). Transfection studies have shown that this fusion protein can cause transformation *in vitro*. In addition to cytogenetic studies this translocation can be reliably detected using RT-PCR, but this requires undegraded RNA and in most cases this means that only fresh tumour tissue is suitable. FISH may be a suitable alternative method of detection and immunocytochemical detection of the fusion protein correlates closely with the presence of t(2;5) (Figure 9.15).

Figure 9.15 The t(2,5). This translocation is found in some nodal anaplastic lymphoma and possibly other T-cell lymphomas. It results in the production of a fusion protein formed from parts of the ALK tyrosine kinase and nucleophosphin.

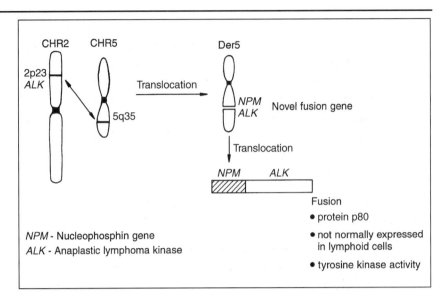

The t(2;5) is present in only approximately 50% of cases of anaplastic large cell lymphoma and it has been suggested that this may define a subgroup of younger patients with a better than average prognosis. It is unclear to what extent the t(2;5) occurs in other types of peripheral T-cell lymphoma without typical anaplastic morphology. If it is common this may lead to a re-evaluation of the validity of recognizing anaplastic lymphoma, based on morphological criteria, as a distinctive disease entity. The available data suggest that t(2;5) probably does not occur in the cutaneous form of anaplastic large cell lymphoma, further emphasizing the distinctiveness of this condition. Despite early reports, the consensus now appears to be that t(2;5) is very rarely, if ever, found in Hodgkin's disease. However, it has recently been suggested that a subtype of B-cell lymphoma may express the ALK kinase protein without a t(2;5).

A common feature of ALC is the apparent deregulation of *p53* as detected by immunohistological techniques, but several studies have shown a low incidence of *p53* mutations. This suggests that an alternative mechanism of *p53* stabilization may be operative. A high incidence of c-*myc* gene abnormalities and overexpression have also been described.

Anaplastic large cell lymphoma often presents with a combination of nodal and extranodal disease

Anaplastic large cell lymphoma occurs in any age group from young children to elderly patients, with a lower mean age of onset than other T-cell lymphomas. Most patients present with bulky stage III or IV nodal disease and extranodal deposits are most common in skin and soft tissues. This must be distinguished from the localized cutaneous variant (discussed in Chapter 10), which has an excellent prognosis. Overt bone marrow infiltration is rare at presentation although occult or minimal disease may be more common. Although ALC lymphoma has the features of a highly aggressive tumour most reports indicate a complete remission rate and overall survival similar to other types of large cell lymphoma of comparable stage following similar treatment. A few patients may present with indolent, localized or even apparently regressing disease.

The differential diagnosis of anaplastic large cell lymphoma includes Hodgkin's disease and metastatic tumours

Before the advent of marker studies it is likely that many cases of anaplastic lymphoma were diagnosed as metastatic tumours of various types. This should now prove less of a problem. In a few cases where CD45 is negative there may be difficulty in distinguishing anaplastic lymphoma from germ cell tumours that also express membrane CD30.

The distinction between anaplastic lymphoma and Hodgkin's disease is based on the pattern of nodal infiltration, the immunophenotype and lack of association of anaplastic lymphomas with EBV (Figure 9.16). The presence of t(2;5) or deregulated expression of the NPM-ALK protein may also prove to be of value in this regard. Particular problems may arise in tumours with the cytological and phenotypical features of anaplastic lymphoma which have a nodular sclerotic pattern of growth.

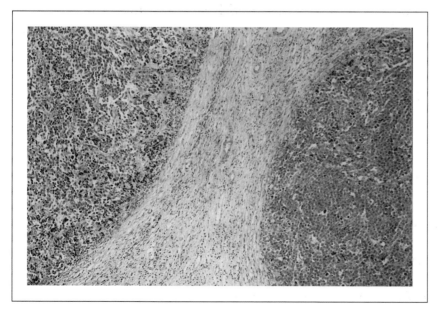

Figure 9.16 Anaplastic large cell lymphoma. This case of anaplastic lymphoma shows a nodular sclerosing pattern similar to nodular sclerosing Hodgkin's disease.

9.3.3 Rare variants of peripheral T-cell lymphoma

Haemophagocytosis may be a dominant clinical feature of some T-cell lymphomas

A group of patients present with cytopenias, fever and other systemic symptoms. On examination of the marrow haemophagocytosis is seen in reactive histiocytes. In some patients this is a transient illness whereas in others there is a fulminant clinical course. In patients with self-limiting

Figure 9.17 Pannaculitic peripheral T-cell lymphoma. This patient presented with a panniculitis and pancytopenia. A subcutaneous tissue biopsy showed extensive infiltration of fat by large atypical T-cells, which were shown by PCR to be monoclonal (a). In some areas there was necrosis of vessel walls (b). The marrow showed haemophagocytosis without overt infiltration by T-cell lymphoma.

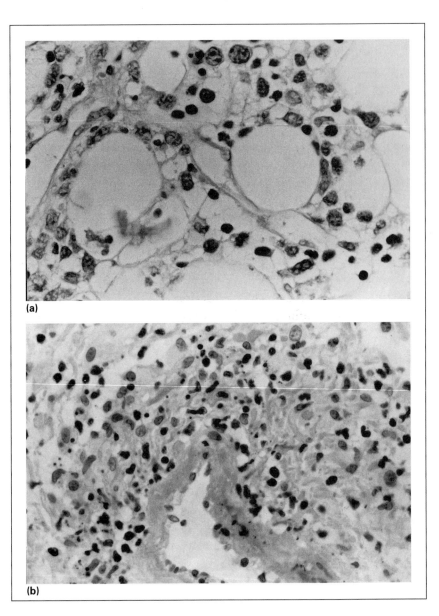

(a)

(b)

disease it appears likely that Parvovirus or a number of other viruses may be the aetiological agent. In adult patients with a progressive course many, if not all, have a T-cell lymphoma. Such patients often have hepatosplenomegaly and/or soft tissue infiltration by lymphoma and tumours of this type have been previously called histiocytic medullary reticulosis. In some patients there is extensive infiltration of subcutaneous fat with clinical features similar to inflammatory causes of panniculitis (Figure 9.17).

There is often a delay in making a definitive diagnosis in these patients, partly because the neoplastic cells may be a relatively inconspicuous feature of the bone marrow and partly because of the confusion that sometimes surrounds the differential diagnosis of marrow haemophago-cytosis. However, the prognosis of patients with haemophagocytosis associated T-cell lymphoma is generally very poor regardless of treatment.

T-cell lymphomas that express TCR1 (gamma/delta) are associated with hepatosplenomegaly

T-cell lymphomas that express TCR1 and show no evidence of TCR2 gene rearrangement appear to be rare. In some of the reported cases the tumour cells have been shown to express CD8 in contrast to the normal TCR1-positive cells found in peripheral blood, which typically lack both CD4 and CD8. At least a proportion of these tumours constitute a distinct clinical entity characterized by predominately liver, spleen and marrow infiltration without significant lymphadenopathy or lymphocytosis. The prognosis in these cases appears to be uniformly poor.

9.4 Key references

Cooke, C. B., Krenacs, L., Stetler-Stevenson, M. *et al.* (1996) Hepatosplenic T-cell Lymphoma: a distinct clinicopathologic entity of cytotoxic gamma/delta T-cell origin. *Blood,* **88,** 4265–4272.

D'Amore, F., Johansen, P., Houmand, A. *et al.* (1996) Epstein–Barr virus genome in non-Hodgkin's lymphomas occurring in immunocompetent patients: highest prevalence in nonlymphoblastic T-cell lymphoma and correlation with a poor prognosis. Danish Lymphoma Study Group, LYFO. *Blood,* **87,** 1045–1055.

Delsol, G., Lamant, L., Mariame, B. *et al.* (1997) A new subtype of large B-cell lymphoma expressing the ALK Kinase and lacking the 2:5 translocation. *Blood*, **89**, 1483–1490.

Foss, H. D., Anagnostopoulos, I., Araujo, I. *et al.* (1996) Anaplastic large-cell lymphomas of T-cell and null-cell phenotype express cytotoxic molecules. *Blood*, **88**, 4005–4011.

Franchini, G. and Streicher, H. (1995) Human T-cell leukaemia virus. *Baillières Clinical Haematology*, **8**, 131–148.

Fujimoto, J., Shiota, M., Iwahara, T. *et al.* (1996) Characterization of the transforming activity of p80, a hyperphosphorylated protein in a Ki-1 lymphoma cell line with chromosomal translocation t(2;5). *Proceedings of the National Academy of Sciences of the United States of America*, **93**, 4181–4186.

Herbst, H., Anagnostopoulos, J., Heinze, B. *et al.* (1995) ALK gene products in anaplastic large cell lymphomas and Hodgkin's disease. *Blood*, **86**, 1694–1700.

Pulford, K., Lamant, L., Morris, S. W. *et al.* (1997) Detection of anaplastic lymphoma kinase (ALK) and nucleolar protein nucleophosmin (NPM)– ALK proteins in normal and neoplastic cells with the monoclonal antibody ALK1. *Blood*, **89**, 1394–1404.

Richards, S., Short, M. and Scott, C. S. (1995) Clonal CD3⁺CD8⁺ Large granular lymphocyte LGL/NK associated NKa expansions: primary malignancies or secondary reactive phenomena? *Leukemia and Lymphoma*, **17**, 303–311.

Weisenberger, D. D., Gordon, B. G., Vose, J. M. *et al.* (1996) Occurrence of t(2;5) (p23:q35) in Non-Hodgkin's lymphoma. *Blood*, **87**, 3860–3686.

Wong, K. F., Chan, J. K., Matutes, E. *et al.* (1995) Hepatosplenic gamma delta T-cell lymphoma. A distinctive aggressive lymphoma type. *American Journal of Surgical Pathology*, **19**, 718–726.

Yamaguchi, K. (1994) Human T-lymphotropic virus type I in Japan. *Lancet*, **343**, 213–216.

Extranodal lymphoproliferative disorders

10

There is, as yet, no clear definition of extranodal lymphoproliferative disorders and this has led to some confusion in comparing results of different studies. Leaving aside the involvement of extranodal sites in advanced stage disease, there are two main groups of extranodal lymphoma.

Firstly, there are tumours that remain essentially localized to their extranodal site of origin, though sometimes with infiltration of local nodes. Spread to distant nodes, blood or marrow does not occur until late in the course of the disease. Many of these tumours are marginal zone lymphoma (MALToma), a type of tumour that rarely presents as nodal disease, or diffuse large B-cell lymphomas. An exception is the skin, where peripheral T-cell lymphomas predominate. A feature of many of these tumours is that they arise in the context of chronic inflammatory reactions in which there is development of organized lymphoid tissue at sites where it is not normally present. Until recently the term pseudolymphoma was in common use, reflecting the lack of clear criteria to distinguish indolent forms of extranodal lymphoma from florid chronic inflammatory reaction. Until the advent of effective marker studies some extranodal lymphomas were misdiagnosed as poorly differentiated carcinomas.

The second main group of extranodal lymphomas comprises tumours that may present as an extranodal mass although on investigation generalized disease is often present or rapidly develops. An example of this type of tumour would be a thymic mass in T-lymphoblastic disease or mantle cell lymphoma of Waldeyer's ring. A number of tumours do not fit neatly into either of these two categories; for example, multiple lymphomatous polyposis is a bowel-centred variant of mantle cell lymphoma that progresses to blood and marrow infiltration at a relatively early stage in the disease.

10.1 Cutaneous lymphoproliferative disorders

Cutaneous lymphomas are the largest group of extranodal lymphomas and are also the most diverse

Unlike other extranodal sites a high proportion of cutaneous lymphomas are of T-cell type. In the past the terminology of skin lymphomas has been daunting and has perhaps inhibited progress in this field. Despite this there is now increasing agreement that there are three main groups of cutaneous lymphomas. These are: classical mycosis fungoides and its variants; lymphomatoid papulosis and cutaneous anaplastic lymphoma, which are linked by immunophenotype; and the relatively rare cutaneous B-cell lymphoma. The skin, of course, can also be involved by many types of systemic leukaemia and lymphoma and a proportion of generalized peripheral T-cell lymphomas initially present with cutaneous nodules.

10.1.1 Mycosis fungoides and its variants

Classical mycosis fungoides is a well defined clinical and pathological syndrome

Mycosis fungoides in its classical form is a disease that affects mainly middle-aged and elderly patients. The initial presentation is usually with

Figure 10.1 Mycosis fungoides. Mycosis fungoides evolves through a series of histological stages. In early disease **(a)** there is a sparse infiltrate of T-cells, which show cytological atypia and in this case are forming intraepidermal aggregates **(b)**. As the tumour progresses the dermal infiltrate becomes more diffuse **(c)**.

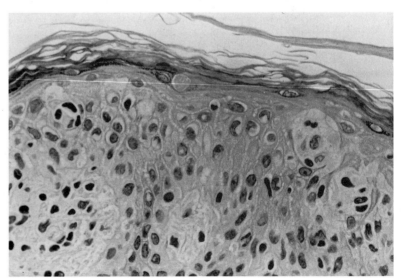

(a)

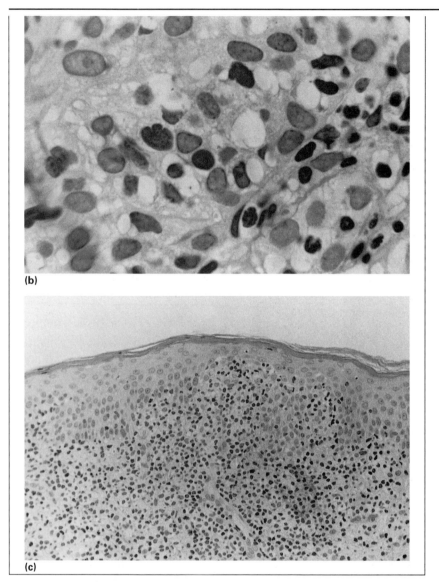

(b)

(c)

a pruritic, flat, scaling patch on the trunk or buttocks. As the disease progresses and the degree of infiltration increases palpable plaques form. As the area of involved skin increases some parts of the plaque may undergo spontaneous involution, creating striking cyclical patterns on the skin. Unlike many inflammatory skin disorders the distribution of mycosis fungoides is often irregular and asymmetrical (Figure 10.1).

If typical clinical appearances are present the histological diagnosis of mycosis fungoides is seldom a problem. A skin biopsy will show a perivascular or a diffuse upper dermal infiltrate of T-cells which are larger than peripheral blood lymphocytes and show elongated, convoluted or folded nuclei. The term 'cerebriform' is sometimes used to describe the nuclear morphology. A few larger blast cells are usually present. The most distinctive histological feature is invasion of the epidermis by neoplastic T-cells and the formation of Pautrier microabscesses. These structures consist of intraepidermal aggregates of atypical T-cells associated with one or more Langerhans cells. The latter can be identified by the presence of S100 protein or by their distinctive nuclear morphology. The degree of cytological atypia of the T-cells is often more easily recognized in the intraepidermal lymphocytes. In all cases accurate diagnosis of mycosis fungoides depends on high quality histological sections; the use of methyl methacrylate embedding is ideal for this purpose.

Mycosis fungoides is a peripheral T-cell lymphoma. In around two-thirds of cases the phenotype is that of normal CD4$^+$ peripheral T-cells. Peripheral T-cells can be distinguished from precursor T-cells by lack of CD1 and Tdt but this is rarely required in the assessment of cutaneous infiltrates. All cases express class II MHC, which is a T-cell activation marker, but expression of CD30 is very rare. The remaining one-third of cases have an abnormal phenotype; in the majority of cases this involves loss of one or more of the pan-T antigens, with CD7 being the most commonly affected. A further immunophenotypical feature is discordance between epidermal and dermal T-cell populations. In some cases of mycosis fungoides the T-cells express the integrin recognized by CD103 and this may correlate with the ability of the neoplastic T-cells to infiltrate the epidermis. In a few cases coexpression of CD4 and CD8 is found; this appears to be more common in progressive disease.

Several problems may arise in the interpretation of T-cell marker studies in mycosis fungoides. In the dermal infiltrate a considerable proportion of CD8$^+$ cells may be seen although these tend to more sparse within the epidermis. There is some preliminary evidence to suggest that increased numbers of CD8$^+$ cells may be an indicator of a more favourable prognosis. A further problem is that Langerhans cells, which may be greatly increased in number, express CD4, and this may confuse interpretation.

The detection of T-cell monoclonality is increasingly used in the diagnosis of cutaneous lymphoid infiltrates. PCR techniques to detect T-cell-receptor-gamma gene rearrangements can be used in the same way as for other forms of T-cell malignancy but it can be difficult to extract tumour DNA from a skin biopsy where the infiltrate is sparse, and a false-negative result may be obtained when large numbers of non-neoplastic

T-cells are present. Unfortunately, these are the circumstances in which histological and immunophenotypical studies may also be equivocal. More importantly, there is as yet insufficient data on the incidence of T-cell monoclonality in inflammatory skin conditions to use it unequivocally for the diagnosis of cutaneous T-cell malignancy.

Classical mycosis fungoides has a predictable clinical course

Classical mycosis fungoides progresses in a relatively predictable way and can be staged using a TNM system modified for this purpose (Table 10.1).

Progression of the disease within the skin is associated with the development of larger and more extensive plaques. Eventually within these plaques tumour nodules develop, which usually consist of larger more atypical T-cells, with a lesser propensity to invade into the epidermis (Figure 10.2).

The lack of epidermotropism may cause confusion if a biopsy is examined without knowledge of the preceding history. An alternative form of progression is the development of a generalized erythroderma with or without tumour nodules. Lymphadenopathy may be seen at a relatively early stage of the disease but in most cases histological examination of the nodes will show a reactive dermatopathic pattern rather than overt lymphoma. This boundary is obscured by the use of immunogenetic techniques, which may show a clonal T-cell population without morphological evidence of tumour (Figure 10.3). The presence of morphologically or

Table 10.1 TNM staging for mycosis fungoides

T1	Limited plaque (< 10% of surface area)
T2	Generalized plaques
T3	Cutaneous tumours
T4	Generalized erythroderma
N1	No adenopathy
N2	Adenopathy – biopsy negative
N3	No adenopathy – biopsy positive
N4	Adenopathy – biopsy positive
M0	No visceral involvement
M1	Visceral involvement
Stage 1:	T1N0M0 or T2N0M0
Stage 2:	T1N1M0 or T2N0M0
Stage 3:	T4N0M0
Stage 4:	T1–4N2M0 or T1–4N0–3M1

Figure 10.2 Mycosis fungoides - tumour phase. In the late stages of mycosis fungoides tumour nodules develop within plaques. These consist of larger, more rapidly proliferating T-cells.

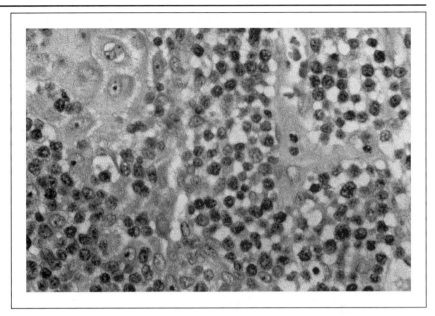

phenotypically detectable mycosis cells in blood or marrow means a late stage of the disease but the use of sensitive PCR-based techniques may demonstrate this somewhat earlier. Only in rare cases of mycosis fungoides does overt leukaemia develop in the terminal phase of the disease.

The term 'Sézary's syndrome' is used to describe the combination of generalized erythroderma and a CD4+ peripheral T-cell leukaemia in which the morphology of the cells seen in the peripheral blood is similar to that seen in skin biopsies (Figure 10.4).

Sézary's syndrome does not necessarily represent the end stage of the disease spectrum of mycosis fungoides and many, possibly the majority, of patients present *de novo* without a preceding indolent phase. These cases of Sézary's syndrome can be considered to have a variant of peripheral T-cell leukaemia with skin homing properties. Patients with Sézary's syndrome have a poor prognosis.

The clinical and pathological distinction between early mycosis fungoides and inflammatory disorders can be difficult

The most common problem in the diagnosis of mycosis fungoides is the recognition of early stages of the disease. Early mycosis fungoides and chronic superficial dermatitis are clinically similar with features of parapsoriasis *en plaque*. Whether cases of chronic dermatitis can progress to lymphoma is an unresolved question. In other patients early lesions have poikilodermatous features in which the epidermis is atrophic with mild dermal oedema and inflammation. This appearance is also seen in a variety of connective tissue disorders such as dermatomyositis. When the clinical features are equivocal it is unlikely that the biopsy will be more than suggestive of the diagnosis and it is uncommon for a definitive diagnosis to be made at this stage. As already described, it would be unwise to make a definitive diagnosis on the finding of a clonal T-cell-receptor gene rearrangement in the absence of supporting morphological

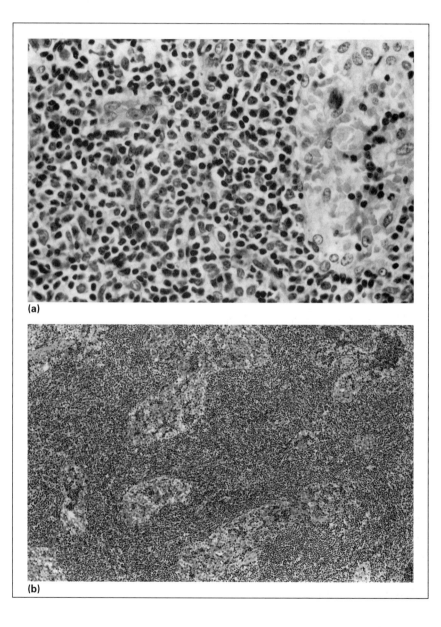

(a)

(b)

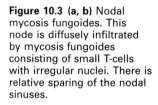

Figure 10.3 (a, b) Nodal mycosis fungoides. This node is diffusely infiltrated by mycosis fungoides consisting of small T-cells with irregular nuclei. There is relative sparing of the nodal sinuses.

Figure 10.4 Sézary's syndrome. This patient presented with lymphocytosis and erythroderma. The peripheral blood contained large numbers of lymphocytes with highly convoluted nuclei. These were CD4+ with an otherwise normal T-cell phenotype. There was no evidence of underlying mycosis fungoides.

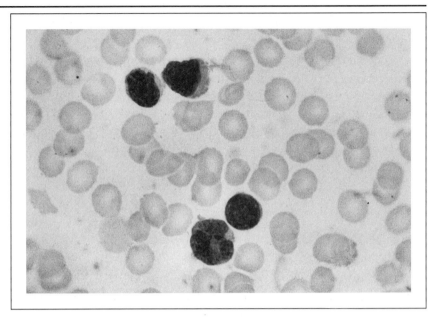

or clinical evidence. Such cases should be followed up closely and their clinical evolution monitored. Treatment at any stage of the disease is not curative and nothing is lost by this conservative approach.

A number of common conditions, such as lupus erythematosus and lichen planus, can also be confused with mycosis in its early stages. These conditions may have large numbers of activated lymphocytes in the cutaneous infiltrate, and morphometric studies have shown that the degree of nuclear irregularity may be similar to that seen in mycosis fungoides. A more significant degree of cytological abnormality – including, rarely, epidermal invasion – may be seen in an atypical reaction to sunlight, which is confusingly known as actinic reticuloid.

There are a number of variants of mycosis fungoides that have distinctive clinical features

In advanced mycosis fungoides a histiocytic infiltrate is common and has been reported as a good prognostic feature. In a few cases granulomas may be present and these may be associated with destruction of elastin fibres, leading to loss of skin elasticity. This is sometimes described as 'granulomatous slack skin disease'.

In a small proportion of cases the neoplastic T-cells preferentially invade the hair follicle epithelium rather than the surface epidermis. This can be associated with the deposition of glycosaminoglycan within the hair follicle, leading to the clinical features of follicular mucinosis. It is uncertain whether all cases of this highly distinctive lesion are due to lymphoma. Other clinical variants include cases in which depigmentation or bulla formation occurs (Figure 10.5).

Pagetoid reticulosis is the term used to describe lesions in which there is an intensely epidermotrophic infiltrate of atypical T-cells, often associated with epidermal hyperplasia and hyperkeratosis. In some cases the T-cell infiltrate appears to express CD8 rather than CD4. In the past some of these cases were mistaken for melanoma or pagetoid spread of carcinoma. The most typical form of Pagetoid reticulosis presents as localized unilesional disease on the limbs. More generalized disease may occur but in these cases the distinction from classical-type mycosis is more difficult. In patients with the localized form of the disease, local radiotherapy may be curative.

Finally, although mycosis fungoides is a disease of the elderly, cases do arise in children and young adults with identical clinical and pathological features. Although the rate of progression may be similar to typical adult cases this, of course, represents a very poor prognosis for a child.

The aim of treatment in mycosis fungoides is effective palliation

Mycosis fungoides is a rare condition with around 3–4 cases per million per year. This has inhibited the development of effective clinical trials and

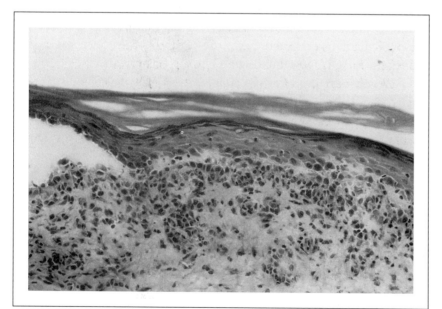

Figure 10.5 Mycosis fungoides – bullous form. In this case epidermal invasion by mycosis fungoides was accompanied by intraepidermal splitting and bulla formation.

there is a lack of consensus in treatment approach. There is no evidence that any form of treatment is curative in the majority of patients and the aim of most therapies is effective palliation. During the early stages of the disease most patients will be treated with a combination of topical steroids or PUVA, which leads to symptomatic improvement in the majority of patients. Topical nitrogen mustard may also be used but is associated with local side effects and possibly carries a risk of secondary malignancy. In patients with both early or more advanced plaque phase disease total body electron therapy can induce complete remissions. Once tumours have developed, the ability of electrons to penetrate deeply is a limiting factor. When remissions are induced, treatment with IFNα may have a role in delaying relapse.

In advanced stage disease local radiotherapy in combination with single-agent or combination chemotherapy will often induce a good initial response, but this is usually short-lived.

10.1.2 Lymphomatoid papulosis and CD30$^+$ cutaneous lymphoma

Lymphomatoid papulosis is a self healing tumour with distinctive histological and immunophenotypical features

Lymphomatoid papulosis is recognized by its distinctive clinical features. Patients are usually aged over 30 years and present with one or more rapidly growing lesions on the trunk or upper body. These lesions grow to around 1 cm, ulcerate and then regress with scarring. Such a relapsing remitting course is typical and continues for many years.

The lesions of lymphomatoid papulosis are pathologically distinctive. Large lesions have a definite structure. Around the periphery of the lesion there is perivascular and diffuse infiltration by small T-cells, which may or may not show a degree of atypia. The central area of the lesion contains a highly pleomorphic population of cells, which includes large atypical lymphoid cells with abundant cytoplasm and an open nuclear chromatin pattern and prominent nucleoli, some of which may have morphological features similar to Reed–Sternberg cells. These cells are mixed with atypical small lymphocytes, macrophages, eosinophils and prominent vessels. The overlying epidermis may be degenerate or ulcerated. The large atypical cells show strong expression of CD30 with a CD4$^+$ peripheral T-cell phenotype, although loss of pan-T antigen such as CD7 is common (Figure 10.6). The small amount of data available

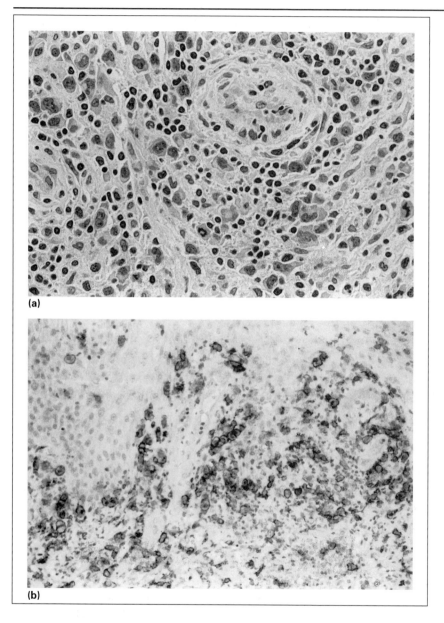

Figure 10.6 Lymphomatoid papulosis. Biopsy of a lesion with clinical features typical of lymphomatoid papulosis. In the centre of the lesion there are large numbers of atypical lymphoid cells some of which have bilobular nuclei (a). These cells showed high levels of CD30 expression (b).

suggest that lymphomatoid papulosis is a clonal T-cell disorder and that recurrent lesions contain the same clone.

In a minority of cases the histological features of lymphomatoid papulosis resemble mycosis fungoides

In the rare type B form of lymphomatoid papulosis the lesion consists of small to intermediate-sized T-cells showing epidermal invasion. These cells are CD4$^+$ peripheral T-cells but CD30 expression is less prominent. Without details of the clinical features these lesions cannot be reliably distinguished from mycosis fungoides.

It now thought likely that cases which in the past were diagnosed as regressing atypical histiocytosis are also part of the spectrum of lymphomatoid papulosis. The differences in clinical and pathological features, if any, are not clear.

Pityriasis lichenoides may be closely related to lymphomatoid papulosis

Pityriasis lichenoides is clinically similar to lymphomatoid papulosis. Patients tend to be young adults who present with recurrent crops of papules that heal by scarring. Lesions vary in their rate of evolution and tendency to ulceration, which defines the acute and chronic clinical variants of this condition.

Histological examination of the more acute lesions of pityriasis lichenoides shows a perivascular and diffuse infiltrate of activated CD4$^+$ and CD8$^+$ T-cells. These cells may show a significant degree of nuclear atypia but the large CD30$^+$ cells seen in lymphomatoid papulosis are not seen or are present in only small numbers. The infiltration of the epidermis is associated with basal cell and keratinocyte injury. In the dermis, vascular damage may be present with extravasation of red blood cells which may become trapped within the epidermis. The pathogenesis of pityriasis lichenoides is uncertain but a small number of reports suggest that the skin is infiltrated by a clonal T-cell population. As discussed above this is not evidence of malignancy and as far as is known pityriasis lichenoides does not progress to overt lymphoma.

Cutaneous CD30$^+$ lymphoma has a much better prognosis than similar tumours in lymph nodes and other sites

A proportion of cases of lymphomatoid papulosis undergo progression to lymphoma but there is uncertainty about the risk, which may be around 5–10% per patient. Transformation is recognized by lesions that continue to grow and do not regress within the expected time. These tumours are CD30$^+$ T-cell lymphomas and most have anaplastic morphology similar to the atypical cells seen in lymphomatoid papulosis (Figure 10.7).

CD30$^+$ large cell lymphomas of this type may also occur as primary tumours in the skin without preceding lymphomatoid papulosis. It has been suggested that a proportion may originate by transformation of

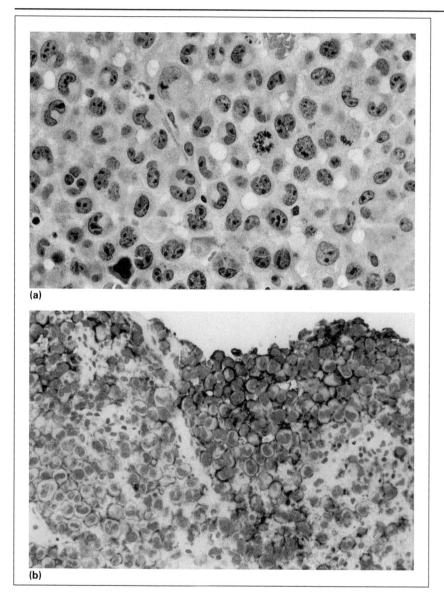

(a)

(b)

Figure 10.7 Cutaneous anaplastic lymphoma. This solitary skin lesion consisted of a diffuse infiltrate of highly pleomorphic large lymphocytes **(a)** that express strong surface CD30. **(b)** CD3 expression was also present.

mycosis fungoides, though this is doubtful. These tumours may be morphologically similar to anaplastic large cell lymphomas found in lymph nodes and other organs but the cutaneous tumours have a more complete T-cell phenotype, do not express epithelial membrane antigen and do not appear to carry the t(2;5). The distinction between primary cutaneous and other types of anaplastic lymphoma is of great importance. Recent studies suggest that primary cutaneous CD30[+] lymphomas have a good prognosis despite the risk of skin recurrence. Only about 25% of patients show systemic progression and many show partial or complete regression. In contrast, nodal CD30$^+$ anaplastic lymphomas are relatively aggressive tumours. In earlier published series this distinction is often lost because of a failure to separate systemic and localized CD30$^+$ lymphomas. The optimum treatment of cutaneous CD30$^+$ lymphomas is unknown.

10.1.3 Cutaneous lymphoid hyperplasia and B-cell lymphoma

Cutaneous lymphoid hyperplasia present as nodules in the head and neck

Some patients present with one or more cutaneous nodules which on biopsy are found to consist of reactive lymphoid tissue. Unless a specific cause is apparent these are best described as cutaneous lymphoid hyperplasia rather than using obsolete terms such as Jessner's lymphocytic infiltrate, Speigler–Fendt sarcoid or lymphocytoma cutis. In the lesions of cutaneous lymphoid hyperplasia the epidermis and the papillary dermis is usually normal. The infiltrate consists of a dense central nodular mass of lymphoid tissue with a perivascular component towards the periphery of the lesion. In most cases markers will show B-cell follicles with follicular dendritic cell networks surrounded by a T-cell zone in which there are prominent vessels and variable numbers of macrophages (Figure 10.8). The T-cells show the range of morphological forms normally seen in the lymph node paracortex, with a mixture of small CD4$^+$ and CD8$^+$ lymphocytes together with larger more irregular activated cells and a few blasts.

These histological features are likely to occur in response to a variety of agents including reactions to insect bites and possibly bacterial colonization of the skin, but in most cases no cause can be found. Some lesions have a predominance of T-cells and examination of multiple sections may show injury to follicular or surface epithelium with epidermal atrophy and follicular plugging suggestive of LE. This group corresponds to many of the lesions previously diagnosed as Jessner's lymphocytic infiltrate. In the older literature, skin involvement by CLL is often cited as a differential diagnosis when infiltrates consist mainly of small lymphocytes. CLL does occasionally affect the skin but can be easily distinguished from cutaneous lymphoid hyperplasia by marker studies, and isolated skin without blood or marrow involvement is very unlikely.

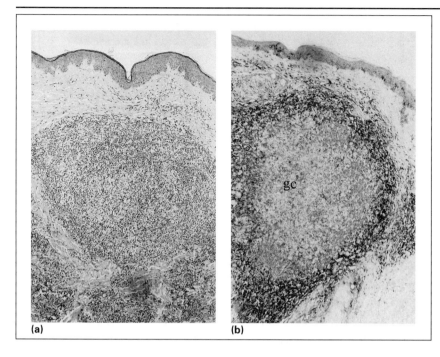

Figure 10.8 Cutaneous lymphoid hyperplasia. This is a solitary lesion from the chest. **(a)** There is a dense multinodular lymphoid infiltrate, which spared the epidermis and upper dermis. **(b)** The nodules show a peripheral zone of T-cells, demonstrated by anti-CD3, surrounding B-cell follicles with reactive germinal centres.

Idiopathic forms of cutaneous lymphoid hyperplasia may recur and there appears to be a risk of transformation to B-cell lymphoma. The incidence of transformation to lymphoma is unknown but appears to be low.

Most cases of primary cutaneous B-cell lymphomas are of diffuse large cell type

Cutaneous B-cell lymphomas are much rarer than cutaneous T-cell lymphomas. They almost always occur on the head and neck and present as solitary nodules (Figure 10.9).

Size and growth rate may be a distinguishing factor but otherwise these tumours clinically resemble cutaneous lymphoid hyperplasia. The majority of cases are diffuse large B-cell lymphomas consisting of cells with morphological features of centroblasts, large centrocytes and immunoblasts. In some cases there may be features suggestive of an underlying lymphoid hyperplasia. Other types of primary cutaneous B-cell lymphoma are very rare. Occasional cases of marginal zone lymphoma (MALToma) may be found (Figure 10.10). These tend to be very indolent, slowly progressive tumours. Primary cutaneous follicle centre lymphoma is described in some classifications of lymphoprolifer-

Figure 10.9 (a, b) Diffuse large B-cell lymphoma – skin. This is a solitary, rapidly growing lesion from the head. There is a multinodular lesion, which consists of a monomorphic population of large lymphoid cells, most of which have centroblastic-type features.

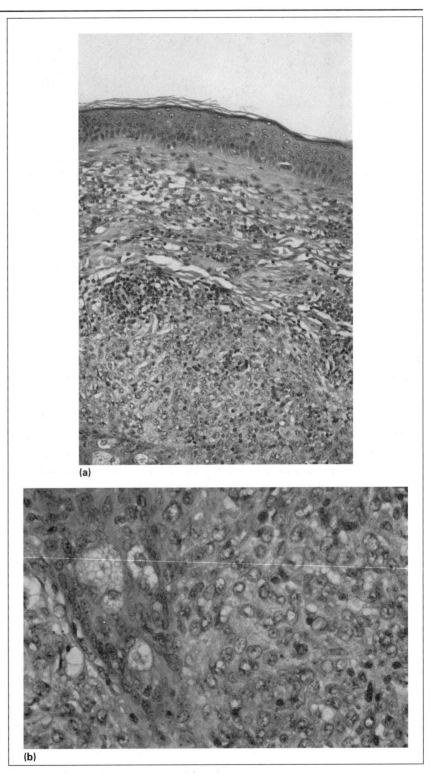

(a)

(b)

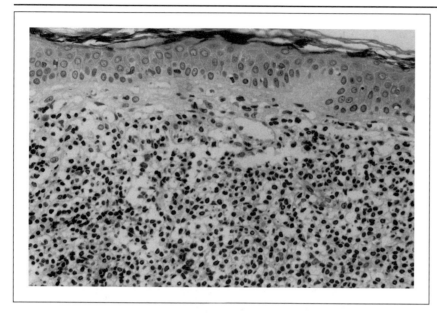

Figure 10.10 Marginal zone lymphoma – skin. Biopsy of an indolent nodular lesion from the face. The epidermis is uninvolved and there is a clear area of upper dermis (Grenz zone). In the deeper dermis there is a dense infiltrate of B-cells, which have centrocyte like or plasmacytoid morphology. In other parts of the lesion there were reactive germinal centres that were partly infiltrated.

ative disorders of the skin. However, this is not universally accepted and the relationship of this entity to nodal follicle centre lymphomas is far from clear.

In a few cases of cutaneous lymphoid hyperplasia there may be small numbers of large atypical B-cells present outwith the context of follicles. It may be possible to demonstrate a clonal B-cell population by PCR in some of these lesions and this may represent the initial stage in evolution of large cell lymphoma.

Tumours on the skin tend to present early as small localized lesions and many cutaneous B-cell lymphomas are fully excised at the time of diagnosis. Many patients will also receive adjuvant local radiotherapy. The prognosis appears to be excellent and death from disease is very rare.

10.1.4 Skin infiltration by leukaemia and non-cutaneous lymphoma

Many types of lymphoma and leukaemia may involve the skin, sometimes at presentation and may cause various diagnostic difficulties. Any type of peripheral T-cell lymphoma may produce skin or subcutaneous nodules and in rare entities such as lymphomatoid granulomatosis (see below) or panniculitic T-cell lymphoma (Chapter 9) extensive infiltration of skin and subcutaneous tissue may be the dominant feature of the disease. Skin involvement by anaplastic large cell lymphoma is relatively frequent and, as described above, it is important to distinguish between primary cutaneous anaplastic lymphoma and secondary involvement. Skin infiltration by B-cell lymphomas appears to be less common than T-cell lymphoma with CLL being the most common (Figure 10.11).

Acute myeloid leukaemia may present with skin infiltration usually in AML M5 and AML M0 types. In most cases the other features of acute

Figure 10.11 Lymphomatoid granulomatosis – vulva. This patient presented with an ulcerating necrotic mass on the vulva. Biopsy showed infiltration and destruction of vessels by T-cells but within the lesion there was a population of highly atypical large cells **(a)** with a B-cell phenotype and expression of the EBV protein Lmp-1 **(b)**.

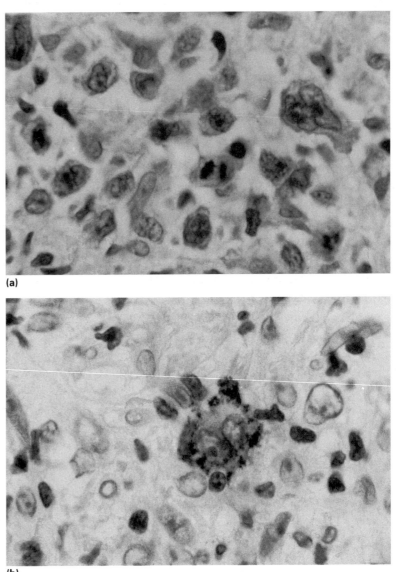

(a)

(b)

leukaemia are present or develop after a few days. Acute leukaemia or myelodysplasia may also present as Sweet's syndrome in which there is a dense granulocytic infiltrate in the dermis.

10.2 Lymphoproliferative disorders of the gastrointestinal tract

Primary extranodal lymphoproliferative disorders occur at any level in the gastrointestinal tract but a high proportion of cases arise in the stomach. Unlike the skin, the majority of gastrointestinal lymphomas are of B-cell type and many of these appear to be marginal zone lymphomas (MALToma), the main exception being intestinal T-cell lymphoma (ITCL).

10.2.1 Lymphomas of the stomach

Organized gastric lymphoid tissue is acquired as a result of *Helicobacter* infection

Apart from a few basally situated small aggregates in the oxyntic mucosa, the human stomach is virtually devoid of lymphoid cells. Organized lymphoid tissue develops in the stomach as a consequence of chronic infection or autoimmune gastritis. Infection by *Helicobacter pylori* appears to be by far the most common infection of the stomach and is thought to play a central role in the pathogenesis of chronic peptic ulceration.

The source of *Helicobacter* infection in the environment remains unknown. It appears likely that the probability of becoming infected correlates with poor socioeconomic conditions. Although the prevalence of chronic *Helicobacter* infection in Western countries may be declining, there remain very large numbers of patients who have gastric colonization by *Helicobacter pylori*. An unknown proportion of these individuals have symptoms related to the infection. Even in patients with chronic dyspepsia who have *Helicobacter* colonization it is not always possible to ascertain that the organism is the cause of the symptoms.

The development of lymphoid tissue in the gastric antral mucosa in response to *Helicobacter* infection had been extensively described. B-cell aggregates develop in the deep mucosa and a variable proportion show germinal centres. A proportion of CD5$^+$ B-cells are also present. Most of the thickness of the mucosa is occupied by T-cells, some of which express activation antigens. In the superficial part of the mucosa plasma cells can be found. This broadly resembles the structure of Peyer's patches in the small bowel although in the stomach a marginal zone is not a prominent feature and specialized M-type epithelial cells, which overlie small-intestinal lymphoid tissue, are not usually apparent. Organized lymphoid tissue in the small intestine has its own pathways of lymphocyte recirculation, which have been extensively studied, and it is suspected that similar pathways may also develop when mucosa-associated lymphoid tissue forms in the stomach. How quickly this gastric lymphoid tissue is lost after treatment of *Helicobacter* infection with antibiotics is unknown.

The evidence for an association between gastric lymphoma and *Helicobacter* infection is now very strong

Several lines of evidence strongly indicate that *Helicobacter pylori* is involved in the pathogenesis of gastric lymphoma. Direct and serological evidence of infection is present in almost all cases of gastric lymphoma. It is possible to induce gastric lymphomas in mice by experimental infection with various *Helicobacter* strains and treatment of some patients with anti-*Helicobacter* therapy has been shown to result in tumour regression.

The mode of action of *Helicobacter* in causing lymphomas is not fully understood. There is some evidence to suggest that *Helicobacter* acts by immune stimulation and that the neoplastic B-cells are dependent on *Helicobacter* stimulated T-cells. Equally there are a number of ways in which *Helicobacter* may generate carcinogens in the gastric mucosa, such as the production of free radicals in the course of periodic episodes of acute inflammation. Why some patients develop carcinoma and others lymphoma is unknown (Figure 10.12).

Lymphomas arising in gastric mucosa-associated lymphoid tissue (MALT) include marginal zone and diffuse large B-cell lymphomas

Indolent gastric lymphomas consist of a polymorphous population of B-cells, which includes variable numbers of cells that resemble the centrocytes of germinal centres, monocytoid B-cells (so-called because of their resemblance to monocytes), plasmacytoid cells, mature plasma cells and a few larger blast cells. The tumour cells express clonal surface IgM, CD19, CD20, CD22, CD32 and CD38

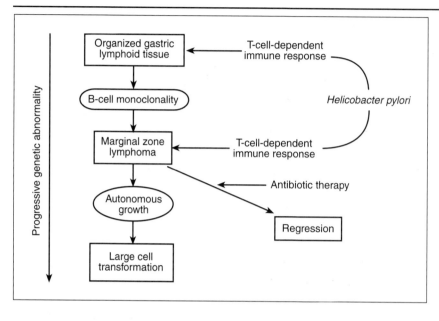

Figure 10.12 The evolution of gastric lymphoma. A number of well defined steps can be identified in the evolution of gastric B-cell lymphoma. Organized lymphoid tissue forms as a result of *Helicobacter* infection and monoclonal B-cell populations may evolve in the absence of lymphoma. The evolution and growth of marginal zone lymphoma depends on the continued presence of *Helicobacter* and this may be mediated through T-cells. As tumour progression occurs, autonomy from *Helicobacter* develops, ending in some cases with large cell transformation. Treatment with anti-*Helicobacter* therapy prior to this stage may result in tumour regression. This process of tumour evolution is associated with progressive genetic change, which may be accelerated by carcinogens produced by *Helicobacter* combined with a failure to eliminate genetically damaged cells.

and lack CD23, CD10, CD5 and IgD expression. The expression of CDw75 is variable. In some cases cytoplasmic granular reactivity with the anti-CD68 antibody KiM1p may be present. The pattern of infiltration of the gastric mucosa is the most characteristic feature (Figure 10.13).

Cells which morphologically resemble centrocytes invade and destroy gastric glands, forming lymphoepithelial lesions. In dense infiltrates this feature is best demonstrated using an anticytokeratin antibody to highlight residual epithelial cells. The neoplastic cells surround and invade reactive germinal centres. When this occurs the tumour may appear to have a nodular growth pattern. The residual germinal centres can be shown using an antibody that reacts with follicular dendritic cells, such as CD21. There is often a broad band of plasma cells underlying the gastric surface epithelium that in most cases does not show obvious light chain restriction, although this does not exclude the possibility that some of the plasma cells are tumour-derived. As the tumour progresses the neoplastic infiltrate extends into the submucosa and muscularis mucosae, and may take the form of scattered nodules rather than continuous tumour.

Clonal immunoglobulin heavy-chain rearrangements have been demonstrated in gastric lymphomas using IgH PCR. However, similar rearrangements can also be demonstrated in a small proportion of *Helicobacter*-associated gastritis in which there is no suspicion of lymphoma. This means that the presence of monoclonality should be used to support a diagnosis of malignancy only if strong morphological evidence is present.

The cells in a gastric marginal zone lymphoma may express *bcl-2* protein but do not appear to show a t(14;18). Using sensitive techniques this translocation may be detected in reactive lymphoid tissue and it is possible that this may account for the small number of cases in which a t(14;18) has been reported in gastric lymphoma. Trisomy 3 is suggested

Figure 10.13 Gastric B-cell lymphoma. Most gastric lymphomas are marginal zone lymphomas or diffuse large B-cell lymphomas, some of which arise by transformation. One of the key features of gastric marginal zone lymphomas is the presence of lymphoepithelial lesions **(a)**, in which neoplastic B-cells infiltrate and destroy gastric glandular epithelium, in this case shown using an anticytokeratin antibody. The majority of symptomatic gastric lymphomas have a large cell component **(b)** in which the wall of the stomach is infiltrated by large lymphoid cells, which may have centroblastic or immunoblastic features. There is strong surface CD20 expression **(c)**.

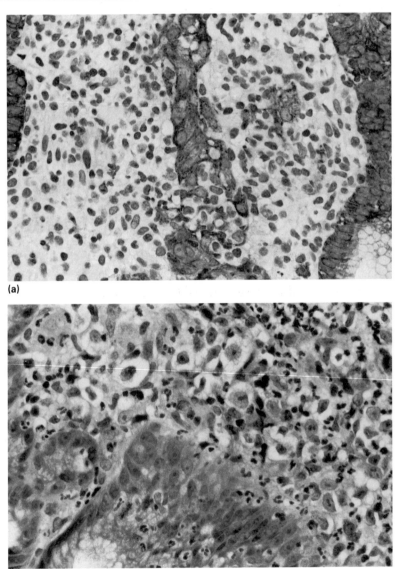

(a)

(b)

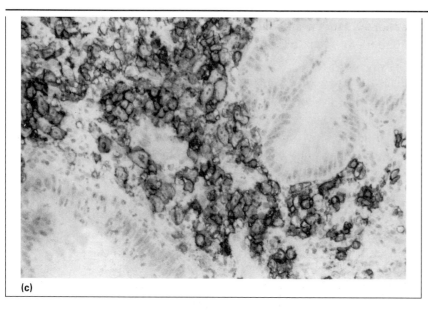

(c)

to be present in about one-third of gastric lymphomas, although the pathogenic significance of this abnormality is not yet known.

Marginal zone tumours of this type account for the minority of symptomatic gastric B-cell lymphomas. In the majority of instances a diffuse large B-cell lymphoma is present. This type of tumour consists of a mixture of cells morphologically resembling centroblasts, immunoblasts or large centrocytes, which invade deeply into the gastric wall. Where adequate histological material is available some, but not all, diffuse large B-cell lymphomas of the stomach will be found to have lymphoepithelial lesions and other features of an underlying marginal zone lymphoma. Where these are not present it is difficult to be certain that the tumour has originated in the stomach and dose not represent secondary spread from an adjacent nodal tumour, although in practice this is relatively rare.

Patients diagnosed as having gastric lymphoma fall into two distinct clinical groups

Upper gastrointestinal endoscopy is now the standard investigation for dyspepsia. In a large centre many thousands of investigations will be carried out each year and around two-thirds will show evidence of *Helicobacter* colonization. In a very small number of patients who have no other specific symptoms a gastric lymphoma will be found. Most of these will be early lesions and will show the typical features of a marginal cell lymphoma. In some of these cases the first biopsy may be suspicious but does not show definitive evidence of lymphoma, and further biopsies may be required.

The second and largest group of patients are those presenting with bleeding, gastric ulceration or outflow obstruction, and tumour is found at endoscopy. In these patients it is very likely that the tumour will be a diffuse large B-cell lymphoma invading deeply into the gastric wall.

Gastric B-cell lymphoma has a typical pattern of spread, which has important implications for treatment

Gastric lymphoma typically spreads within the stomach, to local lymph nodes and sometimes to other mucosal sites (Figure 10.14).

Diffuse large cell lymphomas arising in the stomach may spread vertically through the gastric wall into the serosal tissues. Spread to extraintestinal sites, including the bone marrow, is rare. When gastrectomy specimens have been examined in great detail it has been shown that gastric marginal zone lymphoma is a multifocal disease with foci of tumour which are often not visible macroscopically. This has important implications for treatment by gastrectomy, as partial gastrectomy may fail to remove all of the tumour.

When a large number of nodes are examined from a resection specimen containing a large cell lymphoma it is usual to find one or more nodes involved (Figure 10.15).

The morphological identification of nodal infiltration by large cell lymphoma presents no specific problem. However, early nodal infiltration by marginal zone lymphoma may be more difficult to recognize. In its most characteristic form reactive follicles are surrounded by infiltrating neoplastic B-cells, which may have a monocytoid appearance. As invasion of the node progresses the follicles are replaced and eventually there is diffuse involvement. Gastric marginal zone lymphoma may sometimes spread to involve other mucosal sites, although at least at a clinical level this appears to be quite rare. The bronchus and colon are probably the most commonly involved. In a very few cases, where an anti-idiotype monoclonal antibody is available, it has been possible to show small numbers of gastric lymphoma cells in other organs such as the spleen where bulk tumour is not usually found. It is very rare to detect circulating cells in the blood or marrow.

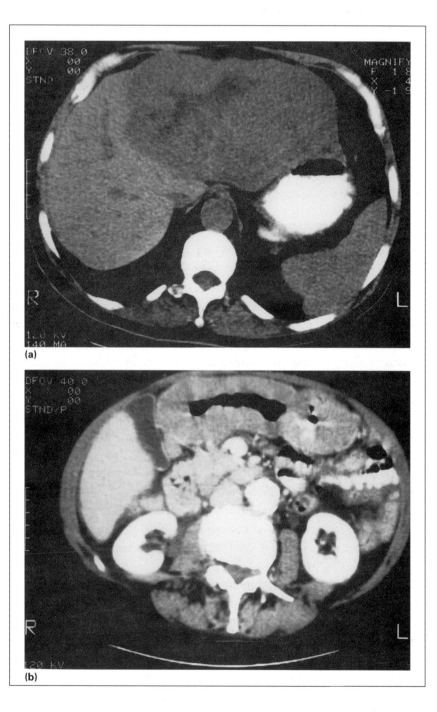

Figure 10.14 Gastric lymphoma – pattern of infiltration. **(a)** Diffuse large B-cell lymphomas of the stomach may cause gastric ulceration, shown in this contrast-enhanced CT scan. **(b)** In other cases there is diffuse infiltration and thickening of the gastric wall.

Figure 10.15 Gastric lymphoma – nodal disease. In this node taken from a gastric resection specimen there is infiltration of a reactive germinal centre by marginal zone lymphoma.

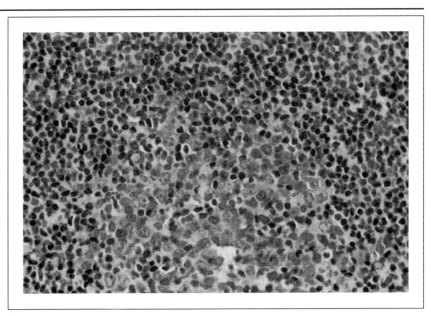

The limitations of the Ann Arbor staging system in non-Hodgkin's lymphoma have been particularly obvious in relation to the assessment of disease of the gastrointestinal tract.

There have been a number of proposed systems that attempt to take due account of the probable prognostic significance of tumour size, depth of invasion and nodal involvement (distinguishing local from more distant 'spread'). One 'consensus approach' takes the Ann Arbor classification as a basic framework but redefines each stage. The subscript 'E' is strictly applied only to indicate extension of gastrointestinal lymphoma with involvement of adjacent organs. Where there is supradiaphragmatic disease, this is considered to represent extensive disease appropriately assigned to stage IV. Hence there is no stage III in this system (Table 10.2).

The optimum treatment of gastric lymphoma is not known

When gastric lymphoma is confined to the stomach the prognosis appears to be relatively good. However, there is no firm consensus as to what constitutes adequate treatment. It has now been clearly shown that some cases of marginal zone lymphoma will respond to anti-*Helicobacter* therapy alone. Where a small lesion is found at endoscopy in a patient being investigated for dyspepsia, it would seem rational to eradicate *Helicobacter* infection and then observe changes in the lesion by

Table 10.2 Staging of gastrointestinal lymphoma

Stage I	Tumour confined to GI tract
	Single 'primary' site or multiple non-contiguous lesions
Stage II	Tumour extending into abdomen from 'primary' site
	Nodal involvement
	II$_1$ local
	e.g. paragastric in gastric lymphoma; paraintestinal in intestinal lymphoma
	II$_2$ distant
	e.g. mesenteric in intestinal lymphoma; para-aortic, paracaval, pelvic, inguinal
Stage IIE	Penetration of serosa to involve adjacent tissues or organs
	e.g. IIE [pancreas]; II$_2$E [posterior abdominal wall]
	(para-aortic and paracaval nodes also involved)
Stage IV	Disseminated extranodal involvement or where there is supradiaphragmatic nodal involvement

endoscopy. Although there is no definitive test which can predict whether a tumour will regress with anti-*Helicobacter* therapy it would not be prudent to rely solely on *Helicobacter* eradication where there is evidence of deep invasion or a large-cell component is present in the tumour.

In tumours that do not respond or are not suitable for treatment by anti-*Helicobacter* therapy the options include surgery, chemotherapy or radiotherapy. There is little doubt that some patients are cured by surgical excision but in comparing the results of studies it is very important to consider the nature of the procedure being used. As described above, marginal cell lymphoma in the stomach is often a multifocal disease and the logical procedure is a total gastrectomy with clearance of gastric lymph nodes. Unlike the more routinely performed partial gastrectomy, this is a major surgical procedure, which carries significant postoperative morbidity and mortality and may represent overtreatment, especially of an indolent localized lesion. The alternative approach is to treat indolent lesions without a large cell component with an alkylating agent and use combination chemotherapy (e.g. CHOP) for those with more aggressive disease. Combination chemotherapy alone or with surgery can produce cures but there is a danger of producing perforation in large lesions, although in practice this appears to be rare. Radiotherapy to the stomach is complicated by the choice and consistency of the field applied and the side effects of irradiating the bowel, and is not generally adopted.

10.3 Lymphoproliferative disorders of the small intestine and colon

Lymphomas that occur in the small intestine are more diverse than those found in stomach and include both T- and B-cell lymphomas. Tumours of all types can present as an abdominal mass or with bleeding, perforation or obstruction.

10.3.1 B-cell lymphomas of the small intestine and colon

Marginal zone lymphomas of the intestine are similar in structure to those in the stomach

Marginal zone lymphomas occur at any site in the small intestine, colon or rectum but are relatively rare. Small localized lesions are much less likely to be symptomatic than in the stomach, although in the distal bowel they may rarely be a cause of rectal bleeding (Figure 10.16). Tumours may be single or multiple and, as in the stomach, larger symptomatic lesions are likely to be associated with a more aggressive large cell lymphoma.

A problem in differential diagnosis of intestinal marginal zone lymphoma is the distinction from reactive lymphoid hyperplasia.

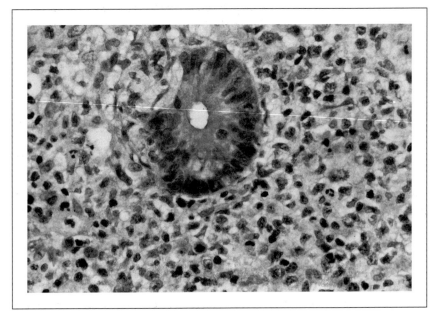

Figure 10.16 Marginal cell lymphoma – rectum. This case presented as rectal bleeding with a nodular lesion found on sigmoidoscopy. The rectum was infiltrated by neoplastic B-cells with marginal zone morphology with lymphoepithelial lesions as a prominent feature.

Hyperplastic lymphoid tissue in the rectum and the terminal ileum may be sufficiently large to cause symptoms. The distinction is made by demonstrating the presence of destructive lymphoepithelial lesions and monoclonality by light-chain restriction, and identifying the range of cells typical of marginal zone lymphoma.

Immunoproliferative disorder of the small intestine (IPSID) is almost certainly a special form of marginal zone lymphoma. It is characterized by infiltration and replacement of the lamina propria by lymphoma in which the majority of cells are clonal IgA-secreting plasma cells. In some cases regression occurs after antibiotic treatment, although the bacterial infection underlying the tumour is not known. IPSID is a disease of the Mediterranean lands and is very rare in north-west Europe.

Mantle cell lymphoma may present with multiple polypoid lesions in intestine

Mantle cell lymphoma in lymph nodes has been extensively characterized. It is a tumour of B-cells with centrocyte-like morphology that express moderate levels of sIg and CD5 and lack CD23. CD43 and IgD are also useful additional markers in fixed tissue. Mantle cell lymphoma is associated with the overexpression of cyclin D1 and t(11;14) and this may soon become a defining feature of the disease. Some patients present with a pattern of disease that is predominately localized to the small intestine. The main manifestation of the tumour is the presence of multiple polypoid lesions usually more frequent in the small intestine (multiple lymphomatous polyposis). These polyps consist of lymphoid tissue that is heavily infiltrated by mantle cell lymphoma. In the early stages of infiltration reactive germinal centres may be spared. Larger lesions involve the full thickness of the wall of the intestine and in a few cases there is apparent large cell transformation.

The distinction between marginal zone lymphoma and mantle cell lymphoma can be difficult in an intestinal biopsy. Both tumours may appear nodular as a result of infiltration and replacement of germinal centres and both may consist predominantly of cells with centrocytic-like features. Lymphoepithelial lesions are specific for marginal zone lymphoma but may not be apparent in a small biopsy. In most cases the immunophenotype will allow accurate diagnosis to be made.

Unlike marginal zone lymphoma, mantle cell lymphoma presenting in the intestine is often disseminated and blood and marrow involvement may be present at presentation or develop later. As with other forms of mantle cell lymphoma the optimum treatment remains unclear for the reasons discussed in Chapter 8 and the prognosis is poor. It has been claimed that in the intestinal variant there is a significant risk of perforation when chemotherapy is given.

The terminal ileum is a common site of diffuse large B-cell lymphoma

A distinctive syndrome seen in elderly patients is infiltration of the caecum and ileum by a diffuse large B-cell lymphoma consisting of cells with mainly centroblastic morphology. This usually presents as obstruction or perforation and at operation a large mass involving bowel, mesentery and nodes is found. It is unclear whether this is a nodal lymphoma arising in a mesenteric node or a primary extranodal lymphoma, as it is very rare to find evidence of associated marginal zone lymphoma. In a few cases an underlying follicle centre cell lymphoma may be present, suggesting a nodal origin.

Burkitt's lymphoma often involves the intestine

The diagnostic features of Burkitt's and Burkitt-like lymphomas have been described in detail in Chapter 8. One of the distinguishing features of this group of tumours is their high propensity to infiltrate the intestine, usually the distal small bowel. These are highly aggressive tumours with a very poor prognosis. Obstruction and treatment-related perforation are major gastrointestinal complications.

10.3.2 T-cell lymphoma of the intestine

Many intestinal T-cell lymphomas are enteropathy-associated

The association of lymphomas with villous atrophy and coeliac disease has been recognized for over 20 years. However, at various times the tumour has been considered to be of histiocytic, B-cell and T-cell lineage. Enteropathy-associated lymphomas of the intestine are now regarded as T-cell lymphomas.

Patients with the typical form of intestinal T-cell lymphoma present with perforation or obstruction

The typical patient with intestinal T-cell lymphoma (ITCL) presents with perforation or obstruction and is found at operation to have an intestinal and mesenteric mass. It should be noted that only a relatively small proportion of patients are diagnosed as having coeliac disease before they present with lymphoma and it is uncertain whether adequate treatment of coeliac disease reduces the risk of subsequent lymphoma.

ITCLs consist of large T-cells with oval or convoluted nuclei and one or more nucleoli. A proportion of the cells may have abundant clear cytoplasm. These cells have a peripheral T-cell phenotype, which is often abnormal, with loss of one or more lineage markers. It is usually possible to demonstrate a clonal T-cell-receptor gene rearrangement. ITCLs often have a large population of reactive cells present including histiocytes, plasma cells and eosinophils. When a perforation or ulcer is present an intense inflammatory infiltrate may confuse the histological features. In some patients enteropathy may be present in the intestine distant from the tumour but in other cases the mucosal changes may be more localized, making the association with coeliac disease less certain.

ITCL spreads by direct invasion of the serosa, mesenteric tissues and local lymph nodes. Systemic spread occurs and involvement of the liver is a typical feature. Patients with ITCL are usually treated with combination chemotherapy such as CHOP. However, there is high early mortality and the prognosis is very poor.

Early lesions of enteropathy-associated T-cell lymphoma are increasingly recognized and may cause diagnostic problems

Small intestinal ulceration may develop in patients with coeliac disease and in some cases may be the presenting problem. In many cases the ulceration is due to ITCL but there is a group of patients with small intestinal ulceration in which detailed examination of a resection specimen shows no convincing evidence of lymphoma. The distinction between lymphoma and benign ulceration may be difficult because of the presence of an intense reactive inflammatory infiltrate that is a feature of both conditions. In some of these cases the use of non-steroidal anti-inflammatory drugs may be a factor in the pathogenesis of ulceration. Even in patients in whom no lymphoma is demonstrated it appears that coeliac-related ulceration is associated with significant mortality.

Examination of resection specimens from patients with ITCL often shows that the intraepithelial lymphocytes in the adjacent intact mucosa are morphologically atypical (Figure 10.17).

An increased number of intraepithelial lymphocytes is one of the key diagnostic features of coeliac disease but in patients with ITCL the lymphocytes may be larger and have more irregular nuclei than normal. In most cases these cells express CD2, CD3, CD5 and CD7 but may lack

CD4 or CD8. Lack of CD4 or CD8 is a feature of TCR-gamma/delta cells which are a normal component of the intramucosal T-cell population. Cases are now being recognized of intramucosal T-cell lymphoma which have extensive involvement of the intestinal mucosa but without a mass lesion. In many cases T-cell monoclonality can be shown but the incidence of monoclonality in isolated coeliac disease is not sufficiently well documented to rely on this feature alone Patients

Figure 10.17 Enteropathy-associated T-cell lymphoma. This patient presented with jejunal ulceration and perforation without a preceding history of coeliac disease. The mucosa adjacent and distant to the lesion showed hyperplastic villous atrophy (a). There was diffuse infiltration of the full thickness of the bowel wall by intermediate to large T-cells (b). Adjacent to the tumour there are large numbers of intraepithelial T-cells, which show a degree of cytological atypia (c).

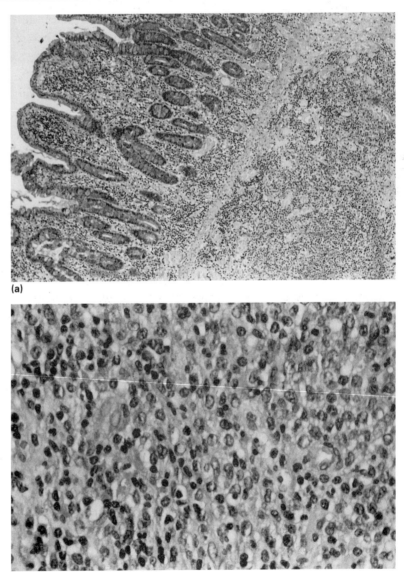

(a)

(b)

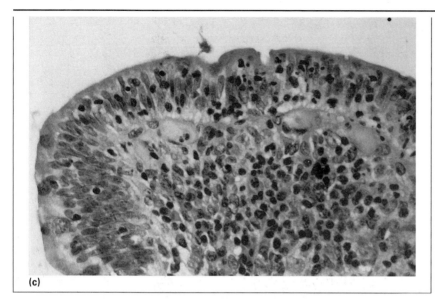

(c)

may be symptomatic with bleeding and erosions. Progression to typical ICTL has been described but there is as yet no consensus as to how these early lesions should be treated.

10.4 Lymphomas of the salivary glands

Primary lymphomas are a rare cause of salivary gland enlargement. Almost all are marginal zone B-cell lymphomas (MALToma). Swelling of major salivary glands may also occur as a consequence of enlargement of intrasalivary lymph nodes due either to reactive hyperplasia or to involvement by lymphoma. Hodgkin's disease, follicle centre or mantle cell lymphoma may all present in this way. The distinction of these systemic lymphomas from primary lymphoma of the salivary gland is of great importance from the point of view of therapy and progress.

Primary lymphomas of the salivary gland are associated with chronic sialadenitis

The normal salivary gland is almost devoid of lymphoid tissue. Chronic inflammation may develop as a consequence of duct obstruction or in so-called autoimmune-type sialadenitis. It is the latter that is associated with the development of lymphoma. Autoimmune-type sialadenitis is characterized by the development of organized lymphoid tissue around ducts and later by extensive infiltration of the lobules by T-cells, which result in the destruction of the specialized secretory cells. In some cases lymphoepithelial lesions develop, which are an admixture of proliferating ductal epithelium, myoepithelium and B-cells with centrocyte-like features. The term myoepithelial sialadenitis (MESA) has been used to describe this lesion. Patients with this type of lesion can have a variety of clinical features ranging from swelling of a single gland to Sjögren's syndrome. Related conditions such as SLE or rheumatoid disease may be present.

The distinction between MESA and marginal zone lymphoma of the salivary gland is very difficult and the precise criteria are not well defined. An important histological feature that is regarded as evidence for the development of lymphoma is a presence of a band of marginal-zone-type cells surrounding the lymphoepithelial lesions. As at other sites, this population may include cells with centrocyte- or monocytoid-like morphology (Figure 10.18).

As the disease progresses this population expands to form more confluent sheets of cells and colonization and replacement of reactive germinal centres may occur. If cryostat sections are available it may be possible to demonstrate light-chain restriction in the B-cell population; however this may be complicated by the presence of reactive germinal centres and plasma cells. Clonality studies based on IgH rearrangement can be performed but there is not yet sufficient data to be able to interpret them as unequivocal evidence of malignancy.

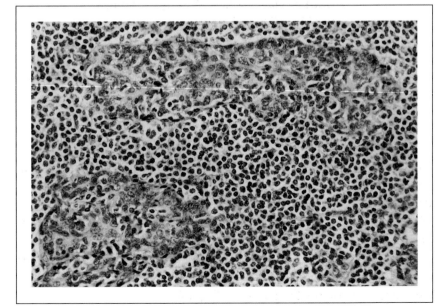

Figure 10.18 Marginal zone lymphoma – salivary gland. This patient presented with a parotid swelling. Large lymphoepithelial lesions were present, surrounded by a diffuse infiltrate of B-cells, many of which had monocytoid features with reactively abundant clear cytoplasm. Monoclonality was demonstrated by PCR.

Lymphomas of the salivary gland present at an early stage because of their anatomical location

Salivary gland lymphomas have a good prognosis and it is less common than at other sites to find evidence of transformation to diffuse large cell lymphoma or nodal involvement. This may be because of early presentation at a stage of low tumour bulk. It is usual to treat primary salivary gland lymphoma with a combination of surgical excision and local radiotherapy and from the relatively small number of series reported this appears to result in a good outcome, though local recurrence can occur and other glands may rarely show involvement.

A small number of patients with salivary gland lymphoma may present with local lymphadenopathy rather than enlargement of the gland. In these cases the lymph nodes show the features seen in nodal infiltration by marginal zone lymphoma. This appears to apply to a high proportion of cases diagnosed as marginal zone lymphoma (monocytoid B-cell lymphoma) in neck lymph nodes.

10.5 Lymphoproliferative disorders of the mediastinum and respiratory tract

10.5.1 Tumours of the mediastinum

Mediastinal involvement is a feature of Hodgkin's disease, T-ALL and primary mediastinal B-cell lymphoma

Many types of lymphoma may involve the mediastinal nodes but there are three types that are likely to give rise to a clinically significant mediastinal mass. By far the commonest is Hodgkin's disease of nodular sclerosing type. The problems associated with the diagnosis and management of mediastinal masses in Hodgkin's disease are discussed in Chapter 7. A thymic and nodal mass is a common feature of T-ALL, but this will almost always be accompanied by some degree of marrow and blood infiltration. Some cases may present as massive mediastinal masses and pleural infiltration and may be diagnosed by mediastinal biopsy or pleural aspirate. Mediastinal B-cell lymphoma may be restricted to the mediastinum at presentation and can be a more difficult diagnostic problem, with a differential diagnosis that includes non-lymphoid tumours such as metastatic carcinoma or thymoma. In most cases mediastinal B-cell lymphoma will require an open biopsy for definitive diagnosis.

Mediastinal B-cell lymphoma is a rapidly growing aggressive tumour that may cause vena caval obstruction or directly invade the chest wall

This tumour occurs more frequently in younger women and early reports suggested that it was more common in Mediterranean countries. This is probably not the case and this tumour is found in all ethnic groups. If an adequate biopsy is obtained the diagnosis of mediastinal B-cell lymphoma should not prove to be difficult. Most diagnostic problems are due to inadequate or crushed needle or mediastinoscopy biopsies.

It is a diffuse large cell lymphoma consisting of cells with centroblastic or immunoblastic features but with many of the cells having a conspicuous amount of clear cytoplasm (Figure 10.19). A highly distinctive feature is the presence of fine collagen bands dividing the cells into small clusters which can be clearly seen in a reticulin preparation, and more extensive fibrosis may be present. However, the cellular morphology should not lead to confusion with Hodgkin's disease.

Mediastinal B-cell lymphomas express pan-B-cell markers CD19 and CD22 but lack CD21. A particular feature of these tumours is lack of sIg expression, although cytoplasmic μ heavy chain may be seen. On the basis of this rather unusual phenotype it has been suggested that this is the malignant counterpart of a normal population of B-cells found in the thymus. In a very few cases thymic tissue may be found in the biopsy specimen.

Figure 10.19 Mediastinal B-cell lymphoma. This patient presented with a rapidly growing anterior mediastinal mass. On biopsy this was shown to be mediastinal B-cell lymphoma consisting of large cells with abundant clear cytoplasm (a). These cells had a B-cell phenotype but lacked surface immunoglobulin expression. A common feature in this type of tumour is extensive pericellular sclerosis (b). Shortly after commencing therapy small intestinal perforation occurred. In this section of jejunum (c) the bowel wall is infiltrated by CD20+ tumour cells.

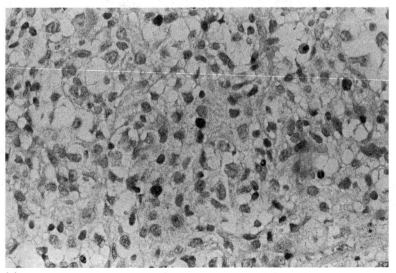

(a)

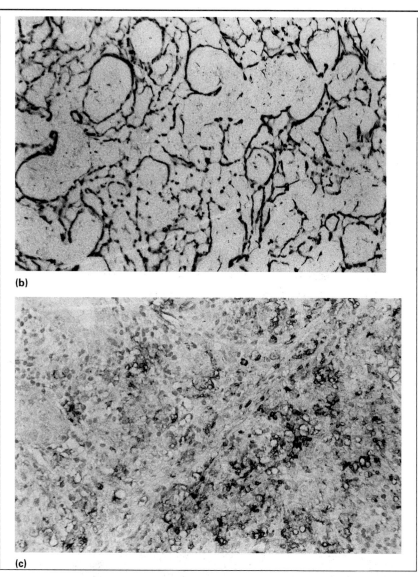

(b)

(c)

Mediastinal B-cell lymphomas are highly aggressive tumours and the prognosis is less favourable than with other diffuse large cell lymphomas. This may in part be due to the poor clinical condition of many patients at diagnosis. Early tumour spread may be to cervical nodes but in some patients lymphoma may occur at unusual sites such as the kidney or small intestine. Initial management is aimed at gaining local control of the mediastinal mass and relieving or preventing the features of superior vena caval obstruction. Combination chemotherapy which may be preceded or followed by radiotherapy is indicated.

10.5.2 Tumours of Waldeyer's ring and the upper respiratory tract

Most lymphomas of Waldeyer's ring are localized diffuse large B-cell lymphomas

The majority of cases of lymphoma of Waldeyer's ring present as a localized rapidly enlarging mass within one tonsil. A smaller group of patients have involvement of lymphoid tissue in the posterior tongue or nasopharynx. The main differential diagnosis is squamous cell carcinoma. Almost all the lymphomas presenting in this way will be diffuse large B-cell lymphomas that infiltrate and replace the normal lymphoid tissue. These tumours consist of a relatively monomorphic population of large lymphoid cells with the morphology of centroblasts or immunoblasts. The tumour cell may be highly cohesive and the distinction from carcinoma can only be made confidently by immunophenotypical marker studies.

In most cases of large B-cell lymphoma of Waldeyer's ring the surrounding lymphoid tissue is normal with no evidence of an underlying indolent lymphoma. However, a small number of well documented cases of marginal zone lymphoma occurring at this site have been reported.

Almost all large B-cell lymphomas of Waldeyer's ring are localized to the site of origin or adjacent lymph nodes and very few have greater than stage II disease at presentation. Radiotherapy will cause rapid tumour regression but, although definitive studies are sparse, combination chemotherapy appears to result in a more durable remission. There is no place for radical surgery in the treatment of these tumours.

Systemic lymphomas may involve Waldeyer's ring

It is rare for tonsillar enlargement to be a presenting feature of systemic lymphoma or to pose a significant clinical problem in its management. The most common tumour found in lesions that are biopsied appears to be mantle cell lymphoma, followed by follicle centre lymphoma. In the case of systemic disease the patient is likely to have more generalized enlargement of nasopharyngeal lymphoid tissue but involvement of this site does not appear to have special prognostic significance.

The nose and nasal sinuses are typical sites of angiocentric necrotizing lymphomas

The term 'lethal midline granuloma' was used in the past to describe a destructive lesion, beginning in the nose or sinuses and involving the face and orbits, which led to extensive necrosis. Vascular destruction was only a feature of these lesions. The pathogenesis of this disorder appears to be ischaemic necrosis due to vascular destruction. It is likely that this clinical syndrome includes several distinct pathological entities, including some cases of inflammatory vasculitic disorders such as Wegener's granulomatosis.

Among the remaining cases is one of the few examples of true NK-cell solid tumours. The incidence of these lesions appears to be higher in the Far East and there is an association with Epstein–Barr virus. The diagnosis of NK-cell tumours depends on the demonstration of NK-associated markers such as CD56 or CD57, together with cytotoxic granules, proteins such as perforin, in the absence of CD3/TCR expression and a germline configuration of the TCR genes. In contrast to most peripheral T-cell lymphomas, CD4 and CD45RO are not expressed by NK cells. Vascular invasion and extensive tissue destruction in the nose and pharynx is not unique to this type of tumour and may be seen in peripheral T-cell and B-cell lymphomas. A small number of cases of lymphomatoid granulomatosis, in which a population of EBV-transformed atypical B-cells is associated with a destructive T-cell infiltrate, may also present at this site. These tumours are considered in more detail below.

10.5.3 Other lymphoid tumours of the upper respiratory tract

Diffuse large B-cell lymphomas occur within the nasal cavity and those arising in the pharyngeal lymphoid tissue may invade the nose and sinuses. Like the tumours of Waldeyer's ring these tend to be localized tumours. It is likely that they are more common than the more extensively studied T-cell and NK-cell lymphomas.

The other tumour typical of the upper respiratory tract is a solitary plasmacytoma. These are rare and consist mainly of mature clonal plasma cells sometimes with small numbers of proliferating blast cells. These tumours are effectively managed by local surgery and radiotherapy and there appears to be no risk of developing myeloma, although a few cases of tumour dissemination have been reported. The nature and origin of these tumours is uncertain; one possibility is that they are a manifestation of marginal zone lymphoma.

10.5.4 Lymphoproliferative disorders of the lungs

Almost all lymphomas arising in the lungs are marginal zone lymphomas

In the past there has been debate about the distinction between pulmonary pseudolymphoma and true lymphoma. The concept of pseudolymphoma is untenable and recent studies indicate that most lesions which were classified as such are marginal zone lymphomas. These are very rare indolent tumours and it is not unusual for tumours to be discovered at the time of routine chest X-ray or after presenting with non-specific minor symptoms such as persistent cough. Most cases show a solitary nodule confined to one lobe although cases with multifocal disease are described. The diagnosis may be suggested on transbronchial biopsy but in the majority of cases an open lung biopsy is performed and if a clearly localized lesion is present the surgeon may opt to perform a lobectomy.

Figure 10.20 Marginal zone lymphoma – lung. This is a resection specimen of an asymptomatic pulmonary mass. There was an extensive interstitial and nodular lymphoid infiltrate **(a)**, which included reactive germinal centres and plasmacytosis. Lymphoepithelial lesions involving bronchial epithelium were present **(b)** and B-cell monoclonality was demonstrated by PCR.

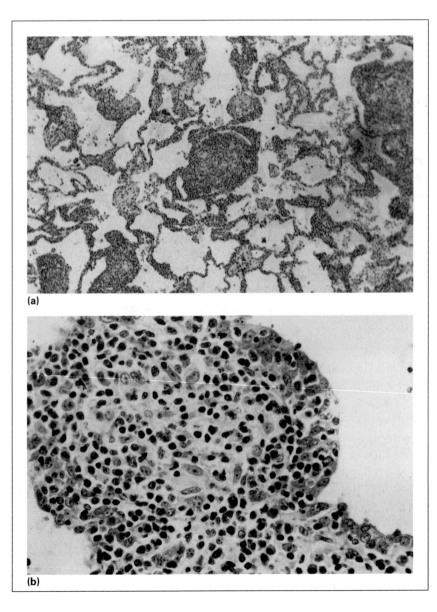

(a)

(b)

The features of pulmonary lymphoma are similar to marginal zone lymphomas at other sites. There is a diffuse infiltrate of centrocyte-like cells, monocytoid B-cells and plasma cells. Plasma cells are often a prominent feature and may appear to be polyclonal by light-chain restriction. In a lobectomy specimen it is usually possible to show lymphoepithelial lesions involving bronchial mucosa (Figure 10.20). There is often a large reactive component with numerous T-cells and hyperplastic germinal centres, suggesting that an inflammatory process may underlie the tumour, although no causative agent has been suggested. Large cell transformation appears to be uncommon in these tumours, although when it occurs invasion of the pleura and chest wall may follow.

There is little reliable data on the management of pulmonary marginal zone lymphoma. In a localized indolent lesion treated by lobectomy it is doubtful whether further treatment is required. Radiotherapy or chemotherapy is indicated for more aggressive lesions.

An important differential diagnosis of pulmonary B-cell lymphoma is lymphocytic interstitial pneumonitis. This condition is associated with systemic autoimmune disorders and is a cause of a restrictive defect in pulmonary function. In most cases multiple lobes are affected with diffuse lymphocytic infiltration of the alveolar septae and larger focal aggregates of lymphoid tissue which may contain organized B-cell follicles. The available evidence indicates that this is a reactive or inflammatory disorder, although some cases with clonal B-cells have been recorded. It has a poor prognosis, with many patients developing progressive respiratory failure and pulmonary fibrosis.

10.6 Other types of lymphoma involving the lungs and pleura

Pulmonary infiltration may occur as the presenting feature or develop in the course of a range of other types of lymphoma. The lung is a classical site of lymphomatoid granulomatosis, which typically also affects skin, brain and other extranodal sites. This is an aggressive disease characterized by necrotizing tumour masses. Until recently, lymphomatoid granulomatosis was regarded as a type of peripheral T-cell lymphoma. However, it is now recognized that in many cases with these clinical features there is a population of atypical Epstein–Barr-virus-infected large B-cells and in some cases a monoclonal immunoglobulin gene rearrangement is present. These cells are in a minority and the predominant population, including the angiodestructive component, consists of activated T-cells. One hypothesis is that these lesions represent a form of hypersensitivity reaction to an expanded population of EBV-infected B-cells.

The lungs and in particular the pleural surfaces may be involved in follicle centre and other disseminated lymphoma. This can be difficult to diagnose since the pleural fluid may contain only reactive T-cells even when the pleura is extensively infiltrated. A small number of HIV-positive patients develop a very aggressive large cell lymphoma associated with HHV8 infection, which primarily affects the pleura and other body cavities.

10.7 Lymphomas of the central nervous system

Lymphomas may arise within the central nervous system or cause neurological problems by infiltration from surrounding structures. This is an important distinction from the point of view of prognosis and treatment.

Primary cerebral lymphoma is an aggressive form of B-cell lymphoma with a poor prognosis

Primary lymphomas of the central nervous system are rare tumours. At least half the cases are associated with immunodeficiency, either post-transplant or HIV-related, but the remainder occur in patients with no history or features of immune dysfunction. Most lymphomas of the central nervous system present with seizures, focal neurological signs, dementia and raised intracranial pressure. In most cases initial investigation by MR or CT scan shows a lesion localized to the cerebral white matter or basal ganglia. This may be unilateral or bilateral. Although the imaging features are typical the diagnosis needs to be confirmed by open brain biopsy and histological examination of the tumour. It is very rarely possible to make the diagnosis on cytological examination of the cerebrospinal fluid.

The most typical feature is the accumulation of B-cells in the specialized connective tissue that surrounds blood vessels in the CNS

The cellular content of primary lymphoma of the CNS varies from small lymphocytes, centrocyte-like cells and plasma cells similar to those seen in other extranodal lymphomas to tumours that contain a more monomorphic population of large lymphoid cells with centroblastic or immunoblastic morphology. These cells express the usual pan-B-cell markers and surface immunoglobulin, which in most cases is IgM. A characteristic feature of cerebral lymphomas is the tendency of the tumour cell to accumulate in the loose connective tissue surrounding blood vessels (the Virchow–Robin space). As the disease progresses there is more diffuse infiltration of the brain, often associated with necrosis (Figure 10.21). In general there is little difficulty in distinguishing lymphomas from gliomas or metastatic carcinoma.

Based on the detection of Lmp-1 expression or by *in situ* hybridization, EBV is present within the tumour cells of about 20% of cerebral lymphoma. This is in contrast to other extranodal lymphomas where EBV is rarely detected. It is possible that this could reflect defects in the local immunity in the CNS, but as yet there is little known about this subject.

The majority of patients with primary cerebral lymphoma present with localized disease. Despite this, few patients survive 2 years and only 5–10% are alive at 5 years. Treatment has generally consisted of radiotherapy, usually to the whole brain with or without a boost to the site of the tumour. The majority of patients die with local recurrence rather than systemic disease. The role of chemotherapy continues to be explored although as yet there is little to suggest that combined modality treatment is any better than radiotherapy alone. One of the major problems has been to devise effective regimens consisting of drugs that cross the blood–brain barrier.

A wide range of lymphoproliferative disorders may invade the CNS from surrounding structures

Secondary infiltration of the CNS is many times more common than primary cerebral lymphoma. The spinal cord is most often affected and patients usually present with cord compression requiring urgent surgical decompression to prevent permanent neurological damage. This can occur by collapse of a vertebral body with extension of the tumour into the meninges and spinal cord, which, in the majority of cases, is due to myeloma or plasmacytoma. Alternatively, tumour within paraspinal nodes may infiltrate surrounding tissues, including the spinal canal. This most often occurs in diffuse large B-cell lymphomas, mantle cell lymphoma or follicle centre lymphomas and is only rarely seen with Hodgkin's disease.

Systemic lymphomas may invade the meninges without evidence of direct spread from bone. This may occur at the base of the brain and present with cranial nerve signs or raised intracranial pressure. In almost every case the patient is known to have lymphoma so the possibility will be considered and the correct diagnosis made. The meninges also are a sanctuary site for the cells of acute lymphoblastic leukaemia and in these cases routine CSF screening and prophylaxis should be undertaken.

Figure 10.21 Primary cerebral B-cell lymphoma. This patient presented with an intracerebral mass. At the edge of the lesion there was a perivascular infiltrate of large B-cells **(a)**. In the central area of the lesion there was a more diffuse infiltrate of larger cells associated with extensive necrosis **(b, c)**.

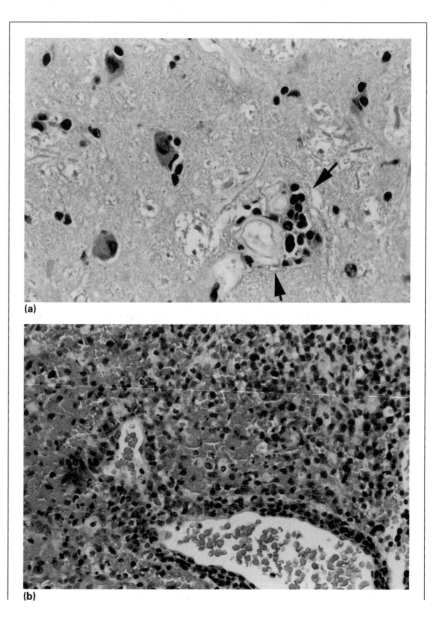

(a)

(b)

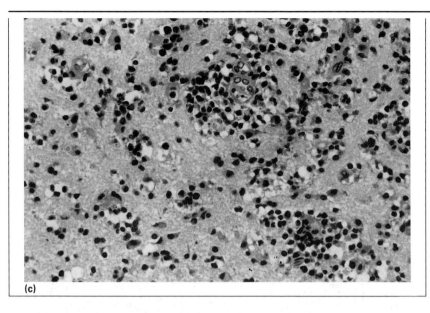

(c)

10.8 Lymphomas of the orbit and related structures

Lymphomas within the eye are very uncommon, although infiltration of the optic nerve and retina may be seen in patients with meningeal involvement by acute lymphoblastic leukaemia. Those occurring within the orbit, eyelids and conjunctiva are less rare and may give rise to considerable diagnostic difficulties. In part this is due to a complex terminology which in the past has led to a lack of discrimination between lymphomas and benign reactive disorders that share the same clinical features. Lymphomas occur mainly in elderly patients and present as a visible mass or with displacement of the eye or proptosis. Detailed imaging studies and clinical examination are needed to accurately document the extent of disease within the orbit (Figure 10.22).

As with other extranodal sites it is now recognized that many conjunctival lymphomas have the typical features of marginal zone lymphoma

These may arise in association with lacrimal glands or acquired conjunctiva-associated lymphoid tissue. The incidence of lacrimal gland lymphomas in relation to Sjögren's syndrome is not known. There is a high incidence of bilateral tumours occurring in patients with marginal zone lymphoma. Large cell transformation at this site is very rare.

Figure 10.22 Orbital lymphoma. This CT scan showed an extensive orbital lesion displacing the eye, which on biopsy was found to marginal zone B-cell lymphoma.

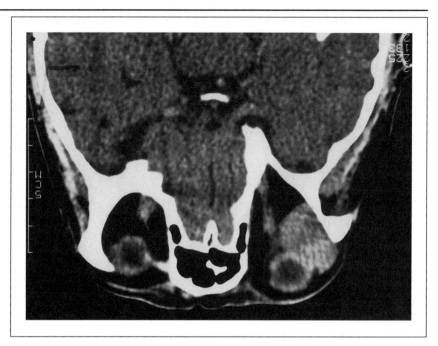

However, a number of studies suggest that a wider range of lymphomas occur in the orbit than is apparent at other extranodal sites. This may in part be a reflection of varying terminology but it appears that follicle centre and mantle cell lymphomas may be found in the orbit and not all are associated with systemic disease (Figure 10.23).

Figure 10.23 Marginal zone lymphoma of the conjunctiva. This patient had diffuse infiltration of the conjunctiva, which on biopsy was shown to a marginal zone type B-cell lymphoma consisting mainly of small cells with centrocyte-like morphology. There were lymphoepithelial lesions affecting glandular and surface epithelium.

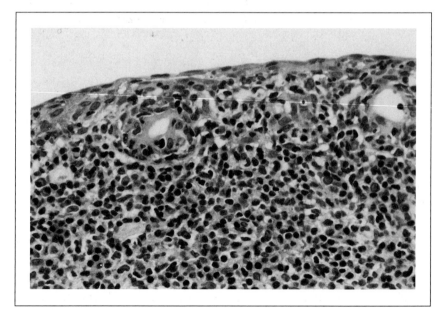

The differential diagnosis of lymphomas of the orbit includes lymphoid hyperplasia and orbital pseudotumour

An intraorbital mass may be due to lymphoid hyperplasia in which there are organized T- and B-cell areas with germinal centres and variable numbers of reactive macrophages and plasma cells, and is probably analogous to cutaneous lymphoid hyperplasia. After specific infections have been excluded most cases remain idiopathic. Marginal zone lymphomas are also found within the orbit and, as with tumours at other sites, they may have a prominent reactive lymphoid component suggesting an origin in lymphoid hyperplasia. The distinction between marginal zone lymphomas and hyperplasia is made using the same criteria as at other sites.

Orbital inflammatory pseudotumour differs from lymphoma and lymphoid hyperplasia in that it occurs in a much wider age distribution and is reported to be a more painful condition. The histological features usually allow this condition to be readily separated from lymphoma. There is a sparse perivascular infiltrate, which consists of lymphocytes, macrophages, plasma cells and granulocytes. As the lesion progresses B-cell follicles and germinal centres may be found. The key feature of this condition is dense fibrosis and in an established lesion the lymphoid component may be relatively slight. A further feature of this condition is that most cases respond rapidly to corticosteroid therapy.

The orbit may also be involved by invasion of lymphomas from the nose and sinuses or by extension of tumours in bone such as myeloma or Langerhans cell histiocytosis. If systemic disease has been excluded orbital lymphomas may be treated with local radiotherapy or by alkylating agents and corticosteroids, and prognosis is generally good.

10.9 Extranodal B-cell lymphomas of the thyroid, breast and testis

Thyroid lymphoma presents with enlarging tumours mainly in middle-aged and elderly women

Some patients presenting with thyroid lymphoma will have a history of hypothyroidism but most will be euthyroid. Before the widespread use of cell marker studies many cases of thyroid lymphoma were diagnosed as anaplastic carcinoma, a diagnosis that is now very rarely made. Thyroid lymphomas have typical marginal zone lymphoma features with lymphoepithelial lesions but most cases at presentation have evidence of large cell transformation. In almost every case there is evidence of underlying chronic thyroiditis, often in a discrete area at the edge of the tumour. Thyroiditis can be distinguished from the lymphoma by the

Figure 10.24 Marginal zone lymphoma of the thyroid. This patient presented with a large mass that was shown on CT scan to arise from the thyroid **(a)**. In the resection specimen the mass consisted mainly of large B-cells **(b)** but in some areas a more polymorphic B-cell infiltrate was present **(c)**, suggesting that the lesion had developed by transformation of an underlying marginal zone lymphoma. In some parts of this lesion there were large numbers of clonal plasma cells **(d)**.

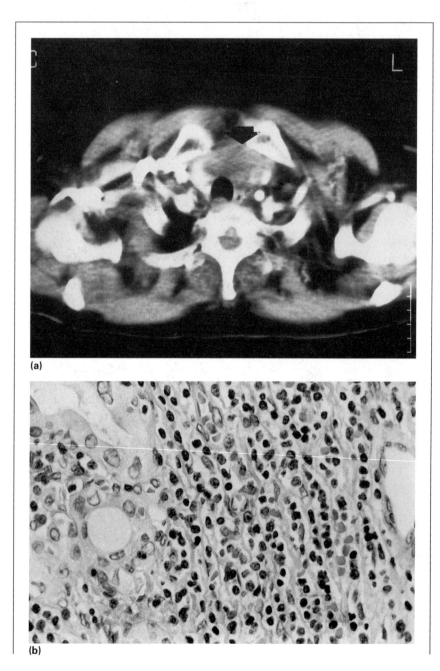

(a)

(b)

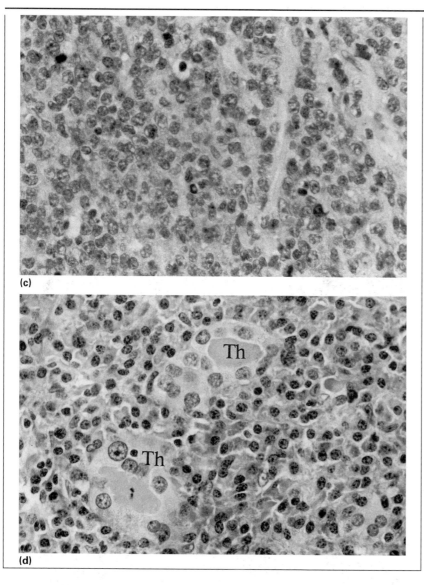

predominance of T-cells and the typical Hurtle cell change in residual thyroid acini (Figure 10.24).

In the majority of cases a partial thyroidectomy will have been performed at diagnosis and it is usual to give adjuvant radiotherapy to treat disease in the residual thyroid and local nodes. In patients with clinically more aggressive disease combination chemotherapy (e.g. CHOP) is also given. The prognosis appears favourable, with few deaths from disease. In a few cases the tumour may spread to other extranodal sites such as gastrointestinal tract.

Figure 10.25 Testicular B-cell lymphoma. This patient presented with a rapidly growing testicular mass. The orchidectomy specimen shows extensive infiltration by lymphoma which had a high component of large B-cells. The seminiferous tubules (ST) are atrophic and surrounded by concentric rings of tumour cells separated by reticulin fibres.

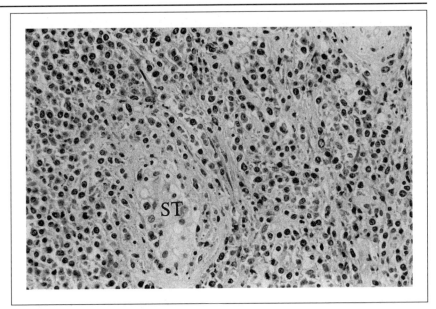

In elderly men lymphomas account for about half of testicular tumours although in absolute terms this is a very small number of cases

As with all testicular tumours lymphomas present with painless testicular swelling. In most cases an orchidectomy will be the diagnostic procedure. Testicular lymphomas show a distinctive pattern of lymphoepithelial

Figure 10.26 B-cell lymphoma of the breast. This patient presented with a mass that was thought likely to be a carcinoma. **(a, b)** On biopsy there was a multifocal lymphoid infiltrate surrounding breast ducts (arrow). This included reactive germinal centres and plasma cells together with a more diffuse of monoclonal B-cells, many of which had centrocyte like features. In some areas there was extensive infiltration of ductular epithelium by these cells **(c)**.

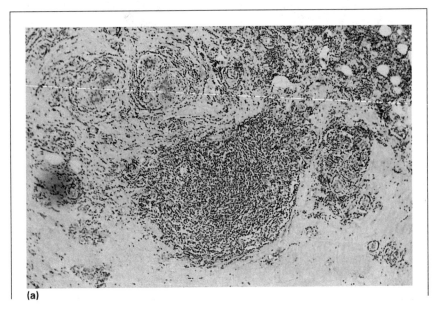

(a)

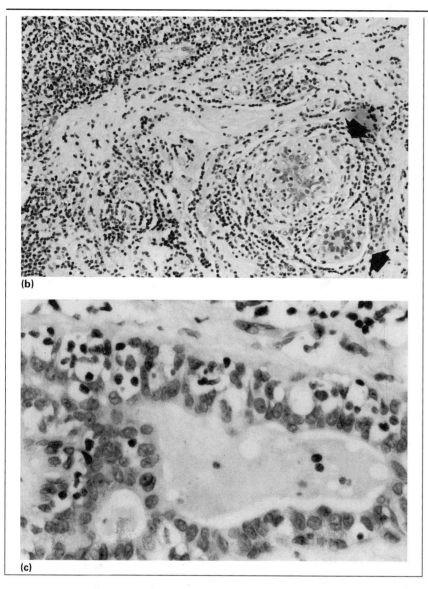

(b)

(c)

lesions. Neoplastic B-cells appear to infiltrate between the Sertoli cells of the seminiferous tubules and the tubular basement membrane. A new basement membrane forms and the process continues, leading to multiple layers of tumour cells admixed with basement membrane around tubules which become atrophic. At presentation almost all testicular B-cell lymphomas consist mainly of diffuse infiltrates of large lymphoid cells (Figure 10.25). The pattern of spread is similar to other testicular tumours, with involvement of retroperitoneal nodes. If the patient is fit enough, treatment is with combination chemotherapy and/ or radiotherapy.

The testis is a site of relapse in ALL but this should not give rise to confusion with primary testicular lymphoma.

Primary lymphoma of the breast is a very rare cause of a breast lump

Breast lymphomas should not be confused with cutaneous lymphomas, including B-cell lymphoma and cutaneous lymphoid hyperplasia, that may involve the skin of the breast. Equally, patients with very aggressive systemic lymphomas and leukaemias may have breast infiltration. Solitary plasmacytomas also occur rarely in the breast.

Primary lymphomas of the breast occur within breast lobules and typically have features of a low-grade marginal zone lymphoma with lymphoepithelial lesions in duct epithelium (Figure 10.26).

In the surrounding breast tissue there may be evidence of lymphocytic lobulitis. Although the exact relationship of lymphoma to this inflammatory condition remains unclear, by analogy with other sites it would not be surprising if breast lymphomas also developed in the context of chronic inflammation. The correct treatment of breast lymphoma is unknown but surgical excision and local radiotherapy appears to be adequate treatment in most cases.

10.10 Key references

10.10.1 Skin

Burns, M. K., Chan, L. S. and Cooper, K. D. (1995) Woringer–Kolopp disease (localized pagetoid reticulosis) or unilesional mycosis fungoides? An analysis of eight cases with benign disease. *Archives of Dermatology*, **131**, 325–329.

DeCoteau, J. F., Butmarc, J. R., Kinney, M. C. and Kadin, M. E. (1996) The t(2;5) chromosomal translocation is not a common feature of primary cutaneous CD30+ lymphoproliferative disorders: comparison with anaplastic large-cell lymphoma of nodal origin. *Blood*, **87**, 3437–3441.

El-Azhary, R. A., Gibson, L. E., Kurtin, P. J. *et al.* (1994) Lymphomatoid papulosis: a clinical and histopathologic review of 53 cases with leukocyte immunophenotyping, DNA flow cytometry, and T-cell receptor gene rearrangement studies. *Journal of the American Academy of Dermatology*, **30**, 210–218.

Herrmann, J. J., Roenigk, H. H. Jr, Hurria, A. *et al.* (1995) Treatment of mycosis fungoides with photochemotherapy (PUVA): long-term follow-up. *Journal of the American Academy of Dermatology*, **33**, 234–242.

Saed, G., Fivenson, D. P., Naidu, Y. and Nickoloff, B. J. (1994) Mycosis fungoides exhibits a Th1-type cell-mediated cytokine profile whereas Sézary syndrome expresses a Th2-type profile. *Journal of Investigative Dermatology*, **103**, 29–33.

Willemze, R., Beljaards, R. C. and Meijer, C. J. (1994) Classification of primary cutaneous T-cell lymphomas. *Histopathology*, **24**, 405–415.

10.10.2 Gastrointestinal tract

Bolin, T. D., Hunt, R. H., Korman, M. G. *et al.* (1995) *Helicobacter pylori* and gastric neoplasia: evolving concepts. *Medical Journal of Australia*, **163**, 253–255.

Domizio, P., Owen, R. A., Shepherd, N. A. *et al.* (1993) Primary lymphoma of the small intestine. A clinicopathological study of 119 cases. *American Journal of Surgical Pathology*, **17**, 429–442.

Durr, E. D., Bonner, J. A., Strickler, J. G. *et al.* (1995) Management of stage IE primary gastric lymphoma. *Acta Haematologica*, **94**, 59–68.

Hussell, T., Isaacson, P. G., Crabtree, J. E. and Spencer, J. (1993) The response of cells from low-grade B-cell gastric lymphomas of mucosa-associated lymphoid tissue to *Helicobacter pylori*. *Lancet*, **342**, 571–574.

Isaacson, P. G. (1994) Gastrointestinal lymphoma. *Human Pathology*, **25**, 1020–1029.

Kumar, S., Kremsac, L., Otsuki, T. *et al.* (1996) Bcl-1 rearrangement and cyclin D1 protein expression in multiple lymphomatous polyposis. *American Journal of Clinical Pathology*, **105**, 737–743.

Parsonnet, J., Hansen, S., Rodriguez, L. *et al.* (1994) *Helicobacter pylori* infection and gastric lymphoma. *New England Journal of Medicine*, **330**, 1267–1271.

Speranza, V., Lomanto, D., Meli, E. Z. *et al.* (1995) Primary gastric lymphoma: a 15-year review. *Hepato-Gastroenterology*, **42**, 371–376.

Wotherspoon, A. C., Doglioni, C., Diss, T. C. *et al.* (1993) Regression of primary low-grade B-cell gastric lymphoma of mucosa-associated lymphoid tissue type after eradication of *Helicobacter pylori*. *Lancet*, **342**, 575–577.

10.10.3 Respiratory tract

Guinee, D. Jr, Jaffe, E., Kingma, D. *et al.* (1994) Pulmonary lymphomatoid granulomatosis. Evidence for a proliferation of Epstein–Barr virus infected B-lymphocytes with a prominent T-cell component and vasculitis. *American Journal of Surgical Pathology*, **18**, 753–764.

Jaffe, E. S., Chan, J. K., Su, I. J. *et al.* (1996) Report of the Workshop on Nasal and Related Extranodal Angiocentric T/Natural Killer Cell Lymphomas.

Definitions, differential diagnosis, and epidemiology. *American Journal of Surgical Pathology,* **20**, 103–111.

Koss, M. N. (1995) Pulmonary lymphoid disorders. *Seminars in Diagnostic Pathology,* **12**, 158–171.

Tao, Q., Ho, F. C., Loke, S. L. and Srivastava, G. (1995) Epstein–Barr virus is localized in the tumour cells of nasal lymphomas of NK, T or B cell type. *International Journal of Cancer,* **60**, 315–320.

Wong, K. F., Chan, J. K. and Ng, C. S. (1994) CD56 (NCAM)-positive malignant lymphoma. *Leukemia and Lymphoma,* **14**, 29–36.

10.10.4 Other sites

Lee, A. H., Millis, R. R. and Bobrow, L. G. (1994) Primary lymphoma of the breast and lymphocytic lobulitis. *Histopathology,* **25**, 297–298.

Tomlinson, F. H., Kurtin, P. J., Suman, V. J. *et al.* (1995) Primary intracerebral malignant lymphoma: a clinicopathological study of 89 patients. *Journal of Neurosurgery,* **82**, 558–566.

Wotherspoon, A. C., Hardman-Lea, S. and Isaacson, P. G. (1994) Mucosa-associated lymphoid tissue (MALT) in the human conjunctiva. *Journal of Pathology,* **174**, 33–37.

Immunodeficiency and lymphoproliferative disorders

11

Immunodeficiency is well recognized as a major risk factor in the development of lymphoproliferative disorders, although there are differences in the magnitude of this risk and the types of tumour associated with different causes of immunodeficiency. Immunodeficiency is classified into primary disorders, where the cause is genetic or unknown, and secondary disorders, where an infective or other cause has been identified.

11.1 Primary immunodeficiency disorders

It is not the aim of this chapter to review the numerous types of primary immunodeficiency, most of which are very rare. Common variable immunodeficiency and ataxia telangiectasia are considered in detail because of their relative frequency and association with lymphoproliferative disorders.

11.1.1 Common variable immunodeficiency

Common variable immunodeficiency is an acquired disorder and is the commonest form of primary immunodeficiency

Common variable immunodeficiency (CVI) is the generic name for a group of acquired idiopathic disorders characterized by low serum immunoglobulin levels in the absence of an identifiable cause such as drugs or lymphoproliferative disorders. This may either be panhypogammaglobulinaemia or selectively affect IgG/IgA or IgG/IgM. The incidence of this disorder has been estimated at 20–40 cases/million, and there are currently around 1000 patients known in the UK, although there is almost certainly a population of asymptomatic undiagnosed individuals.

The clinical features of CVI are mainly related to chronic or persistent infection. Infections of the respiratory tract and nasal sinuses with *Streptococcus pneumoniae* or *Haemophilus influenzae* are the most common complications and in the untreated patient may progress to bronchiectasis. In the gastrointestinal tract infection with *Giardia lamblia*, *Campylobacter jejuni* or *Salmonella typhi* are associated with CVI and may be resistant to normal antibiotic therapy. There is also evidence for a high incidence of joint or urinary tract infections with *Mycoplasma* or *Ureaplasma* species and in the case of *Mycoplasma* this may lead to chronic arthropathy. In contrast to bacterial infection, viral infection other than iatrogenic hepatitis C is uncommon (Table 11.1).

There are two important clinical features of CVI. Firstly, about one in five patients have autoantibodies despite the presence of a defect in antibody production. This may be asymptomatic or associated with idiopathic thrombocytopenic purpura (ITP), haemolytic anaemia or other autoimmune disorders. Secondly, some patients present with recurrent lymphadenopathy and the possibility of CVI should be considered in patients presenting with lymphadenopathy, especially when granulomas are present in the node without an identifiable cause such as mycobacterial infection or toxoplasmosis.

The cause and pathogenesis of CVI is poorly understood but it is considered to be an acquired state, possibly as a sequel of common viral

Table 11.1 Common variable immunodeficiency

- Infection of the Respiratory Tract
  - Otitis media and sinusitis
  - Bronchitis and bronchiectasis
- Infection of the gastrointestinal tract
  - *Giardia lamblia*
  - *Cryptosporidium*
- Arthropathy
- Lymphadenopathy
  - Granulomas
  - Lymphoproliferative disorders
- Panhypogammaglobulinaemia or selective reduction in IgG, IgA or IgM

infections with onset in adulthood. There is a possibility that in some cases there may be a genetic component because an increased incidence in first-degree relatives has been noted. The interaction between genetic predisposition, possibly at the level of class II MHC genes affecting the response to viral infections such as EBV is an area of current interest. It is clear that the pathogenesis of this disorder is more complex than a simple failure of B-cells to secrete antibody and that different mechanisms may operate in different patients. In many patients there is an absolute lymphopenia, with low numbers of circulating T-cells, but an absence of B-cells is present in only a few patients. Experimental evidence suggests that in most cases B-cells are capable of secreting immunoglobulin, suggesting that the defect may lie at the level of T-cell/B-cell interaction and may be related to abnormal cytokine secretion. There is current interest in the therapeutic use of IL-2, with early results suggesting that this may restore immunoglobulin production.

There is a high relative risk of lymphoma in patients with CVI

The relative risk of lymphoma in patients with CVI is estimated to be around 30, although this must be qualified in view of the relatively small numbers of patients studied and the uncertainty about the incidence of subclinical disease in the population. A further problem is that after a diagnosis of lymphoma has been made and treatment commenced it is impossible to make a retrospective diagnosis of CVI although it may be suspected if there is a convincing clinical history of recurrent infection.

The lymphomas that develop in CVI are of B-cell lineage and it has been suggested that they include indolent extranodal tumours, some of which may be associated with EBV infection. However, the data at present are sparse, with most series reporting only a few cases. The definitive diagnosis of lymphoma in patients with CVI may be very difficult. The nodal architecture may be abnormal, with disorganization of normal B-cell follicles and possibly a clonal population detected by IgH PCR (Figure 11.1). A granulomatous element can also be present. These changes can persist as a relatively stable state without progression to overt malignancy and a failure to appreciate this may have led to an overestimation of the incidence of lymphoma associated with CVI in older studies.

CVI is treated by immunoglobulin replacement

Patients with CVI are treated by lifelong intravenous immunoglobulin replacement therapy and treatment of infections if they occur. The aim of

Figure 11.1
Lymphadenopathy associated with CVI. The patient had lymph-adenopathy and bronchi-ectasis. Investigation showed hypogammaglobulinaemia and failure of response to test vaccines. Repeated node biopsies showed disorganized architecture with abnormal follicles, lack of plasma cells and a granulomatous infiltrate. The same clonal IgH rearrangement was present. However, the patient remains well on immunoglobulin therapy and has no evidence of progressive lymphoma.

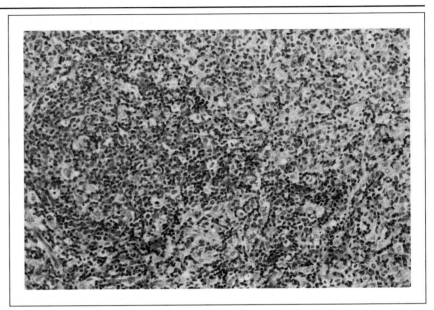

therapy is to achieve trough Ig levels in the normal range, which has been shown to prevent progression of lung disease and reduce infections. The main complication of this therapy is Hepatitis C infection and there remains uncertainty as to the criteria for the selection of donor plasma and its preparation in order to prevent this. Even if the immunoglobulin deficit is corrected in this fashion there is no evidence to suggest that it is beneficial in reducing the risk of developing lymphoma.

11.1.2 Ataxia telangiectasia

Ataxia telangiectasia is the commonest inherited form of primary immunodeficiency associated with lymphoma

Abnormal cell-mediated immunity and impaired antibody production are part of the ataxia telangiectasia (AT) syndrome, which also includes cerebellar ataxia, cutaneous telangiectasia and gonadal dysgenesis. It is an autosomal recessive condition with a relatively high incidence of heterozygotes estimated at around 1:100. AT is the most common condition reported to specialist registries of immunodeficiency-associated malignancy and it is estimated that by early adulthood around 5–10% of patients with AT will have developed a lymphoproliferative disorder with a median age of onset of 9 years. AT differs from other types of

Table 11.2 Clinical features of ataxia telangiectasia

- Cerebellar ataxia
- Telangiectasia of skin and eye
- Infertility
- Immunodeficiency
- Chromosomal breaks
- Risk of malignancy – mainly T-ALL

immunodeficiency in that there is a high preponderance of T-cell malignancy which includes both lymphoblastic leukaemia and peripheral T-cell lymphomas (Table 11.2).

Ataxia telangiectasia is characterized by genetic instability and it has been estimated that 10% of all T-cells in patients homozygous for AT show the presence of chromosomal abnormalities, the most common of which are breakpoints in chromosomes 7 and 14. These defects are also sometimes seen in the T-cells of normal individuals at a much lower frequency. In a few AT-affected individuals it has been possible to trace the evolution of the T-cell leukaemia through the progressive acquisition of chromosomal abnormalities. These abnormalities are similar to those seen in T-cell neoplasms in non-AT-affected patients and the study of AT patients may provide an important opportunity to understand the pathogenesis of these tumours.

Recently the *AT* gene on chromosome 11q22–23 has been cloned. The protein product of this gene appears to be similar to the family of phosphotidylinositol-3 kinases which are involved in signal transduction and cell cycle control. Although the detailed pathogenesis of AT is far from understood, one function of the *AT* gene product may be in the detection of DNA damage and, through p53 activation, induction of cell cycle arrest or cell death.

Given the incidence of AT heterozygotes an important question is whether the presence of a single mutated *AT* gene results in an increased incidence of malignant disease. Some studies indicate an increased risk of breast cancer in heterozygotes. These results await confirmation and at present it is not known whether heterozygotes are at increased risk of lymphoid malignancy.

11.1.3 The investigation of suspected primary immunodeficiency

Only a small number of patients with recurrent infection or persistent reactive lymphadenopathy will be found to have CVI or other forms of primary immunodeficiency. The complexity and expense of detailed immunological investigations means that selection according to clinical features and the use of staged protocol investigations beginning with screening tests is essential. The more suggestive clinical features include arthropathy, autoimmunity and autoantibodies, a family history and hepatosplenomegaly.

The total serum globulin concentration may be reduced only in patients with severe antibody deficiency and normal levels do not exclude a disorder of antibody production. IgG subclass deficiency may also occur in the presence of a normal or even elevated total immunoglobulin level. Patients who have low levels of an IgG subclass should have test immunizations and those who respond normally are unlikely to have a clinically significant defect.

The presence of an absolute lymphopenia without apparent cause is a good screening test for T-cell defects. However, transient changes in T-cell subset counts may occur in many circumstances and it should be stressed that absolute T-cell or CD4 counts should never be used as a definitive test of immunodeficiency or a surrogate for HIV/AIDS serology. In adults and older children a positive delayed-type hypersensitivity response to intradermal injection of *Candida albicans* almost excludes any T-cell defect and as such is a highly cost-effective and simple screening test. The clinical features of complement deficiency include recurrent meningococcal disease or primary disease with an unusual serotype and atypical SLE (antinuclear-antibody-negative, anti-Ro-positive and skin disease). Red cell lysis tests are used to screen for defects in the alternative or classical pathways. Recurrent staphylococcal, Gram-negative or fungal infections are the classical clinical features of phagocyte defect with chronic granulomatous disease being the commonest example. Defective oxygen-mediated cell killing, which is the basic defect in this condition, can be detected using the Nitroblue Tetrazolium test.

11.2 Secondary immunodeficiency disorders

The two most common and clinically important forms of secondary immunodeficiency are HIV infection and drug-induced immunosuppression in transplant patients. In both of these conditions there is a considerable increase in the risk of lymphoma. The clinical features of HIV are well known and the discussion of the extensive literature on the pathogenesis and treatment of HIV infection is beyond the scope of this chapter.

Latent Epstein–Barr virus infection is a central feature in the pathogenesis of many lymphoproliferative disorders associated with secondary immunodeficiency

Epstein–Barr virus is a Herpesvirus that is one of the most common human infections, a high proportion of the world's population showing evidence of past infection. The virus is acquired by droplet spread and enters the circulation, where it is highly trophic for B-cells. This specificity is partly mediated by CD21 but other factors may be involved. During the acute phase of the infection up to 10% of B-cells may be infected but this proportion is rapidly reduced by a cytotoxic T-cell response. In many individuals cells containing latent EBV persist for long periods of time and are controlled by an active T-cell response.

At least a proportion of B-cells containing latent EBV have the capacity for immortal growth in culture and may produce tumours when injected into immunocompromised animals. A number of viral genes have been found to be important in mediating immortalization. These include: genes that encode two nuclear proteins, EBNA1, which appears to be involved in viral DNA replication, and EBNA2, which is a transcription factor; BHRF1, which is an antiapoptotic protein of the Bcl-2 family, and a membrane protein, Lmp-1 (Figure 11.2). In cultured cells immortalization by EBV produces blast cells expressing the activation markers CD23 and CD30, which are protected against apoptosis by expression of Bcl-2 and its viral homologue. The specific

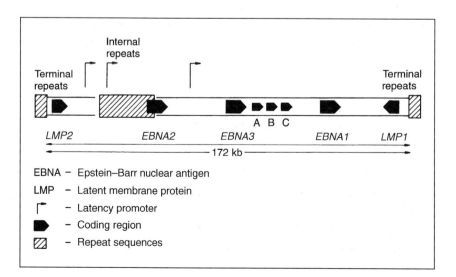

Figure 11.2 EBV genome. Schematic representation of the Epstein–Barr virus genome showing the major genes involved in pathogenesis of infection. The pattern of gene expression varies between tumour types.

role of Lmp-1 in upregulation of Bcl-2 remains unclear with apparent difference in cells *in vivo* and *in vitro*.

The presence of latent EBV within cells can be readily demonstrated in clinical specimens using *in situ* hybridization detection of *EBER1* and *EBER2*, which are very abundant species of viral RNA. Variation in the number of terminal repeats between viral particles can be used as a marker to show that infection preceded clonal expansion. When virus is demonstrated within tumours using these methods it is clear that there are tumour-type-specific differences in the expression of the viral proteins, which are thought to be important in inducing the immortal B-cell phenotype *in vitro*. The pattern seen in *in vitro* infected cells of EBNA1 and EBNA2 and Lmp-1 expression is commonly seen in post-transplant lymphoproliferative disorders. At the other end of the spectrum African Burkitt's lymphoma cells usually only express EBNA1. It is possible that EBNA1 may interact and potentiate the effects of c-*myc* deregulation, resulting in transformation without the requirement for the other EBV proteins to be expressed. Minimal expression of viral proteins, particularly those on the cell membrane, may make the cell less immunogenic and able to escape surveillance by cytotoxic T-cells. Most cases of Hodgkin's disease have an intermediate pattern with strong expression of EBNA1 and Lmp-1 but not EBNA2. Many questions remain to be answered about the interaction between latent EBV infection and other transforming genetic abnormalities in a number of types of lymphoma.

11.2.1 Lymphoproliferative disorders associated with therapeutic immunosuppression

Therapeutic immunosuppression results in a heterogeneous group of EB-driven lymphoproliferative disorders

The recipients of organ transplants treated with immunosuppressive drugs have long been recognized as being at risk of developing lymphoproliferative disorders. The general mechanism underlying these disorders appears to be failure of normal anti-EBV cytotoxic T-cell responses, which result in expansion of EBV immortalized B-cells. As described above, the pattern of EBV gene expression closely resembles that seen in *in vitro* infection but the clinical and pathological features of these lesions are very heterogeneous.

There have been a number of attempts to classify post-transplant lymphoproliferative disorders in a clinically meaningful way but a general consensus may now be emerging. At the most benign end of the spectrum there may be significant enlargement of lymphoid tissue but retention of normal architecture with a large expansion of late B-cells showing plasmacytoid features, together with mature plasma cells and usually hyperplasia of germinal centres. Clonal immunoglobulin gene rearrangements are rarely found in this group although the detection of clones containing a single form of EBV may be more common. This is probably the least common type of post-transplant disorder to be seen in routine biopsy material.

At the opposite end of the spectrum of disease are a group of lesions that have the features of diffuse large B-cell lymphomas, are classified as immunoblastic lymphoma and consist of a monomorphic population of large pleomorphic immunoblasts or plasmablasts. These highly aggressive and disseminated tumours often involve extranodal sites. They are clonal by both IgH rearrangements and EBV type and often have a range of other genetic abnormalities such as *p53* or *ras* mutations.

Between these extremes lie a more varied group of lesions, which are classified as polymorphic B-cell lymphoproliferative disorders. These occur in nodes and extranodal sites and show replacement of normal lymphoid architecture by mixture of plasmacytoid cells, lymphocytes, immunoblasts and plasma cells. These have been subdivided into a hyperplastic variant and a lymphomatous variant, based on the presence of necrosis numbers of immunoblasts and cytological atypia. This distinction can be difficult and is of doubtful clinical value. Almost all of these lesions appear to be monoclonal both by IgH rearrangements and EBV type and there is a strong argument for regarding the polymorphic lymphoproliferative lesions as a single group (Figures 11.3–11.6).

There are two further factors that need to be considered in the diagnosis and classification of post-transplant lymphoproliferative disorders. Firstly, some patients have multiple lesions that originate from different clonal populations of EBV-infected lymphocytes. These may show different histological features. Secondly, in a number of cases it can be shown using microsatellite techniques that the tumour may have originated from donor rather than host lymphocytes. This is mainly confined to recipients of allo-BMT although it has occasionally been described in transplantation of solid organs. Following allo-BMT, T-cells derived from the engrafted stem cells are processed in the host thymus and may be incapable of recognizing EBV viral antigen in association with donor MHC molecules. The probability of this occurring will depend on the extent of donor–recipient mismatch.

Figure 11.3 Post-transplantation lymphoproliferative disorder – brain. This patient developed cerebral lesions several years after a renal transplant. The infiltrate, which was shown to be monoclonal, is highly polymorphic and includes cells with irregular cleaved nuclei, nucleolated blast cells and plasmacytoid cells.

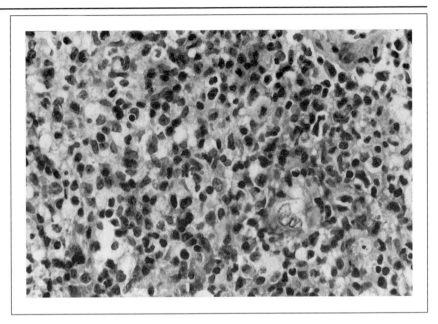

The feature of this group of disorders that has attracted most attention is the regression of some lesions when immunosuppression is reduced. In patients with polymorphic lymphoproliferative disorders or overt large cell lymphomas there are no pathological features that are reliably predictive of response to reduced immunosuppressive therapy. Most

Figure 11.4 Post-transplantation lymphoproliferative disorder – abdomen. This patient on immunosuppressive therapy after a renal transplant presented with a rapidly growing abdominal mass. The tumour consisted of large lymphoid cells with a high rate of proliferation and apoptosis.

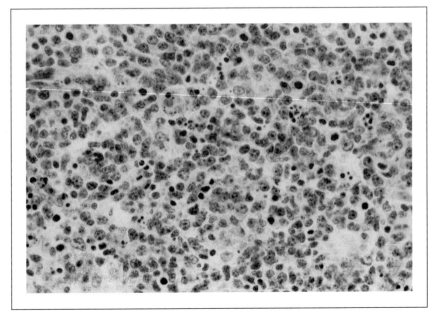

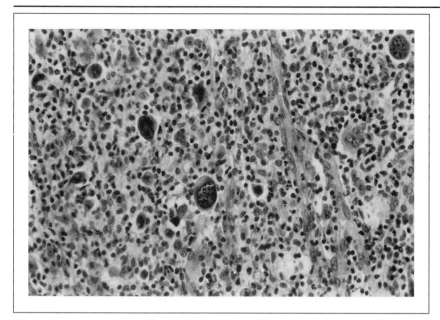

Figure 11.5 Post-transplantation lymphoproliferative disorder – node. This patient developed a very large axillary mass after a cardiac transplant. Most of the mass consisted of polymorphic B-cells, which were shown to be clonal and expressed EBV-associated markers. In addition, there were scattered CD30+ Reed–Sternberg-like cells.

patients will not achieve a complete response and will receive combination chemotherapy or local surgery and radiotherapy based on clinical assessment of disease progression. In a number of relatively small series published the overall prognosis appears to be relatively poor with a low complete remission rate in comparison to other types of large cell

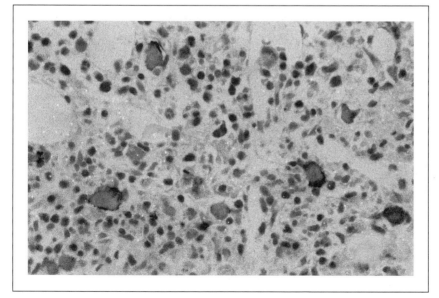

Figure 11.6 Post-transplantation lymphoproliferative disorder – bone marrow (anti-Lmp-1). This patient presented with marrow failure several years after a renal transplant. The marrow was partially replaced by a highly pleomorphic infiltrate, which included numerous large Reed–Sternberg cells that expressed Lmp-1. There was no evidence of tumour at other sites and the patient responded completely to treatment.

lymphoma. A novel and interesting approach to the treatment of this condition is the use of cloned donor cytotoxic lymphocytes with specificity against EBV.

11.2.2 Lymphoproliferative disorders and AIDS

HIV/AIDS is associated with a diverse group of lymphoproliferative disorders

The development of malignant lymphoma is a major feature of AIDS, with around 10% of patients affected. This figure may be an underestimate as some tumours may be undiagnosed in terminally ill patients with multiple infective and other problems. The range of lymphomas seen in AIDS patient is much greater than in patients with post-transplant lymphoproliferative disorders. The majority of tumours are aggressive B-cell lymphomas, which can be classified into two main groups. In most studies the largest group are diffuse large B-cell lymphomas, which contain varying proportions of cells with immunoblastic or centroblastic morphology and occur at a variety of nodal or extranodal sites (Figure 11.7).

Some of these tumours may appear to be polyclonal by IgH PCR techniques. This group has the highest incidence of detectable EBV and

Figure 11.7 HIV-associated diffuse large B-cell lymphoma. This patient, who was known to be HIV-positive, presented with a rapidly progressive lymphadenopathy. The lymph node biopsy showed a diffuse large B-cell lymphoma associated with pericellular fibrosis.

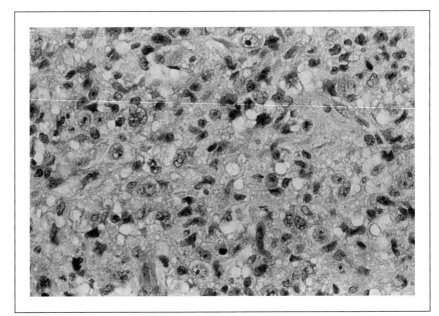

shows expression of EBNA1 and Lmp-1, but differs from the post-transplant lymphoproliferative disorders in usually lacking EBNA2 expression. A subtype of these tumours that occurs frequently in AIDS patients is diffuse large B-cell lymphoma of the brain. Very low CD4 T-cell count appears to be a major risk factor for the development of this type of tumour.

The second main group of B-cell lymphomas have Burkitt's-like features with very high rates of proliferation and apoptosis (the difficulties implicit in using the term 'Burkitt's lymphoma' have been discussed in Chapter 8). EBV is detectable in around one-third of these cases by ISH and, as in the case with typical African Burkitt's lymphoma, Lmp-1 expression is not usually present. As might be expected, there is a high incidence of t(8;14) with c-*myc* deregulation, often in conjunction with abnormalities of *p53*.

There are three other types of lymphoma that occur in AIDS patients at much lower frequency. In a number of series a proportion of the tumours express CD30 and are classified as morphologically anaplastic large cell lymphoma. Tumours with T-, B- and null-cell phenotype have all been described. Most of these cases have detectable EBV with expression of Lmp-1, unlike their equivalent in the non-HIV-infected host. It is not yet known whether HIV-related anaplastic lymphoma contains the t(2;5). Hodgkin's disease is also reported as occurring with increased frequency in patients with HIV/AIDS, although it is not yet accepted as part of the syndrome. Cases of Hodgkin's disease occurring in HIV-positive patients have a strong association with EBV. Small numbers of cases have been reported of a highly aggressive large B-cell lymphoma that tends to primarily involve pleural, pericardial and peritoneal cavities. This body-cavity-based B-cell lymphoma is very strongly associated with infection with HHV-8, the Herpesvirus that is involved in the pathogenesis of Kaposi's sarcoma and possibly multiple myeloma.

With the possible exception of Hodgkin's disease, all types of lymphoma occurring in AIDS patients have a very poor prognosis irrespective of treatment.

11.3 Key references

Ansari, M. Q., Dawson, D. B., Nador, R. *et al.* (1996) Primary body cavity-based AIDS-related lymphomas. *American Journal of Clinical Pathology,* **105**, 221–229.

Filipovich, A. H., Mathur, A., Kamat, D. *et al.* (1994) Lymphoproliferative disorders and other tumors complicating immunodeficiencies. *Immunodeficiency*, 5, 91–112.

Gatti, R. A. (1995) Ataxia-telangiectasia. *Dermatologic Clinics*, 13, 1–6.

Hanto, D. W. (1995) Classification of Epstein–Barr virus-associated posttransplant lymphoproliferative diseases: implications for understanding their pathogenesis and developing rational treatment strategies. *Annual Review of Medicine*, 46, 381–394.

Herndier, B. G., Kaplan, L. D. and McGrath, M. S. (1994) Pathogenesis of AIDS lymphomas. *AIDS*, 8, 1025–1049.

Kaplan, M. A., Ferry, J. A., Harris, N. L. and Jacobson, J. O. (1994) Clonal analysis of posttransplant lymphoproliferative disorders, using both episomal Epstein–Barr virus and immunoglobulin genes as markers. *American Journal of Clinical Pathology*, 101, 590–596.

Knowles, D. M., Cesarman, E., Chadburn, A. *et al.* (1995) Correlative morphologic and molecular genetic analysis demonstrates three distinct categories of posttransplantation lymphoproliferative disorders. *Blood*, 85, 552–565.

Moore, P. S., Gao, S. J., Dominguez, G. *et al.* (1996) Primary characterization of a herpesvirus agent with Kaposi's sarcoma. *Journal of Virology*, 70, 549–558.

Morrison, V. A., Dunn, D. L., Manivel, J. C. *et al.* (1994) Clinical characteristics of post-transplant lymphoproliferative disorders. *American Journal of Medicine*, 97, 14–24.

Nador, R. G., Ceserman, E., Chadburn, A. *et al.* (1996) Primary effusion lymphoma; a distinct clinicopathological entity associated with Kaposi's sarcoma-associated Herpes virus. *Blood*, 88, 645–656.

Papadopoulos, E. B., Ladanyi, M., Emanuel, D. *et al.* (1994) Infusions of donor leukocytes to treat Epstein–Barr virus-associated lymphoproliferative disorders after allogeneic bone marrow transplantation. *New England Journal of Medicine*, 330, 1185–1191.

Rabkin, C. S. (1994) Epidemiology of AIDS-related malignancies. *Current Opinion in Oncology*, 6, 492–496.

Raphael, M. M., Audouin, J., Lamine, M. *et al.* (1994) Immunophenotypic and genotypic analysis of acquired immunodeficiency syndrome-related non-Hodgkin's lymphomas. Correlation with histologic features in 36 cases. French Study Group of Pathology for HIV-Associated Tumors. *American Journal of Clinical Pathology*, 101, 773–782.

Rea, D., Delecluse, H. J., Hamilton-Dutoit, S. J. *et al.* (1994) Epstein–Barr virus latent and replicative gene expression in post-transplant lymphoproliferative disorders and AIDS-related non-Hodgkin's lymphomas. French Study Group of Pathology for HIV-associated Tumors. *Annals of Oncology*, 5(Suppl. 1), S113–S116.

Rea, D., Fourcade, C., Leblond, V. *et al.* (1994) Patterns of Epstein–Barr virus latent and replicative gene expression in Epstein–Barr virus B cell lymphoproliferative disorders after organ transplantation. *Transplantation*, **58**, 317–324.

Sander, C. A., Medeiros, L. J., Weiss, L. M. *et al.* (1992) Lymphoproliferative lesions in patients with common variable immunodeficiency syndrome. *American Journal of Surgical Pathology*, **16**, 1170–1182.

Shibata, D. (1994) Biologic aspects of AIDS-related lymphoma. *Current Opinion in Oncology*, **6**, 503–507.

Sparano, J. A. (1995) Treatment of AIDS-related lymphomas. *Current Opinion in Oncology*, **7**, 442–449.

Taylor, A. M., Metcalfe, J. A., Thick, J. and Mak, Y. F. (1996) Leukemia and lymphoma in ataxia telangiectasia. *Blood*, **87**, 423–438.

Index

Page numbers appearing in **bold** refer to figures and page numbers appearing in *italic* refer to tables.